Neuropeptide Y and Drug Development

Neuropeptide Y and Drug Development

edited by

Lars Grundemar
Department of Clinical Pharmacology,
Lund University Hospital,
S-221 85 Lund, Sweden

and

Stephen R. Bloom
Division of Endocrinology and Metabolism,
Royal Postgraduate Medical School,
University of London, Hammersmith Hospital,
London, UK

Academic Press
San Diego   London   Boston
New York   Sydney   Tokyo   Toronto

Academic Press, Inc.
525 B Street, Suite 1900, San Diego, California 92101-4495, USA
http://www.apnet.com

Academic Press Limited
24–28 Oval Road, London NW1 7DX, UK
http://www.hbuk.co.uk/ap/

ISBN 0-12-304990-3

A catalogue record for this book is available from the British Library

Typeset by Servis Filmsetting Ltd, Manchester
Printed in Great Britain by Hartnolls Ltd, Bodmin, Cornwall

97 98 99 00 01 02 EB 9 8 7 6 5 4 3 2 1

Front cover: Autoradiography showing the distribution of Y1-binding sites (top) and Y2-binding sites
(bottom) at the level of the hippocampal formation of the monkey brain (see Dumont *et al.*, Chapter 4).

Back cover: Serendipity means the faculty of making fortunate discoveries by accident. The word comes from
the Persian fairy tale 'The Three Princes of Serendip' (from Persian Sarandip, former name of Sri
Lanka), the heroes of which were . . . 'always making discoveries, by accident and sagacity, of things they
were not in quest of', and the expression serendipity was coined by the English author Horace Walpole
in 1754. Serendipity is sometimes used in the pharmaceutical process of drug development in order to
illustrate the random discovery of drugs and the often unpredictable ways they undergo to their final
therapeutical niche (see also Preface).

Contents

Contents

A colour plate section appears between pages 148 and 149

Contributors

Annette G. Beck-Sickinger Federal Institute of Technology (ETH), Department of Pharmacy, Winterthurer Str. 190, CH-8057 Zurich, Switzerland

Stephen R. Bloom Division of Endocrinology and Metabolism, Royal Postgraduate Medical School, University of London, Hammersmith Hospital, Du Cane Road, London W12 0NN, UK

Marvin R. Brown Department of Pharmacology, Alanex Corporation, 3550 General Atomics Court, San Diego, CA 92121, USA

Alejandro J. Daniels GlaxoWellcome, Department of Metabolic Diseases, 3030 Cornwallis Road, Research Triangle Park, NC 27709, USA

Henri N. Doods Division of Preclinical Research, Dr Karl Thomae GmbH, Birkendorfer Str. 65, D-88397 Biberach an der Riss, Germany

Yvan Dumont Department of Psychiatry, Douglas Hospital Research Centre, McGill University, 6875 LaSalle Blvd., Verdun, Quebec, Canada H4H 1R3

Wolfgang Eberlein Division of Preclinical Research, Dr Karl Thomae GmbH, Birkendorfer Str. 65, D-88397 Biberach an der Riss, Germany

Wolfhard Engel Division of Preclinical Research, Dr Karl Thomae GmbH, Birkendorfer Str. 65, D-88397 Biberach an der Riss, Germany

Robert Feinstein Department of Computational Chemistry, Alanex Corporation, 3550 General Atomics Court, San Diego, CA 92121, USA

Vlad Gregor Department of Medicinal Chemistry, Alanex Corporation, 3550 General Atomics Courts, San Diego, CA 92121, USA

Lars Grundemar Department of Clinical Pharmacology, Lund University Hospital, S-221 85 Lund, Sweden

Cristin Hagaman Department of Pharmacology, Alanex Corporation, 3550 General Atomics Court, San Diego, CA 92121, USA

Dennis Heyer GlaxoWellcome, Department of Medicinal Chemistry, Research Triangle Park, NC 27709, USA

Yufeng Hong Department of Medicinal Chemistry, Alanex Corporation, 3550 General Atomics Court, San Diego, CA 92121, USA

Danielle Jacques Department of Psychiatry, Douglas Hospital Research Centre, McGill University, 6875 LaSalle Blvd., Verdun, Quebec, Canada H4H 1R3

Galina Krokhina Department of Medicinal Chemistry, Alanex Corporation, 3550 General Atomics Court, San Diego, CA 92121, USA

Dan Larhammar Department of Medical Pharmacology, Uppsala University, Box 593, S-751 24, Uppsala, Sweden

Anthony Ling Department of Medicinal Chemistry, Alanex Corporation, 3550 General Atomics Court, San Diego, CA 92121, USA

Nurit Livnah Department of Medicinal Chemistry, Alanex Corporation, 3550 General Atomics Court, San Diego, CA 92121, USA

Jan M. Lundberg Division of Pharmacology, Department of Physiology and Pharmacology, Karolinska Institute, S-171 77 Stockholm, Sweden

Rickard E. Malmström Division of Pharmacology, Department of Physiology and Pharmacology, Karolinska Institute, S-171 77 Stockholm, Sweden

John Marvin May Department of Pharmacology, Alanex Corporation, 3550 General Atomics Court, San Diego, CA 92121, USA

Anatoly Mazurov Department of Medicinal Chemistry, Alanex Corporation, 3550 General Atomics Court, San Diego, CA 92121, USA

Donal O'Shea Division of Endocrinology and Metabolism, Royal Postgraduate Medical School, University of London, Hammersmith Hospital, Du Cane Road, London W12 0NN, UK

Alexander Polinsky Department of Computational Chemistry, Alanex Corporation, 3550 General Atomics Court, San Diego, CA 92121, USA

Rémi Quirion Department of Psychiatry, Douglas Research Centre, McGill University, 6875 LaSalle Blvd., Verdun, Quebec, Canada H4H 1R3

Alexandr Rabinovich Department of Medical Chemistry, Alanex Corporation, 3550 General Atomics Court, San Diego, CA 92121, USA

Klaus Rudolf Division of Preclinical Research, Dr Karl Thomae GmbH, Birkendorfer Str. 65, D-88397 Biberach an der Riss, Germany

Claudine Serradeil-Le Gal Sanofi Recherche, Exploratory Research Department, 195 Route d'Espagne, 31036 Toulouse Cedex, France

Andrew Spaltenstein GlaxoWellcome, Department of Medicinal Chemistry, Research Triangle Park, NC 27709, USA

Jaques-André St-Pierre Department of Psychiatry, Douglas Research Centre, McGill University, 6875 LaSalle Blvd., Verdun, Quebec, Canada H4H 1R3

M.D. Turton Division of Endocrinology and Metabolism, Royal Postgraduate Medical School, University of London, Hammersmith Hospital, Du Cane Road, London W12 0NN, UK

Eileen Valenzuela Department of Medicinal Chemistry, Alanex Corporation, 3550 General Atomics Court, San Diego, CA 92121, USA

Heike A. Wieland Division of Preclinical Research, Dr Karl Thomae GmbH., Birkendorfer Str. 65, D-88397 Biberach an der Riss, Germany

Helmut Wittneben Division of Preclinical Research, Dr Karl Thomae GmbH, Birkendorfer Str. 65, D-88397 Biberach an der Riss, Germany

Preface: the search for new therapeutic approaches

'New beauty pill – lose pounds on a once-a-day tablet'. Such newspaper headlines announce yet another spurious breakthrough in a field over-ripe with expectation. The first genuinely safe and effective oral therapy that can be taken over decades will be the world's first trillion dollar drug.

Neuropeptide Y (NPY) causes hypertension, increased food intake, inhibits sexual function, inhibits growth and causes sedation, amongst several other actions. The mythical NPY-blocked man would be thin, tall, vivacious and very interested in sex. Certainly a profitable image.

More seriously, many drugs acting on neuro–hormonal targets modulate the transmission in monoamine transmitter systems, like dopamine, noradrenaline and serotonin. These drugs include antiparkinsonism drugs, neuroleptics, antidepressants and antihypertensive drugs and the principles of how these drugs act are well understood. The launch of such therapeutics in the 1950s and 1960s represented breakthrough achievements in the treatment of many disorders. Ironically, several of these drugs were introduced clinically before they were recognized as important neuropharmacological tools with which it was possible to delineate the significance of monoamines as transmitters in various physiological processes and pathological states.

Developments during the last two decades resulted in the discovery of many novel transmitter types, such as the neuropeptides and polypeptide hormones. Although, there are obvious differences between monoamine transmitters and peptide transmitters in molecular size and processing, monoamines and neuropeptides have many features in common. In fact, transmitters from both chemical groups are often co-stored and co-released from nerve terminals, act on the same neurons through activation of distinct and specific receptors, and affect the same ion channels and signal transduction pathways. Vasopressin and oxytocin analogues, ACTH and some other polypeptide agonists have been used clinically in substitution therapy and other conditions for a number of years. However, for clinical use, peptides suffer from poor pharmacokinetic properties, such as low oral bioavailability and rapid degradation.

Most neuropeptides, like many other neurotransmitters, activate G-protein-coupled receptors. Characteristic of this receptor superfamily are the seven transmembraneous spanning domains, which are linked together by extracellular and intracellular loops, of which the third intracellular loop is known to modulate the function of the G-protein.

It has sometimes been argued that neuropeptides act merely as modulators or that they are redundant in mammalian physiology. The rapidly increasing body of knowledge about the various neuro/hormonal peptide systems in the brain and periphery suggests that many of them indeed play a role in controlling important physiological processes and that several of the peptide receptors are promising therapeutic targets. Although the cloning of monoamine receptors has shown that they consist of many more receptor types than expected, the multitude of neuropeptides and their many receptors offer a large number of additional and attractive drug targets. Much effort has been taken to identify the pharmacophore of several neuropeptides (and other transmitters) and the parts of the receptor that recognize the ligand. This knowledge, in addition to high throughput screening techniques, has been beneficial in the search for non-peptide ligands acting on peptide receptors. Thus, it appears that the obstacle of constructing non-peptide receptor antagonists can be overcome and, for example, the angiotensin II (AT1)-receptor antagonist losartan has recently been approved for use in hypertension in several countries. In many neuropeptide receptor systems there is a search for new therapeutic approaches and they include, for instance, modulation of opioid-, tachykinin-, cholecystokinin-, neurotensin- and NPY receptor systems.

NPY is a member of a family of peptides, which also includes the structurally related gut hormones peptide YY (PYY) and pancreatic polypeptide (PP). Since the isolation and identification of NPY in 1982, several thousand publications have examined various aspects of this neuropeptide. NPY has received much attention because it is ubiquitous in the mammalian nervous system and because numerous physiological functions in the brain and periphery have been attributed to the peptide. Interestingly, the NPY molecule is remarkably well conserved through evolution and appears to be the oldest member in this peptide family, suggestive for an important physiological role of this peptide. For instance, NPY is one of the most potent stimuli of food intake known and it occurs in hypothalamic nuclei known to regulate feeding behaviour. The peptide has been implicated in disorders related to altered energy balance, like obesity and anorexia/bulimia. In the periphery, the peptide occurs in perivascular sympathetic nerve fibres and it is co-released with noradrenaline upon high sympathetic nerve activity. NPY is a potent vasoconstrictor, being several orders of magnitude more potent than noradrenaline and the peptide has been implicated in various cardiovascular disorders.

Very recently Erickson and coworkers presented results on functional consequences of embryonic NPY gene knock out in mice (*Nature* (1996) **381**, 415–418). Such mutated mice appeared to have a normal food intake and body weight, but were more sensitive to weight loss following leptin treatment. Besides an increased susceptability to epileptic seizures, these mice did not show any other gross anomalies and were able to reproduce. These seemingly disappointing results on the importance of NPY in feeding behaviour and other physiological processes should naturally be interpreted with caution. The fundamental system(s) that regulates feeding behaviour consists of many parallel neurotransmitter pathways in a highly complex manner. Conceivably, these results illustrate an embryonic dynamic plasticity, resulting in compensatory mechanisms that are not necessarily apparent in the mature individual. A temporary blockade of NYP effects in the adult animal is probably required to elucidate this issue.

NPY and its congeners act at multiple receptor types, belonging to the family of G-protein-coupled receptors. Several of the NPY-receptor types are promising targets for drug development and many pharmaceutical companies are carrying out research on this peptide. The rational approach of designing non-peptide receptor antagonists by identifying peptide pharmacophores using minimization of polypeptides, followed by the construction of small non-peptide ligands has generated useful NPY-receptor antagonists. The most promising areas for application of NPY-receptor antagonists appear to be in the treatment of obesity and perhaps cardiovascular disorders.

An irrational but important factor in the drug discovery and development is serendipity. Often it is difficult to predict the clinical value of a drug candidate based solely on recognized pharmacological effects. For instance, who could have foreseen the widespread use of β-adrenoceptor antagonists in the treatment of hypertension and other cardiovascular disorders? The pharmacological history of drug development illustrates the fact that important breakthroughs are often associated with accidental findings, and that many drugs on the market are used today on indications quite distinct from those originally predicted. In the case of NPY, it is important first to elucidate the physiological and pathophysiological significance of the peptide. With the use of newly developed NPY receptor antagonists, such knowledge is about to emerge. This knowledge can then be used to increase our understanding of how these agents can best be used in a clinical context. It is not unlikely that future studies will discover novel clinical applications of NPY-receptor antagonists distinct from those already proposed. However, an area that is not discussed in this book is the possible utility of NPY-receptor agonists, which perhaps may be beneficial in nasal congestion, diarrhoea, anxiety, epilepsia and pain. More studies are required to assess the role of NPY in these conditions and it is generally difficult to construct non-peptide agonists with acceptable pharmacodynamic and kinetic properties compared with non-peptide antagonists.

Previous books about NPY have been either proceedings from symposia and meetings, or have aimed to cover wide aspects of the whole NPY/PYY/PP family. This book discusses why NPY-receptors represent promising therapeutic targets and describes the latest progress in NPY pharmacology, molecular biology of receptors, characteristics of newly developed NPY-receptor antagonists, and focuses on physiological systems where the use of such antagonists might offer new therapeutic approaches. Efforts have been made to link basic experimental knowledge with areas of possible clinical importance.

Lars Grundemar, Department of Clinical Pharmacology, Lund University Hospital, Sweden.
Stephen R. Bloom, Division of Endocrinology and Metabolism, University of London, Hammersmith Hospital, Du Cane Road, London, UK.

CHAPTER 1

MULTIPLE RECEPTORS AND MULTIPLE ACTIONS

Lars Grundemar

Table of Contents

1.1 Multiple receptor types

This chapter summarizes the pharmacological properties, functional effects and distribution of the various receptors in the neuropeptide Y (NPY) family. It was observed early on that the entire NPY, and peptide YY (PYY), molecule was necessary to evoke vasoconstriction, whereas N-terminally truncated forms of NPY (and PYY) were quite effective in suppressing sympathetic nerve activity. These findings indicated the existence of two NPY/PYY receptor types, referred to as Y1 and Y2 (Wahlestedt *et al.*, 1986). The receptors in the NPY family have been identified and characterized using a range of truncated and substituted peptide analogues in various functional and binding assays (e.g. Grundemar *et al.*, 1992, 1993a,c, 1996; Kahl *et al.*, 1994). The importance of the various parts of the NPY molecule for receptor recognition is discussed by Beck-Sickinger in this volume.

Cloning studies have confirmed the existence of Y1 and Y2 receptors as distinct entities (Eva *et al.*, 1990; Herzog *et al.*, 1992; Larhammar *et al.*, 1992; Gerald *et al.*, 1995; Rose *et al.*, 1995). There is also pharmacological evidence to suggest the existence of an NPY-specific Y3 receptor, present both in the CNS and periphery (Grundemar *et al.*, 1991a; Grundemar and Håkanson, 1994). It is characteristic of Y1, Y2 and Y3 receptors that they do not recognize pancreatic polypeptide (PP). Very recently, a cDNA encoding a PP receptor, referred to as PP1 (Lundell *et al.*, 1995) or

Table 1 Rank order of potency of NPY and related peptides at receptors in the NPY family

Receptor	Peptides	Tissue
Y1	[Pro^{34}]NPY=NPY=PYY>>NPY 13–36>>PP	Blood vessels Brain
Y2	PYY≥NPY>NPY 13–36>>[Pro^{34}]NPY, PP	Nerve endings Kidney Brain
Y3	NPY≥[Pro^{34}]NPY≥NPY 13–36>>PYY, PP	Brainstem Adrenal glands Colon Heart
PP1/Y4	PP>>PYY>NPY	Brain Pancreas Intestine
Y5 rat	NPY=PYY=NPY 2–36=hPP>>rPP	Brain
Y5 mouse	NPY=PYY=NPY 2–36>>hPP	Hypothalamus Kidney

Y4, has also been cloned and expressed (Bard *et al.*, 1995). Most recently, hypothalamic receptors referred to as Y5 have been cloned from different species (Gerald *et al.*, 1996; Weinberg *et al.*, 1996). In this volume Larhammar discusses the characteristics of cloned NPY/PYY/PP receptors.

The rank order of potency of NPY and related peptides on the various receptor types in the NPY family is shown in Table 1. The recent design of a series of specific and potent peptide and non-peptide NPY receptor antagonists has provided important tools, not only to assess the physiological significance of NPY receptors, but also to discriminate between different NPY receptor types. The properties of such antagonists are described in four separate chapters in this volume. All receptors in the NPY family are G-protein-coupled, and the various receptor types can suppress stimulated adenylate cyclase activity or increase intracellular calcium concentrations (Tables 2–5). The distribution of the various NPY receptor types in the brain is discussed by Dumont and co-workers in this volume.

1.2 Y1 receptors

Y1 receptors are numerous in various regions of the brain and their distribution appears to be species specific. In the periphery, Y1 receptors occur in many arteries and veins, where they are associated with vasoconstriction and the potentiation of effects of other vasoconstrictors. In the rat the anxiolytic-sedative effect of NPY seems to be Y1 receptor mediated. In support of this contention, central injection into the rat of an antisense oligonucleotide directed against Y1 receptor mRNA was found to cause anxiety-like effects (opposite to those induced by Y1 receptor activation) and a subsequent binding analysis revealed a reduced number of Y1, but not Y2 receptors, in the brain (Wahlestedt *et al.*, 1993). Table 2 shows the effects that are associated with activation of Y1 receptors.

The most notable features of the Y1 receptor are the rapid loss of potency upon elimination or substitution of merely one or two N-terminal amino-acid residues. Substitutions in the C-terminus have been introduced without loss of potency. Thus, [Pro^{34}]NPY or variants thereof have been shown to be useful Y1 receptor agonists (Schwartz *et al.*, 1990; Grundemar *et al.*, 1992, 1993b) (Table 1). Using various substituted NPY analogues, it has been suggested that, although the hairpin loop *per se* is not essential, it promotes binding to the Y1 receptor by bringing the N- and C-terminal ends of the NPY molecule in close apposition (Schwartz *et al.*, 1990; Grundemar and Håkanson, 1993; Grundemar *et al.*, 1993a).

Eva *et al.* (1990) isolated a rat brain clone corresponding to a G-protein-coupled receptor, which subsequently was identified as a Y1 receptor. Also the human Y1 receptor cDNA has been isolated and expressed in transfected cells. It was confirmed that the human Y1 receptor is very stringent in its demands on the N-terminal part of the ligand (Herzog *et al.*, 1992; Larhammar *et al.*, 1992). Whether this receptor is identical with the 'atypical' Y1 receptor, which mediates feeding, is at present unknown.

In addition, Y1 receptor heterogeneity has been suggested in the brain (see Dumont *et al.*, this volume) and, recently, also in the periphery, as revealed by the use of different NPY receptor antagonists (Grundemar and Ekelund, 1996; Palea *et al.*, 1995) or agonists (Kirby *et al.*, 1995). Moreover, Nakamura *et al.* (1995) have isolated two different forms of mouse Y1 receptors, which originate from a single gene and are generated by alternative RNA splicing. The so-called Y1-α receptor is thought to correspond to the cloned human Y1 receptor, while the so-called Y1-β receptor is an embryonic and a bone marrow form, which differs in the seventh transmembraneous domain and C-terminal tail.

1.3 Y2 receptors

The Y2 receptor is the predominant NPY receptor type in the rat brain and such receptors are particularly numerous in the hippocampus (Dumont *et al.*, 1992). Many Y2 receptor-mediated effects have been linked to suppression of transmitter release. For instance, the release of glutamate from terminals synapsing on to rat hippocampal CA1 neurons is inhibited by activation of Y2 receptors. Peripheral Y2 receptors are associated with suppression of transmitter release from sympathetic, parasympathetic and sensory C-fibres. Table 3 summarizes these effects.

Y2 receptors are characterized by their propensity to accept also N-terminally truncated forms of NPY and PYY (Colmers *et al.*, 1991; Grundemar and Håkanson, 1993; Grundemar *et al.*, 1993a). The C-terminal part of the ligand is of crucial importance

3

Table 2 Effects associated with Y1 receptors

Effect	Target	References
Vasoconstriction	Various blood vessels	Wahlestedt et al. (1986); Fuhlendorff et al. (1990), Grundemar et al. (1992, 1993a)
Potentiation of vasoconstriction	Various blood vessels	Wahlestedt et al. (1986), McAuley and Westfall (1992)
Anxiolysis-sedation	Rat amygdala	Heilig et al. (1993), Wahlestedt et al. (1993)
HRH secretion	Hypothalamus	Kalra et al. (1990)
Inhibition of adenylate cyclase	Transfected cells	Herzog et al. (1992), Larhammar et al. (1992)
Elevation of intracellular calcium	Transfected cells	Herzog et al. (1992), Larhammar et al. (1992)

for Y2 receptor recognition and [Pro^{34}]NPY is inactive (Table 1). Using various substituted NPY analogues, it could be shown that there is a gradual loss of potency with progressive N-terminal truncation; the key to recognition by the Y2 receptor is the C-terminal hexapeptide. It appears that, while the C-terminus is essential for binding, the hairpin loop is not, although it may help to create a steric conformation of the C-terminal hexapeptide amide that is favourable for Y$_2$ receptor recognition (Schwartz *et al.*, 1990; Grundemar and Håkanson, 1993; Grundemar *et al.*, 1993a; Kahl *et al.*, 1994).

The relative potencies of various NPY analogues (versus NPY) have been shown to differ in several tissues proposed to contain Y2 receptors, indicating the existence of several Y2 receptor subtypes (Grundemar *et al.*, 1993a). A PYY-preferring receptor, displaying some characteristics similar to the Y2 receptor has been proposed in the instestine (Laburthe *et al.*, 1986) and may also indicate heterogeneity among Y2 receptors. Finally, since many binding and functional studies have demonstrated the presence of Y2 receptors in various peripheral tissues, the lack of hybridization of the recently cloned human Y2 receptor mRNA in the periphery may also support the existence of several Y2 receptor subtypes (Gerald *et al.*, 1995; Rose *et al.*, 1995; see also, Dumont *et al.*, this volume).

1.4 Y3 receptors

A number of studies have described a receptor that recognizes NPY but not PYY, and which displays a rank order of potency for NPY-related peptides that differs markedly from those of the known Y1/Y2 receptors (Table 1). Such receptors are referred to as Y3 receptors (Grundemar *et al.*, 1991a,b; Grundemar and Håkanson, 1994). Central effects associated with Y3 receptor activation are hypotension, bradycardia (Figure 1) and inhibition of glutamate effects in response to unilateral injection of NPY into the nucleus tractus solitarius (NTS) of the rat. Bilateral stimulation of Y3 receptors in the NTS results in elevated blood pressure and attenuated baroreceptor reflex. Very recently, we have shown that NPY, but not PYY (or PP) can suppress inhibitory post-synaptic currents in slices of the rat dorsomedial NTS, further supporting the existence of Y3 receptors in this nucleus (Figure 2). In the periphery, NPY binding sites corresponding to Y3 receptors seem to occur in the bovine adrenal medulla (Wahlestedt *et al.*, 1992) and it appears that such receptors suppress the nicotine-stimulated release of catecholamines (Higuchi *et al.*, 1988). Table 4 summarizes effects associated with Y3 receptors. A bovine cDNA corresponding to a G-protein-coupled receptor has been claimed to encode the Y3 receptor (Rimland *et al.*, 1991). However, subsequent studies using the corresponding human cDNA have refuted this proposal (Jazin *et al.*, 1993).

1.5 PP1/Y4 receptors

PP occurs in endocrine cells in the pancreatic islets (Alumets *et al.*, 1978), and the peptide inhibits pancreatic exocrine secretion and gall bladder contraction (Schwartz,

Table 3 Effects associated with Y2 receptors

Effect	Target	References
Suppression of transmitter release	Sympathetic nerve fibres	Wahlestedt et al. (1986), Grundemar and Håkanson (1990), McAuley and Westfall (1992)
Suppression of transmitter release	Parasympathetic nerve fibres	Potter et al. (1989), Stjernquist and Owman (1990)
Suppression of transmitter release	Sensory C-fibres	Grundemar et al. (1990a, 1993b)
Antisecretory effect	Rat intestine	Cox and Cuthbert (1990)
Inhibition of lipolysis	Canine lipocytes	Castan et al. (1992)
Vasoconstriction	Certain blood vessels	McAuley and Westfall (1992), Modin et al. (1991)
Inhibition of mucociliary activity	Rabbit maxillary sinus	Cervin (1992)
Enhanced memory retention	Rat hippocampus	Flood and Morley (1989)
Suppression of glutamate release	Rat hippocampus	Colmers et al. (1991)
Suppression of noradrenaline release	Rat locus coeruleus	Illes et al. (1993)
Inhibition of consumatory behaviour	Rat hypothalamus	Leibowitz and Alexander (1991)
Inhibition of adenylate cyclase	Transfected cells	Gerald et al. (1995), Rose et al. (1995)
Elevation of intracellular calcium	Transfected cells	Gerald et al. (1995), Rose et al. (1995)

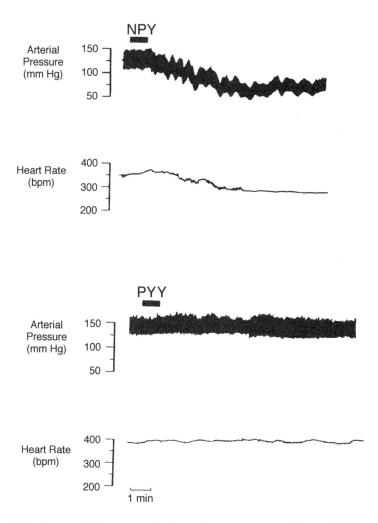

Figure 1 Activation of Y3 receptors in the rat brainstem. (Top) Effects of NPY (90 pmol) injected into nucleus tractus solitarius on arterial pressure and heart rate in the anaesthetized rat. Characteristic of this receptor is that, in contrast to Y1 and Y2 receptors, it is not activated by PYY (90 pmol) (bottom). The black box indicates unilateral injection of peptide. Reproduced from Grundemar and Håkanson (1993) with permission.

1983). Functional PP receptors seem to occur also in the rat vas deferens (Jörgensen *et al.*, 1990). Although, the peptide is not present in the CNS, binding sites for PP have been found in circumventricular nuclei, such as the area postrema (Whitcomb *et al.*, 1990). Very recently, the human PP receptor has been cloned, and it was shown that PP binds to this receptor in a picomolar range, while both NPY and PyY bind in the low to high nanomolar range depending on the type of radio labelled ligand (Bard *et*

7

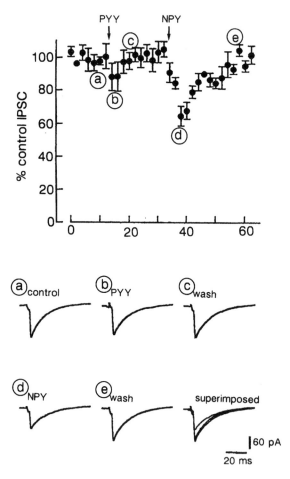

Figure 2 Y3 receptors reversibly inhibit synaptic transmission in the rat nucleus tractus solitarius. (Top) A dot plot illustrating running 2 min (mean ± SEM) of inhibitory post-synaptic currents evoked at 0.1 Hz by electrical stimulation in the ipsilateral tractus solitarius in the presence of AMPA and NMDA receptor antagonists, and recorded with CsCl electrodes at Vhold = –80 mV. Bath application of PYY (500 nM, 90 s, arrow) failed to significantly inhibit IPSCs, whereas NPY (50 nM, 90 s, arrow) potently and reversibly reduced the IPSC. The IPSC amplitude was normalized to the running mean IPSC amplitude recorded over 6 min immediately prior to the plot. (Bottom) Averaged (3) consecutive sweeps of IPSCs recorded from cell A at time points indicated (Glaum, Miller and Grundemar, unpublished).

al., 1995; Lundell *et al.*, 1995) (Tables 1 and 5). This receptor is also coupled to inhibition of cAMP accumulation (Lundell *et al.*, 1995) and to mobilization of intracellular calcium (Bard *et al.*, 1995). *In situ* hybridization studies on human tissue have shown expression of Y4 receptor mRNA in the brain, gut, pancreas and other peripheral tissues (Bard *et al.*, 1995). Also a cDNA encoding the rat PP receptor has recently been cloned (Lundell *et al.*, 1996).

Table 4 Effects associated with Y3 receptors

Effect	Target	References
Increase/decrease in arterial blood pressure and bradycardia	Rat nucleus tractus solitarius	Grundemar et al. (1991a,b)
Inhibition of glutamate effects and baroreceptor reflex	Rat nucleus tractus solitarius	Grundemar et al (1991a,b)
Inhibition of postsynaptic currents	Rat nucleus tractus solitarius	Glaum et al. to be published
Inhibition of catecholamine release	Bovine adrenal medulla	Higuchi et al. (1988), Nörenberg et al. (1995)
Release of aldosterone	Rat adrenal cortex	Bernet et al. (1994)
Contraction	Rat colon	Dumont et al. (1993)
Inhibition of calcium currents	Rat superior cervical ganglia	Foucart et al. (1993)
Inhibition of adenylate cyclase	Rat cardiac membranes	Balasubramaniam et al. (1990)
Elevation of intracellular calcium	Bovine chromaffin cells	Wahlestedt et al. (1992)

Table 5 Effects associated with PP1/Y4 receptors

Effect	Target	References
Inhibition of exocrine secretion	Pancreas	Schwartz (1983)
Inhibition of contraction	Gall bladder	Schwartz (1983)
Suppression of stimulated contractions	Rat vas deferens	Jørgensen et al. (1990)
Inhibition of calcium currents	Rat superior cervical ganglia	Foucart et al. (1993)
Inhibition of adenylate cyclase	Transfected cells	Bard et al. (1995), Lundell et al. (1995)
Elevation of intracellular calcium	Transfected cells	Bard et al. (1995)

1.6 Several Y5 receptors

Pharmacological studies have suggested that the hypothalamic NPY receptor involved in the stimulation of food intake is distinct from the conventional NPY receptor types (Stanley et al., 1992) and it has been referred to as a Y1-like receptor. Very recently, rat, mouse and human hypothalamic NPY receptors have been cloned and termed Y5 (Gerald et al., 1996, Weinberg et al., 1996, Herzog, personal communication). The rat Y5 receptor mRNA is primarily expressed in the brain, including hypothalamic nuclei, such as paraventricular nuclei, lateral hypothalamus and arcuate nucleus. Y5 mRNA has also been detected in hippocampus and thalamic nuclei (Gerald et al., 1996). The rat Y5 receptor has been claimed to be identical with the NPY receptor that stimulates feeding, because it displays a pharmacological profile, which resembles that observed in studies of ingestive behaviour (Gerald et al., 1996, Table 1). The rat Y5 receptor seems to be coupled to inhibition of adenylate cyclase activity (Gerald et al., 1996).

The mouse Y5 receptor mRNA seems to be expressed only in hypothalamic areas and in the kidney (Weinberg et al., 1996). The sequence of the mouse Y5 receptor displays homology to Y1 receptors from several species, whereas the sequence of the rat Y5 receptor is divergent from Y1, Y2 and PP1/Y4 receptors (Larhammar, personal communication). Thus, it is clear that the published mouse and rat Y5 clones correspond to separate genes and encode distinct receptor types. Although rat and mouse Y5 receptors have certain pharmacological features in common there also appears to be some differences (Table 1). While the human PP is equipotent with NPY on rat Y5 receptors, it is not recognized by the mouse Y5 receptor (Gerald et al., 1996, Weinberg et al., 1996). Moreover, no receptor corresponding to that of the mouse Y5 receptor seems to be expressed in the rat (Weinberg, personal communication). The definite classification of Y5 receptors remains to be established. Additional studies are required to elucidate whether these receptors are involved in feeding behaviour. The significance of hypothalamic NPY receptors in energy-metabolic homeostasis and associated disorders is discussed by Turton and coworkers in this volume.

1.7 Other receptors and targets

Receptors in the NPY family with ligand requirements distinct from the conventional Y1–Y4 receptors have been suggested in several tissues, such as neuronal cell lines (Inui et al., 1992; Cox and Tough, 1995), guinea-pig colon (Sawa et al., 1995) and rat brain (Bouali et al., 1994; see also Dumont et al., this volume). Additional studies are required to assess whether they constitute novel receptor types.

Moreover, intravenous injections of NPY and several of its analogues have been shown to induce histamine release from mast cells and long-lasting hypotension in the rat, probably through a non-receptor-mediated mechanism (Grundemar et al., 1990b, 1994; Grundemar and Håkanson, 1991; Mousli et al., 1995). Whether this effect is physiological is not clear, but should, nonetheless, be considered when novel NPY receptor ligands are designed.

Acknowledgements

Lars Grundemar wishes to thank D.R. Gehlert, H. Herzog, D. Larhammar, B.G. Stanley and D. Weinberg for their helpful comments.

References

Alumets, J., Håkanson, R. & Sundler, F. (1978) Distribution, ontogeny and ultrastructure of pancreatic polypeptide (PP) cells in pancreas and gut of the chicken. *Cell Tissue Res.* **194**, 377–386.

Balasubramaniam, A., Sheriff, S., Riegel, D.F. & Fischer, J.E. (1990) Characterization of neuropeptide Y binding sites in rat cardiac ventricular membranes. *Peptides* (1990) **11**, 545–550.

Bard, J.A., Walker, M.W., Branchek, T.A. & Weinshank, R.L. (1995) Cloning and functional expression a human Y4 subtype receptor for pancreatic polypeptide. *J. Biol. Chem.* **270**, 26 762–26 765.

Bernet, F., Maubert, E., Bernard, Montel V. & Dupouy, J.P. (1994) In vitro steroidogenic effects of neuropeptide Y (NPY 1–36), Y1 and Y2 receptor agonists (Leu^{31}, Pro^{34} NPY), NPY (18–36) and peptide YY (PYY) on rat adrenal capsule/zona glomerulosa. *Regul. Peptides* **52**, 187–193.

Bouali, S.M., Fournier, A., St-Pierre, S. & Jolicoeur, B. (1994) In vivo central actions of NPY (1–30), an N-terminal fragment of neuropeptide Y. *Peptides* **15**, 799–802.

Castan, I., Valet, P., Vosin, T., Quitean, N., Laburthe, M. & Lafontan, M. (1992) Identification and functional studies of a specific peptide YY-preferring receptor in dog adipocytes. *Endocrinology* **131**, 1970–1976.

Cervin, A. (1992) Neuropeptide Y 16–36 inhibits mucociliary activity but does not affect blood flow in the rabbit maxillary sinus. *Regul. Peptides* **39**, 237–246.

Colmers, W.F., Klapstein, G.J., Fournier, A., St-Pierre, S. & Treherne, K.A. (1991) Presynaptic inhibition by neuropeptide Y in rat hippocampal slice in vitro is mediated by a Y2 receptor. *Br. J. Pharmacol.* **102**, 41–44.

Cox, H.M. & Cuthbert, A.W. (1990) The effects of neuropeptide Y and its fragments upon basal and electrically stimulated ion secretion in rat jejunum mucosa. *Br. J. Pharmacol.* **101**, 247–252.

Cox, H.M. & Tough, I.R. (1995) Functional characterization of receptors with affinity for PYY, NPY, [Leu^{31}, Pro^{34}] NPY and PP in a human colonic epithelial cell line. *Br. J. Pharmacol.* **116**, 2673–2678.

Dumont, Y., Martel, J.-C., Fournier, A., St-Pierre, S. & Quirion, R. (1992) Neuropeptide Y and neuropeptide Y receptor subtypes in brain and peripheral tissues. *Progr. Neurol.* **38**, 125–167.

Dumont, Y., Satoh, H., Cadieux, A., Taoudi-Benchekroun, M., Pheng, L.H., St-Pierre, S., Fournier, A. & Quirion, R. (1993) Evaluation of truncated neuropeptide Y analogues with modifications of the tyrosine residue in position 1 on Y1, Y2 and Y3 receptor sub-types. *Eur. J. Pharmacol.* **238**, 37–45.

Eva, C., Keinänen, K., Monyer, A., Seeburg, P. & Sprengel, R. (1990) Molecular cloning of a novel G-protein-coupled receptor that may belong to the neuropeptide receptor family. *FEBS Lett.* **271**, 80–84.

Foucart, S., Bleakman, D., Bindokas, V.P. & Miller, R.J. (1993) Neuropeptide Y and pancreatic polypeptide reduce calcium currents in acutely dissociated neurons from adult rat superior cervical ganglia. *J. Pharmacol. Exp. Ther.* **265**, 903–909.

Fuhlendorff, J., Gether, U., Aakerland, L., Langeland-Johansen, J., Thogersen, H. Melberg, S.G., Bang-Olsen, U., Thastrup, O. & Schwartz, T.W. (1990) [Leu^{31}, Pro^{34}] Neuropeptide Y – a specific Y1 receptor agonist. *Proc. Natl Acad. Sci. USA* **187**, 182–186.

Gerald, C., Walker, M.W., Vaysse, P.J.J., He, C.G., Branchek, T.A. & Weinshank, R.L. (1995) Expression cloning and pharmacological characterization of a human hippocampal neuro-peptide Y peptide YY Y2 receptor subtype. *J. Biol. Chem.* **270**, 45, 26758–26761.

Gerald, C., Walker, M.W., Criscione, L., Gustavson, E.L., Batzi-Hartmann, C., Smith, K.E., Vaysse, P.J.J., Durkin, M.M., Laz, T.M., Linemeyer, D.L., Schaffhauser, A.O., Whitebread, S., Hofbauer, K.G., Taber, R.L., Branchek, T.A. & Weinshank, R.L. (1996). A receptor subtype involved in neuropeptide Y-induced food intake. *Nature* **382**, 168–171.

Grundemar, L. & Ekelund, M. (1996) Effects of neuropeptide Y (NPY)-receptor antagonist BIBP3226 on vascular NPY receptors with different ligand requirements. *Pharmacol & Toxicol.* (in press).

Grundemar, L. & Håkanson, R. (1990) Effects of various neuropeptide Y/peptide YY fragments on electrically-evoked contractions of the rat vas deferens. *Br. J. Pharmacol.* **100**, 190–192.

Grundemar, L. & Håkanson, R. (1991) Neuropeptide Y, peptide YY and C-terminal fragments release histamine from rat peritoneal mast-cells. *Br. J. Pharmacol.* **104**, 776–778.

Grundemar, L. & Håkanson, R. (1993) Multiple neuropeptide Y receptors are involved in cardiovascular regulation. Peripheral and central mechanisms. *Gen. Pharmacol* **24**, 785–796.

Grundemar, L. & Håkanson, R. (1994) Neuropeptide Y effector systems. Perspective for the development of new drugs. *Trends Pharmacol. Sci.* **15**, 153–159.

Grundemar, L., Grundström, N., Andersson, R.G.G., Johansson, I. & Håkanson, R. (1990a) Suppression by neuropeptide Y of capsaicin-sensitive sensory nerve-mediated contraction in guinea pig airways. *Br. J. Pharmacol.* **99**, 473–476.

Grundemar, L., Wahlestedt, C., Shen, G.H., Zukowska-Grojec, Z. & Håkanson, R. (1990b) Biphasic blood pressure response to neuropeptide Y in anesthetized rats. *Eur. J. Pharmacol.* **179**, 83–87.

Grundemar, L., Wahlestedt, C. & Reis, D.J. (1991a) Long-lasting inhibition of the cardiovascular responses to glutamate and the baroreceptor reflex elicited by neuropeptide Y injected into the nucleus tractus solitarius. *Neurosci. Lett.* **122**, 135–139.

Grundemar, L., Wahlestedt, C. & Reis, D.J. (1991b) Neuropeptide Y acts at an atypical receptor to evoke cardiovascular depression and to inhibit glutamate responsiveness in the brainstem. *J. Pharmacol. Exp. Ther.* **258**, 633–638.

Grundemar, L., Mörner, S.E.J.N., Högestätt, E.D., Wahlestedt, C. & Håkanson, R. (1992) Characterization of vascular neuropeptide Y receptors. *Br. J. Pharmacol.* **105**, 45–50.

Grundemar, L., Krstenansky, K.L. & Håkanson, R. (1993a) Activation of Y1 and Y2 receptors by substituted and truncated neuropeptide Y analogs: identification of signal epitopes. *Eur. J. Pharmacol.* **232**, 271–278.

Grundemar, L., Wahlestdt, C. & Wang, Z.-Y. (1993b) Neuropeptide Y suppresses the neurogenic inflammatory response in the rabbit eye; mode of action. *Regul. Peptides* **43**, 57–64.

Grundemar, L., Sheikh, S.P. & Wahlestedt, C. (1993c) Characterization of receptors for neuropeptide Y and related peptides. In *The Biology of Neuropeptide Y and Related Peptides* (eds Colmers, W.F. & Wahlestedt, C.), pp. 197–239. Totowa, NJ, Humana Press.

Grundemar, L., Krstenansky, J.L. & Håkanson, R. (1994) Neuropeptide Y (NPY) and truncated NPY analogs release histamine from rat peritoneal mast cells. A direct effect on G proteins? *Eur. J. Pharmacol.* **258**, 163–166.

Grundemar, L., Kahl, U., Langel, U., Callreus, T. Bienen, & Beyermann, M. (1996) Ligand binding and functional effects of systematic double D-amino-acid residue substituted neuropeptide Y analogs on Y1 and Y2 receptors *Regul. Peptides* **62**, 131–136.

Heilig, M., MacLeod, S., Brot, M., Heinrichs, S.C., Menzaghi, F., Koob, G.F. & Britton, K.T. (1993) Anxiolytic-like action of neuropeptide Y: Modulation by Y1-receptors in amygdala, and dissociation from food intake. *Neuropsychopharmacol.* **8**, 357–363.

Herzog, H., Hort, Y.I., Ball, H.J., Hayes, G., Shine, J. & Selbie, L.D. (1992) Cloned human neuropeptide Y receptor couples to different second messenger systems. *Proc. Natl Acad. Sci. USA* **89**, 5794–5798.

Higuchi, H., Costa, E., Yang, W.-Y.T. (1988) Neuropeptide Y inhibits the acetylcholine-mediated release of catecholamines from bovine adrenal chromaffin cells. *Pharmacol. Exp. Ther.* **244**, 468–474.

Illes, P., Finta, E.P. & Nieber, K. (1993) Neuropeptide Y potentiates via Y2-receptors the inhibitory effect of noradrenaline in rat locus coeruleus neurones. *Naunyn Schmiedebergs Arch. Pharmacol.* **348**, 546–548.

Inui, A., Sano, K., Miura, M., Hirosue, Y., Nakajima, M., Okita, M., Baba, S. & Kasuga, M. (1992) Evidence for further heterogeneity of the receptors for neuropeptide Y and peptide YY in tumor cell lines derived from neural crest. *Endocrinol.* **131**, 2090–2096.

Jazin, E., Yoo., H., Blomquist, A.G., Yee, F. & Walker, M.W., *et al.* (1993) A proposed bovine neuropeptide Y (NPY) receptor and its human homologue, described herein, do not confer NPY binding sites nor NPY responsiveness on transfected cells. *Regul. Peptides* **47**, 247–258.

Jørgensen, J.Ch., Fuhlendorff, J. & Schwartz, T.W. (1990) Structure–function studies on neuropeptide Y and pancreatic polypeptide – evidence for two PP-fold receptors in vas deferens. *Eur. J. Pharmacol.* **186**, 105–114.

Kahl, U., Langel, Ü., Bartfai, T. & Grundemar, L. (1994) Functional effects and ligand binding of chimeric galanin-neuropeptide Y (NPY) peptides on NPY and galanin receptor types. *Br. J. Pharmacol.* **111**, 1129–1134.

Kalra, S.P., Sahu, A. & Kalra, P.S. (1990) Hypothalamic neuropeptide Y: a circuit in the regulation of gonadotropin secretion and feeding behaviour. *Ann. N. York Acad. Sci.* **611**, 273–283.

Kirby, D.A., Koerber, S.C., May, J.M., Hagaman, C., Cullen M.J., Pelleymounter, M.A. & Rivier, J.E. (1995) Y1 and Y2 receptor selective neuropeptide Y analogues: Evidence for a Y1 receptor subclass. *J. Med. Chem.* **38**, 4579–4586.

Laburthe, M., Chenut, B., Rouyer-Fessard, C., Tatemoto, K., Couvineau, A., Servin, A. & Amiranoff, B. (1986) Interaction of peptide YY with rat intestinal epithelial plasma membranes: binding of the radioiodinated peptide. *Endocrinology* **118**, 1910–1917.

Larhammar, D., Blomqvist, A.G., Yee, F., Jazin, E., Yoo, H. & Wahlestedt, C. (1992) Cloning and functional expression of a human neuropeptide Y/peptide YY receptor of the Y1 type. *J. Biol. Chem.* **267**, 10 935–10 938.

Lundell, I., Blomqvist, A.G., Berglund, M.M., Schober, D.A., Johnson, D., Statnick, M.A., Gadski, R.A., Gehlert, D.R. & Larhammar, D. (1995) Cloning of a human receptor of the NPY receptor family with high affinity for pancreatic polypeptide and peptide YY. *J. Biol. Chem.* **270**, 29 123–29 128.

L. Grundemar

Lundell, I., Statnick, M.A., Johnson, D., Schober, D.A., Starbäck, R., Gehlert, D. & Larhammar, D. (1996) The cloned rat pancreatic polypeptide receptor exhibits profound differences to the orthologous human receptor. *Proc. Natl Acad. Sci USA* **93**, 5111–5115.

McAuley, M.A. & Westfall, T.C. (1992) Possible location and function of neuropeptide Y receptor subtypes in the rat mesenteric arterial bed. *J. Pharmacol. Exp. Ther.* **261**, 863–868.

Modin, A., Pernow, J. & Lundberg, J.M. (1992) Evidence for two neuropeptide Y receptor subtypes mediating vasoconstriction. *Eur. J. Pharmacol.* **203**, 165–171.

Mousli, M., Trifilieff, A., Pelton, J.T. & Landy, Y. (1995) Structural requirements for neuropeptide Y in mast cell and G protein activation. *Eur. J. Pharmacol.* **289**, 125–133.

Nakamura, M., Sakanaka, C., Aoki, Y., Ogasawara, H., Tsuji, T., Kodama, H., Matsumoto, T., Shimizu, T. & Noma, M. (1995) Identification of two isoforms of neuropeptide Y-Y1 receptor generated by alternative splicing. *J. Biol. Chem.* **270**, 30 102–30 110.

Nörenberg, W., Bek, M., Limberger, N., Takeda, K. & Illes, P. (1995) Inhibition of nicotininic acetylcholine receptor channels in bovine adrenal chromaffin cells by Y3-type neuropeptide Y receptors via the adenylate cyclase/protein kinase A system. *Naunyn Schmiedebergs Arch. Pharmacol.* **351**, 337–347.

Palea, S., Rimland, J.M. & Trist, D.G. (1995) Discrimination by benextramine between the NPY-Y1 receptor subtypes present in rabbit isolated vas deferens and saphenous vein. *Br. J. Pharmacol.* **115**, 3–10.

Potter, E.K., Michell, L., McCloskey, M.J., Tseng, A., Goodman, A.E., Shine, J. & McCloskey, D.I. (1989) Pre- and postjunctional actions of neuropeptide Y and related peptides. *Regul. Peptides* **25**, 167–177.

Rimland, J.R., Vin, W., Sweetnam, P., Saijoh, K. & Nestler, E.J. (1991) Sequence and expression of a neuropeptide Y receptor. *Mol. Pharmacol.* **40**, 869–875.

Rose, P.M., Pabhavathi, R., Lynch, J.S., Frazier, S.M., Kodukula, K., Kienzle, B. & Seethala, R. (1995) Cloning and functional expression of a cDNA encoding a human type 2 neuropeptide Y receptor, *J. Biol. Chem.* **270**, 22 661–22 2264.

Sawa, T., Mameya, S., Yoshimura, M., Itsuno, M., Makiyama, K., Niwa, M. & Taniyama, K. (1995) Differential mechanism of peptide YY and neuropeptide Y in inhibiting motility of guinea pig colon. *Eur. J. Pharmacol.* **276**, 223–230.

Schwartz, T.W. (1983) Pancreatic polypeptide a hormone under vagal control. *Gastroenterology* **85**, 1411–1425.

Schwartz, T.W., Fuhlendorff, J., Kjems, L.L., Kristensen, M.S. & Vervelde, M., *et al.* (1990) Signal epitopes in the three-dimentional structure of NPY interaction with Y1, Y2 and PP receptors. *Ann. N. York Acad. Sci.* **611**, 35–47.

Stanley, B.G., Magdalin, W., Seirafi, A., Nguyen, M.M. & Leibowitz, S.F. (1992) Evidence for neuropeptide Y mediation of eating produced by food deprivation and a variant of the Y1 receptor mediating this peptide's effect. *Peptides* **13**, 581–587.

Stjernquist, M. & Owman, C. (1990) Further evidence for a prejunctional action of neuropeptide Y on cholinergic motor neurons in the rat uterine cervix. *Acta Physiol. Scand.* **138**, 95–96.

Wahlestedt, C., Yanaihara, N. & Håkanson, R. (1986) Evidence for different pre- and postjunctional receptors for neuropeptide Y and related peptides. *Regul. Peptides* **13**, 307–318.

Wahlestedt, C., Regunathan, S. & Reis, D.J. (1992) Identification of cultured cells selectively expressing Y1-, Y2- or Y3-type receptors for neuropeptide Y/peptide YY. *Life Sci.* **50**, PL7–PL12.

Wahlestedt, C., Pich, E.M., Koob, G.F., Yee, F. & Heilig, M. (1993) Modulation of anxiety and neuropeptide Y-Y1-receptors by antisense oligodeoxynucleotides. *Science* **259**, 528–531.

Weinberg, D.H., Sirinathsinghji, D.J.S., Tan, C.P., Shiao, L.-L., Morin, N., Rigby, M.R., Heavens, R.H., Rapoport, D.R., Bayne, M.L., Cascieri, M.A., Strader, C.D., Linemeyer, D.L. & MacNeil, D.J. (1996) Cloning and expression of a novel neuropeptide Y receptor. *J. Biol. Chem.* **271**, 16 435–16 438.

Whitcomb, D.C., Taylor, I.L. & Vigna, S.R. (1990) Characterization of saturable binding sites for circulating pancreatic polypeptide in rat brain. *Am. J. Physiol.* **259**, G687–G691.

CHAPTER 2

CENTRAL EFFECTS OF NEUROPEPTIDE Y WITH EMPHASIS ON ITS ROLE IN OBESITY AND DIABETES

M.D. Turton, D. O'Shea and S.R. Bloom

Table of Contents

2.1 Introduction

Since its discovery from extracts of porcine brain in 1982 (Tatemoto *et al.*, 1982), the involvement of neuropeptide Y (NPY) in the physiological regulation of various autonomic and endocrine functions has been extensively studied. NPY has a diverse range of effects within the central nervous system (CNS) (Table 1). These include the stimulation of feeding, luteinizing hormone (LH) and adrenocorticotrophic hormone (ACTH) secretion, a reduction in growth hormone (GH) release and the regulation of peripheral metabolism. Its physiological role in the regulation of feeding behaviour will form the main focus of this review.

NPY is clearly implicated in the pathophysiology of eating disorders, in particular obesity and its associated non-insulin-dependent diabetes mellitus (NIDDM). Existing pharmacological strategies for the treatment of obesity are largely ineffective (Leibel *et al.*, 1995). To develop effective new treatments, we must elucidate the relationship

Neuropeptide Y and Drug Development
ISBN 0-12-304990-3

Table 1 Summary of the central effects of NPY with their appropriate references

Effect	Reference
Feeding	Clark *et al.* (1984), Levine and Morley (1984), Stanley and Leibowitz (1984, 1985)
Anxiolysis	Heilig *et al.* (1993), Wahlestedt *et al.* (1993)
Gonadotrophin release	Kalra and Crowley (1984, 1992), Sahu *et al.* (1989), Bauer Dantoin *et al.* (1992), Kalra (1993)
Lipoprotein lipase activity	Billington *et al.* (1991, 1994)
CRF and ACTH release	Wahlestedt *et al.* (1987), Haas and George (1989), Tsagarakis *et al.* (1989), Koenig (1990)
Growth hormone secretion	McDonald *et al.* (1985), Härfstrand *et al.* (1987), Rettori *et al.* (1990a,b), Okada *et al.* (1993), Pierrroz *et al.* (1996)
Insulin release	Moltz and McDonald (1985), Dunbar *et al.* (1992), van Dijk *et al.* (1994), Wilding *et al.* (1995)
Thermogenesis	Menendez *et al.* (1990), Billington *et al.* (1991, 1994), Egawa *et al.* (1991)
Temperature regulation	Inui *et al.* (1989), Ruiz de Elvira and Coen (1990), Bouali *et al.* (1995), Jolicoeur *et al.* (1995)

between the transmitters within the brain that regulate feeding, energy storage and expenditure. There appear to be a multitude of receptors mediating the many central effects of NPY. Thus characterization of the receptor types is clearly essential for the development of selective NPY receptor antagonists for the treatment of obesity.

The recent finding that an NPY knockout mouse maintained a normal phenotype (Erickson *et al.*, 1996) may indicate that when NPY is absent from an embryonic stage, alternative pathways can compensate for such a deficiency.

Many neurotransmitters have been hypothesized to play a role in the regulation of feeding. Experimentally an abundance of inhibitors of feeding exist, although few have been demonstrated to be physiologically relevant. Two such examples are the recently discovered product of the obese gene, leptin (Zhang *et al.*, 1994) and the hypothalamic neuropeptide GLP-1 (7–36) amide (GLP-1) (Turton *et al.*, 1996). Leptin, produced exclusively in white adipose tissue (Rink, 1994), is a circulating hormone which is thought to form a feedback loop to the hypothalamus, conveying information about body fat and thus participating in the regulation of food intake (Scott, 1996).

The full sequence receptor for leptin is expressed in the hypothalamus, which would support this hypothesis (Lee *et al.*, 1996). A physiological role for central GLP 1 in the termination of feeding has recently been demonstrated (Turton *et al.*, 1996). GLP-1 is thought to be a neurotransmitter released within the brain as feeding proceeds, thus preventing further food intake. Stimulation of feeding on the other hand has been reported with very few transmitters, namely, noradrenaline (NA) or adrenaline (ADR) (Leibowitz, 1978; Matthews *et al.*, 1978), γ-aminobutyric acid (GABA) (Kelly *et al.*, 1977), growth-hormone releasing hormone (GHRH) (Vaccarino *et al.*, 1985), galanin (Kyrkouli *et al.*, 1986; Tempel *et al.*, 1988) and opioid peptides (Grandison and Guidotti, 1977; Morley *et al.*, 1982). The most powerful stimulator of food intake yet discovered is NPY. It has a potent effect on feeding lasting for hours when injected centrally, even in satiated animals (Clark *et al.*, 1984; Levine and Morley, 1984; Stanley and Leibowitz, 1984, 1985).

The control of feeding is highly complex. The hypothalamus, which lies at the base of the forebrain, plays a vital role in controlling and co-ordinating vital functions such as eating behaviour and the maintenance of energy balance (Williams and Bloom, 1989). It receives and integrates signals from a multitude of factors (food-related, environmental, humoral and endocrine), which it in turn regulates, forming a continuous feedback loop with other areas of the body. NPY is found in abundance in this region of the brain (Allen *et al.*, 1983), and endogenous NPY has been hypothesized to be involved in energy balance (Leibowitz, 1990). NPY not only stimulates feeding, but also exerts direct effects on energy metabolism (Leibowitz, 1991). In fact many of the metabolic effects observed following injection of NPY are similar to those seen in genetically obese rodents (Beck *et al.*, 1992; Zarjevski *et al.*, 1993). Alterations in central NPY have been shown to precede disturbances in feeding in these animals (Beck *et al.*, 1993), supporting a role for NPY in the development of obesity and NIDDM. Indeed, increased NPYergic activity within the hypothalamus has been linked to the development of insulin resistance (Schwartz *et al.*, 1993; Vettor *et al.*, 1994; Zarjevski *et al.*, 1994).

Interactions between NPY and the various other stimulatory and inhibitory transmitters known to be involved in the regulation of feeding will provide us with a better understanding of the neuronal pathways involved. Physiological inhibitors of feeding such as leptin or GLP-1 are possible targets for the development of novel anti-obesity agents.

A putative role for leptin in the control of feeding and metabolism through an action on hypothalmic NPY was reported recently. It is known that hypothalamic NPY gene expression is elevated in two genetic models of obesity, obese (*ob*/*ob*) and diabetic (*db*/*db*) mice (Wilding *et al.*, 1993a and Chua *et al.*, 1991, respectively), which may contribute to the development of obesity and metabolic disorders observed in such animals. Chronic administration of leptin to *ob*/*ob* mice significantly reduced body weight, and neuronal expression of NPY mRNA within the arcuate nucleus of the hypothalmus of these mice was markedly decreased (Stephens *et al.*, 1995; Schwartz *et al.*, 1996). In the *db*/*db* mouse, believed to have a defect in the leptin receptor, leptin had no effect (Stephens *et al.*, 1995; Schwartz *et al.*, 1996). Leptin was also reported to significantly reduce NPY release from rat hypothalami *in vitro* (Stephens *et al.*, 1995). These data suggest that the effects of leptin may be, at least in part, through the inhibition of hypothalamic NPY synthesis and release. NPY knockout

Table 2 Distribution of NPY-like immunoreactivity in the rat brain. Adapted from Allen *et al.* (1983)

Brain region	NPY immunoreactivity (pmol g^{-1} wet tissue)
Olfactory bulb	82.2±4.2
Cortex	180±30
Preoptic hypothalamus	729.8±164
Periventricular hypothalamus	980±162
Nucleus accumbens	891.4±80.9
Amygdala	714.7±56.2
Thalamus	103.4±20.9
Cerebellum	27±5.2
Hippocampus	205.2±31.6

mice, however, maintain normal body weight and an intact response to leptin (Erickson *et al.*, 1996), suggesting that compensatory mechanisms may exist to counteract the deficiency of NPY. Antagonism of the central GLP-1 system increases the feeding response to NPY (Turton *et al.*, 1996). However the extent of the interaction between the GLP-1 and NPY systems remains to be determined.

NPY as a powerful stimulator of feeding remains a potentially better target for the development of anti-obesity agents than inhibitors since the development of specific antagonists is favoured over the development of chemical mimics.

2.2 Pathways mediating the central effects of neuropeptide Y

NPY is predominantly located within neurons of the central and sympathetic nervous systems (Lundberg *et al.*, 1984; Miyachi *et al.*, 1986), with widespread distribution throughout the CNS. NPY has been identified in the hypothalamus (Chronwall *et al.*, 1985; de Quidt and Emson, 1986). The concentrations of NPY in this region are compared with other central sites in Table 2.

The arcuate nucleus (ARC) is the main site of NPY synthesis within the hypothalamus (Bai *et al.*, 1985). The NPYergic neurons arising from the ARC project to the paraventricular nucleus of the hypothalamus (PVN) where it is released (de Quidt and Emson, 1986). An intracerebroventricular (ICV) injection of NPY activates expression of the immediate early gene *c-fos*, a well-established marker of neuronal activation (Sagar *et al.*, 1988), within the PVN (Li *et al.*, 1994; Lambert *et al.*, 1995) and other forebrain regions involved in the regulation of feeding such as the amygdala and brainstem (Xu *et al.*, 1995). Thus it appears that several regions of the CNS are involved in mediating the actions of NPY. Subsequent observation of its potent appetite stimulating effect following central administration (Clark *et al.*, 1984; Levine and Morley, 1984; Stanley and Leibowitz, 1984, 1985) led to the suggestion that NPY may play a key role in normal eating behaviour and body weight regulation. The research which has led to these conclusions is discussed here.

2.3 Neuropeptide Y and the regulation of feeding

NPY is localized in high concentrations within the hypothalamus, in particular the PVN (Chronwall *et al.*, 1985). The PVN is innervated by NPYergic neurons projecting from the arcuate nucleus (Bai *et al.*, 1985), the primary site of NPY synthesis (Gehlert *et al.*, 1987; Morris, 1989), and from brainstem catecholaminergic neurons, which contain NPY as a co-transmitter (Sawchenko *et al.*, 1985; Sahu *et al.*, 1988b). Neonatal monosodium glutamate treatment destroys neurons of the arcuate nucleus resulting in hypophagia and obesity (Scallet and Olney, 1986). Among the neurons affected are those containing NPY, which results in a marked decrease in NPY fibres in the PVN (Kerkerian and Pelletier, 1986; Kagotani *et al.*, 1989). The PVN has an established role in the regulation of feeding behaviour (Gold *et al.*, 1977; Leibowitz, 1988), and it is the abundance of NPY in this region (Chronwall *et al.*, 1985), which led to studies on the effect of NPY on feeding. It has been demonstrated that destruction of the PVN leads to hyperphagia and obesity (Leibowitz *et al.*, 1981). NPY has also been shown to inhibit adenylyl cyclase activity *in vitro* (Michel, 1991; Garlind *et al.*, 1992). These observations led to the suggestion that NPY may stimulate feeding through the inhibition of an inhibitory factor. This may well explain the observed latency to eat in animals injected with NPY, in most cases greater than 10 min (Clark *et al.*, 1985; Stanley and Leibowitz, 1985), which is not seen with other stimulants of feeding such as galanin and NA. Candidate neurotransmitters have been proposed as the inhibitory factor through which NPY may ultimately act, but the evidence is inconclusive.

When administered ICV or directly into the hypothalamus of rats at low doses, NPY produces a robust and sustained increase in feeding, even in satiated animals (Clark *et al.*, 1984; Levine and Morley, 1984; Stanley and Leibowitz, 1984, 1985). The abundance of NPY in the PVN and the greater potency of its effect on feeding when injected directly into this nucleus rather than into the ventricles of the brain suggested that the PVN may be the primary locus for its effects on feeding. Microinjection studies into various regions of the hypothalamus have shown that the PVN is no more sensitive to the orexigenic effect of NPY than other sites such as the ventromedial hypothalamus and lateral hypothalamus (Stanley *et al.*, 1985a; Morley *et al.*, 1987). In an attempt to reveal a site-specific pattern of effect, a more extensive and accurate cannula mapping study was conducted by Stanley and colleagues. Microinjection of NPY, in minute volumes (20 nl) to minimize diffusion, into discrete areas of the hypothalamus was used. This revealed that the perifornical hypothalamus (PFH) was the most sensitive site to the orexigenic effect of NPY (Stanley *et al.*, 1993), providing evidence in favour of the PFH, as opposed to the PVN, as the primary locus of NPY action. It is possible that the greatest abundance of NPY feeding receptors may be located in this region. This is supported by receptor autoradiography, which revealed high concentrations of PYY binding sites in this region (Quirion et al., 1990; see also Dumond et al., this volume).

NPY-treated animals have been reported to show strong preference for carbohydrate when pure macronutrient diets are available, with little or no effect on fat or protein intake (Stanley et al., 1985b; Tempel and Leibowitz, 1990). This had led to the suggestion that NPY may be involved in mediating the consumption of carbohydrate, which is the macronutrient of choice at the start of the active feeding period in rats (Tempel et al., 1989). Indeed, peak levels of NPY are detected in the hypothalamus at this time (Jhanwar Uniyal et al., 1990; McKibbin et al., 1991b). Others have failed to reproduce this carbohydrate selection in food preference studies, and it is possible that palatability and caloric content of diets may account for reported effects on macronutrient selection.

Until recently the orexigenic effect of NPY was thought to be mediated by the Y1 receptor (Kalra et al., 1991a). Both Y1 and Y2 receptors are present within the CNS. However few Y1 receptors have been identified within the hypothalamus (Larsen et al., 1993). Using a more extensive range of NPY analogues, Stanley and colleagues were the first to hypothesize that NPY's effect on feeding was not mediated by a classical Y1 receptor, but by an atypical Y1 receptor. This was based on findings that the NPY fragment NPY 2–36 was as potent an inducer of feeding as NPY itself at a given dose (Stanley et al., 1992), despite its poor binding at the classical Y1 receptor (Grundemar et al., 1992; Beck Sickinger and Jung, 1995a). Further evidence in support of this concept has since emerged from studying the effect of a multitude of NPY analogues on food intake. Kirby and colleagues recently reported that a cyclic analogue of NPY, whilst fully active at the Y1 receptor in vitro, was inactive at stimulating feeding (Kirby et al., 1995). It has been shown that the full Y1 receptor agonist [Pro^{34}]NPY elicits only 50% of the maximum feeding response to NPY, and that deletion of either one or two of its N-terminal amino acids does not result in a loss of potency to stimulate feeding, despite poor affinities for the Y1 receptor (O'Shea et al., in press, Endocrinology). This offers support to the hypothesis that the receptor mediating the orexigenic effect of NPY is not the classical Y1 receptor, and is referred to here as the feeding receptor (YFR). Administration of even a high dose of the Y2 receptor agonist NPY 13–36 had minimal effect alone and failed to augment the maximum feeding response induced by [Pro^{34}]NPY, which led to the suggestion that maximal stimulation of feeding by NPY is fully independent of Y2 receptor activation (O'Shea et al., in press, Endocrinology). A recent paper by Gerald and co-workers reports the cloning of a novel rat hypothalamic NPY receptor, termed Y5, which they suggest may be the feeding receptor (YFR). This is based on its ligand binding profile and the stimulation of feeding by [D-Trp^{32}]NPY, a selective agonist at this receptor (Gerald et al., 1996). The failure of NPY(13–36) to stimulate feeding (Kalra et al., 1991a) despite its ability to activate their Y5 receptor casts some doubt on this proposal. A further Y5 receptor has been cloned from the mouse hypothalamus which has a different pharmacological profile and is less well characterized than the rat Y5 receptor (Weinberg et al., 1996).

NPY is one of the few appetite stimulants shown to have a physiological role in the regulation of feeding. Administration of an NPY antibody to fasted (Lambert *et al.*, 1993) and freely feeding rats (Dube *et al.*, 1994) reduced their food intake, suggesting that endogenous NPY drives feeding. In support of this, hypothalamic NPY and NPY mRNA are known to increase upon fasting, and these changes are reversed by refeeding (Sahu *et al.*, 1988a). Fasting also increases the levels of NPY mRNA in the arcuate nucleus of the hypothalamus (Brady *et al.*, 1990). Indeed, increased appetite for food as a result of fasting has been shown to be accompanied by an increase in hypothalamic release of NPY (Kalra *et al.*, 1991b; Lambert *et al.*, 1994). These increased extracellular levels of NPY return to baseline when food is made available (Kalra *et al.*, 1991b). The administration of insulin has also been demonstrated to prevent the elevation in NPY mRNA and peptide content observed in fasted (Schwartz *et al.*, 1992) and hyperphagic diabetic rats (Sipols *et al.*, 1995). Such changes in the NPY system may be a consequence of a direct action of circulating insulin on the brain, as it is thought to signal body adiposity.

The strongest support for NPY's role in feeding is the observation that it produced persistent hyperphagia in rats when administered chronically by any of three means: continuous infusion by means of an osmotic mini-pump; repeated injection into the third ventricle; or injection into the PVN (Stanley *et al.*, 1986, 1989; Beck *et al.*, 1992; Zarjevski *et al.*, 1993). The increase in feeding was accompanied by a significant gain in body weight. NPY is unique in this respect as there appears to be no tolerance to its appetite stimulating effect. Tolerance does develop to other known stimulators of feeding (Smith *et al.*, 1994). The gain in body weight following chronic administration of NPY was disproportionate to the caloric consumption of the animals, suggesting an effect of NPY on peripheral metabolism separate from its orexigenic properties. Further studies have revealed a diverse range of actions of NPY including effects on themogenesis and lipogenesis, independent of its effect on feeding. Such observations have led to the suggestion that NPY may be involved in the pathophysiology of eating disorders such as obesity, which is discussed later in this chapter.

2.4 NPY and fat deposition

Food intake, body weight homeostasis and thermogenesis (basal metabolic rate) are all closely related. Alterations in one or all of these functions can lead to an excess deposition of fat and consequently to obesity. NPY also appears to be involved in the regulation of energy intake and storage.

2.4.1 Thermogenesis

NPY injection into the PVN of the hypothalamus causes a decrease in brown adipose tissue (BAT) thermogenesis as indicated by the measurement of BAT mitochondrial GDP binding and uncoupling protein mRNA (Billington *et al.*, 1991, 1994). This occurs even when NPY-treated animals are pair-fed, which involves allowing

NPY-treated animals access to the same amount of food consumed by control-treated animals. This reduction in thermogenic activity may be due to decreased activity of the BAT sympathetic innervation (Egawa et al., 1991). The potent orexigenic effect of NPY in addition to a reduction in BAT thermogenesis further facilitates weight gain. An increase in thermogenesis normally accompanies an increase in food intake in cafeteria feeding as a means of expending surplus energy (Glick et al., 1981; Rothwell and Stock, 1981; Rothwell et al., 1982; Tulp et al., 1982). BAT has been proposed as the tissue responsible for the relative resistance of rodents to diet-induced obesity (Rothwell and Stock, 1979). This mechanism is defective in genetically obese animals. The obese (ob/ob) mouse and the Zucker (fa/fa) rat are unable to increase their thermogenic activity as a consequence of increases in feeding or cold exposure (Himms Hagen and Desautels, 1978; Holt et al., 1983). Indeed a recent study demonstrated that a reduction in the mass of BAT (by toxigene-mediated ablation) increases susceptibility to diet-induced obesity and its accompanying disorders such as insulin resistance and hyperlipidemia (Hamann et al., 1996). NPY injection (30–156 pmol) elevated the respiratory quotient, which is indicative of oxidation of carbohydrate, and storage of energy as fat (Menendez et al., 1990).

2.4.2 Carbohydrate metabolism/insulin resistance

It has been hypothesized that NPY may have a specific role in regulating carbohydrate metabolism. Injection of NPY into various regions of the CNS such as the third ventricle (Moltz and McDonald, 1995), the PVN (van Dijk et al., 1994), and the nucleus tractus solitarius (NTS) (Dunbar et al., 1992) raises circulating insulin levels, independent of food consumption (van Dijk et al., 1994). Plasma glucose levels remained unchanged. However, a time-dependency profile, which may have revealed any transient change was not performed. A rise in plasma insulin with no change in glucose in response to NPY suggests either an increase in hepatic glucose output or a reduction in peripheral sensitivity to insulin. To address this issue, tritiated glucose was used as a tracer following ICV injection of NPY in rats fasted for 6 h and subjected to a hyperinsulinaemic euglycaemic clamp. An increase in hepatic glucose output was found to precede a rise in insulin. Conversely peripheral glucose uptake increased during the clamp, suggesting an increase in insulin sensitivity. These changes were accompanied by a small rise in glucagon (Wilding et al., 1995). Studies that have suggested a role for central NPY in increasing insulin sensitivity have suffered from not performing a time-dependency profile and do not really provide evidence to prove such a claim. The precise mechanisms underlying the profound effects of NPY on islet hormone secretion and glucose homeostasis remain unclear. These observations are consistent with a role for NPY in carbohydrate metabolism and the promotion of fat deposition.

2.4.3 Lipid metabolism

The central effect of NPY on lipid metabolism has not been extensively investigated. Intracerebral injection of NPY has been shown to augment both the expression and activity of lipoprotein lipase (Billington *et al.*, 1991, 1994), promoting white fat lipid storage. No correlations with plasma insulin levels or food intake were observed, at least in acute experiments (Billington *et al.*, 1991), thus the mechanism of this effect remains unknown. Interestingly, genetically obese rodents such as the Zucker (*fa/fa*) rat have higher lipoprotein lipase activity than their lean counterparts (Horwitz *et al.*, 1984).

Thus, NPY exhibits potent effects on carbohydrate metabolism, brown fat thermogenesis and white fat lipid storage in addition to its potent effect on feeding, emphasizing an important role for NPY in energy balance. The effects of NPY on energy metabolism would promote energy conservation when food is in short supply. However, in satiated models NPY promotes carbohydrate metabolism and its storage as fat, and increases circulating levels of insulin. Thus, the effect of NPY injection is totally different depending on the model used. A possible hypothesis is that when food is available NPY levels are increased. This may increase insulin release and direct metabolism to storage of energy as fat. When food is scarce, elevated levels of NPY may promote energy conservation by reducing thermogenic activity. Increased activity of the hypothalamic NPY system, in particular within the PVN, may be an important conversatory mechanism designed to promote fat deposition for times of food shortage, and may be responsible at least in part for the defective metabolism observed in genetically obese rodents.

2.5 NPY and pituitary function

NPY antagonists for the treatment of obesity should be without effects on the hypothalamic–pituitary–adrenal (HPA) and growth hormone (GH) axes. There is increasing evidence that the receptors mediating NPY effects on feeding and pituitary function are different, but further research is needed to clarify this.

2.5.1 NPY and the growth hormone axis

Several studies have shown that NPY has an effect on the regulation of the growth-hormone releasing factor (GRF)/somatostatin–GH axis. Early studies in rats revealed a potent effect of NPY in reducing circulating levels of GH (McDonald *et al.*, 1985; Härfstrand *et al.*, 1987). These initial results were confirmed by the observation that administration of an antibody to NPY caused a rise in the levels of GH in both ovariectomized female and normal male rats (Rettori *et al.*, 1990a). GH pulsatility was also partially restored by the central administration of NPY antibody following a 72-h fast (Okada *et al.*, 1993).

It is thought that the effect of NPY on GH is not direct, rather it is mediated through its ability to stimulate the release of hypothalamic somatostatin. Synaptic associations exist between NPY containing and somatostatin containing neurons within the hypothalamus (Hisano *et al.*, 1990). Low doses of NPY stimulate the release of somatostatin from hypothalamic fragments *in vitro* (Rettori *et al.*, 1990a). Pituitary responsiveness to somatostatin is unaltered in rats treated with ICV NPY antiserum, suggesting a hypothalamic mechanism of action on GH levels (Rettori *et al.*, 1990b). Others have suggested a direct effect of NPY on somatotroph secretion, however, results from such studies provide conflicting evidence. For example, GH secretion occurs in response to treatment with NPY in perifused rat anterior pituitary cells (McDonald *et al.*, 1985) and goldfish anterior pituitary (Peng *et al.*, 1990, 1993). However, treatment of somatotropic tumour cells with NPY leads to inhibition of both basal and GRF-stimulated GH secretion (Adams *et al.*, 1987). Such discrepancies may well be the result of species differences. In response to food deprivation or diabetes when hypothalamic NPY levels are high, rats display reduced levels of GH (Tannenbaum *et al.*, 1979; Tannenbaum, 1981). In human obesity, where high hypothalamic levels of NPY are predicted, a reduction in GH levels is found (Ferini Strambi *et al.*, 1991). This further supports a role for NPY in the regulation of GH secretion at the level of the hypothalamus. Of interest is the observation that in animal models of altered metabolism the regulation of hypothalamic GRF expression is opposite to that of NPY (Bruno *et al.*, 1990; Olchovsky *et al.*, 1990).

Strong evidence in favour of a regulatory role between NPY and GRF was recently observed by Pierroz and co-workers. They found that chronic administration of NPY completely abolished normal pulsatile secretion of GH and consequently halved plasma IGF-1 levels in the intact adult male rat within the 7 days of the experiment (Pierroz *et al.*, 1996).

In conclusion, most of the published data provides evidence consistent with a primary effect of NPY to inhibit GH secretion through an action on the release of somatostatin from the hypothalamus.

2.5.2 NPY and the hypothalamic–pituitary–adrenal axis

NPY gene expression is regulated by glucocorticoids (Corder *et al.*, 1988; Barnea *et al.*, 1991; Wilding *et al.*, 1993b); however, NPY also appears to regulate the HPA axis. Central administration of NPY is known to stimulate the secretion of corticosterone in the rat (Wahlestedt *et al.*, 1987; Leibowitz *et al.*, 1988; Albers *et al.*, 1990). This effect is thought to be mediated primarily via the hypothalamus, as NPY also stimulates release of corticotrophin-releasing factor (CRF) (Wahlestedt *et al.*, 1987; Tsagarakis *et al.*, 1989). This in turn stimulates ACTH secretion from the anterior pituitary. This in turn raises circulating corticosterone levels by acting on the adrenal glands. Indeed NPY-containing neurons are known to be in close anatomical association with (actually synapse on) CRF-containing neurons within the PVN (Liposits *et al.*, 1988). However, it has also been postulated that NPY may have a direct effect on the pituitary to stimulate ACTH secretion in synergy with CRF (Koenig, 1990). Studies which have examined the dependency of NPY-induced CRF release on noradrenergic input provide conflicting evidence. β- and α_1-adrenoceptor antagonists fail to block the effect of NPY at doses which block noradrenaline-induced ACTH secretion from rat hypothalami *in vitro* (Tsagarakis *et al.*, 1989). On the other hand, the α_2-adrenoceptor agonist clonidine stimulated CRF release with no alteration in synthesis. The same effect was observed in 6-hydroxydopamine-treated rats injected with NPY, suggesting that α_2-adrenoceptors may mediate NPY stimulation of the HPA axis (Haas and George, 1989). Unlike the stimulation of insulin secretion, which is thought to regulate NPY gene expression negatively, glucocorticoids appear to form a positive feedback loop with NPY in that they have a facilitatory effect on NPY gene expression within the hypothalamus (Higuchi et al., 1988; Akabayashi et al., 1994; Larsen et al., 1994).

It has been suggested that the full sequence of NPY is necessary for activation of the HPA axis. This suggestion was based solely on findings that in comparison to NPY, desamidated NPY or NPY (19–36) were inactive at stimulating ACTH release (Miura et al., 1992). Further studies are needed to characterize the receptor type involved.

2.5.3 NPY and reproductive function

NPY has a profound effect on LH secretion in rats. In addition to the adrenergic neurotransmitters, it is one of the most widely studied of all hypothalamic stimulators of LH secretion (Kalra and Crowley, 1984, 1992). It is involved in the regulation of hypothalamic LHRH secretion, in particular the stimulation of gonadotrophin-releasing hormone (GnRH) neurons necessary to initiate the preovulatory LH surge in female rats (Bauer Dantoin et al., 1992; Kalra, 1993). Sex steroids are essential for the facilitatory effect of NPY on LH secretion through the regulation of both secretion (Sahu et al., 1989, 1992a) and post-synaptic activity (Kalra and Crowley, 1984) of hypothalamic NPY. The complex nature of the interaction which exists between NPY and LH cannot be fully addressed in this chapter. Readers are therefore advised to consult the following reviews by Kalra for a more detailed explanation (Kalra and Crowley, 1992; Kalra, 1993).

A recent paper by Pierroz and colleagues examined the effect of chronic ICV infusion of NPY on the pituitary testicular axis in intact male rats (Pierroz et al., 1996). Administration of NPY for 7 days caused a significant reduction in both seminal vesicle and testis weight. Plasma levels of LH, FSH and testosterone were also reduced. However, pair-feeding was not carried out to eliminate the effects of hyperphagia and consequent body weight gain on such parameters in the NPY treated animals. The Y2 receptor agonist NPY 13–36 had no effect on the pituitary testicular axis. From these observations the authors concluded that the effect of NPY on the gonadotropic axis may be mediated by NPY Y1 receptors. This evidence is insufficient to imply Y1-type receptors in the control of LH release, and no conclusions should be drawn until the effects of a more extensive range of NPY fragments and analogues on reproductive function have been tested.

At present it is not known if the receptor mediating the effect of NPY on feeding is pharmacologically distinct from the receptor mediating the effect of NPY on LH secretion. Further studies are certainly needed to characterize fully the receptor type mediating the effect of NPY on LH release. This is an important consideration if selective NPY receptor antagonists for the treatment of obesity are to be developed devoid of any effect on reproductive function in humans.

2.6 Other central effects of NPY

In addition to its effects on feeding, peripheral metabolism and pituitary function, NPY also displays a diverse range of other effects thought to be mediated through an action within the hypothalamus.

2.6.1 NPY and temperature regulation

Neuropeptide Y immunoreactivity is high in the preoptic area, a region of the hypothalamus known to be involved in the regulation of body temperature. This led to the suggestion that NPY may play a role in thermoregulation. NPY has been shown to attenuate prostaglandin-induced hyperthermia in dogs (Inui et al., 1989). In rats, however, the effect of NPY on body temperature is not consistent, and varies according to the hypothalamic site into which it is injected (Ruiz de Elvira and Coen, 1990; Bouali et al., 1995; Jolicoeur et al., 1995). An ICV dose of 10 μg NPY or more induces a decrease in rectal temperature (Jolicoeur et al., 1991b). Deletion of the N-terminal residue Tyr of NPY resulted in a five-fold loss of potency for decreasing rectal temperature despite being equipotent to NPY on feeding (Jolicoeur et al., 1991a). NPY 1–30 has half the potency of NPY at inducing hypothermia but is inactive at stimulating feeding (Bouali et al., 1994). These findings suggest that the receptors mediating the effects of NPY on feeding and body temperature are distinct from each other.

In conclusion, the effect of NPY on thermoregulation appears to be site-specific and dose-dependent. These studies present strong evidence for the involvement of multiple receptor subtypes in mediating the various central effects of NPY.

2.6.2 NPY and anxiolysis

Observations in experimental animals have led to the suggestion that endogenous NPY may be a potent anxiolytic. ICV NPY is known to display potent anxiolytic-like activity in several rat models of anxiety but its powerful orexigenic effect makes this activity difficult to interpret. Microinjection of NPY into the central nucleus of the amygdala, however, resulted in anxiolytic activity without an increase in feeding. The Y1 receptor agonist [Pro^{34}]NPY was equipotent to NPY, whereas the Y2 receptor agonist NPY 13–36 had no effect, suggesting mediation of anxiolytic activity by Y1 receptors in this region (Heilig et al., 1993). Cortical Y1 receptors have also been implicated. ICV administration of antisense to the N-terminus of the Y1 receptor revealed behavioural signs of anxiety in rats, which were shown to have a reduction in the density of cortical Y1 receptors (Wahlestedt et al., 1993).

2.7 NPY and obesity

Obesity is implicated in the development of NIDDM, ischaemic heart disease, hypertension and stroke. Its prevalence in Western society is steadily increasing. It is a multifactorial disease, which makes the design of effective anti-obesity agents difficult. Indeed, no single treatment has been proven to promote sustained weight loss in obese humans. This is probably as a result of a multitude of counter-regulatory mechanisms that naturally exist to conserve one's body weight, 'over-riding' the anorectic effect of such agents and thus rendering them ineffective in long-term weight control. Ideally treatment would be targeted at more than one system involved in the regulation of feeding. Continuing research in this area will inevitably reveal potential targets for the design of effective pharmacological agents to treat obesity.

Body weight and metabolism are regulated by the hypothalamus. In experimental animals diabetes, insulin resistance and dyslipidaemia can be corrected by weight loss (Brownell et al., 1986; Brindley and Russell, 1995), and this has recently been demonstrated in humans (Benotti and Forse, 1995). Increased activity of the hypothalamic NPY system may contribute to the development of obesity in animals. The abnormalities seen in genetically obese rodents can be mimicked by central injection of NPY (Zarjevski et al., 1993).

The involvement of NPY in the pathophysiology of obesity is supported by the fact that alterations in the hypothalamic NPY system precede the disturbances in feeding of genetically obese rodents (Beck et al., 1993). The obese (ob/ob) mouse, diabetic (db/db) mouse and Zucker (fa/fa) rat are such models, and are characterized by hyperphagia and hyperinsulinaemia. Elevations in the levels of NPY mRNA and peptide within the hypothalamus of these models have been found (Chua et al., 1991; Williams et al., 1991; Wilding et al., 1993a), and these changes are associated with an increase in the release of hypothalamic NPY, as measured by push–pull perfusion (Dryden et al., 1995). Obese Zucker rats exhibit higher levels of NPY and NPY mRNA in the arcuate nucleus of the hypothalamus, and higher levels of NPY within the PVN than their lean counterparts (Beck et al., 1990; Sanacora et al., 1990; Pesonen et al., 1991). They are also refractory to the orexigenic effect of centrally administered NPY (Brief et al., 1992). Obese Zucker rats also have elevated levels of circulating insulin and corticosterone (Zucker and Antoniades, 1972; Fletcher et al., 1986). This is consistent with the stimulatory effects of centrally administered NPY on insulin and corticosterone secretion in normal rats (Wahlestedt et al., 1987; Leibowitz et al., 1988; Albers et al., 1990). These results, in combination with the striking similarities between the observed effects on feeding and metabolic activity, and the hyperphagia and defective metabolism observed in obese animals, lend credibility to a role for NPY in the pathophysiology of obesity.

Genetically obese rodents have altered regulation of their NPY system. Elevated levels of hypothalamic NPY mRNA observed in these animals cannot be reversed by an ICV injection of insulin (Schwartz et al., 1991, 1992) and this has been proposed as one mechanism for the increase in NPY synthesis observed in these rodents (Schwartz et al., 1991). This lends support to the hypothesis that these animals have a 'central resistance' to the action of insulin, and that insulin is at least in part a regulator of hypothalamic NPY. Additional support is provided by the finding that animals made obese and consequently hyperinsulinaemic by feeding a highly palatable diet for 6 weeks also display higher levels of hypothalamic NPY than those maintained on standard laboratory chow (Wilding et al., 1992).

It is well known that repeated injection of NPY into the third ventricle or PVN of rodents results in sustained hyperphagia and consequent obesity (Stanley *et al.*, 1986, 1989; Beck *et al.*, 1992). Zarjevski and colleagues examined the effects of chronic ICV NPY infusion on energy, carbohydrate and lipid metabolism (Zarjevski *et al.*, 1993). Pair-feeding was used to separate the direct metabolic effects of NPY from those occurring as a consequence of weight gain. Both *ad libitum* and pair-fed animals chronically treated with NPY had elevated serum triglyceride, insulin and corticosterone levels, and increased body fat compared to controls. Blood glucose levels remained unchanged, however, suggesting an increase in peripheral insulin resistance in NPY-treated animals. Glucose utilization was increased in white adipose tissue, as was *de novo* lipogenesis and lipoprotein lipase activity. On closer examination, glucose utilization in fat was increased in association with an increase in GLUT 4 protein and mRNA. Insulin resistance in muscle was found to increase, however, no change in GLUT 4 was observed. The exact mechanism for this decrease in insulin sensitivity in muscle remains unknown.

2.8 NPY, bulimia and anorexia nervosa

A severe restriction in eating with a massive loss of body weight characterizes anorexia. Body weight loss can sometimes be so severe as to be fatal. Bulimia is characterized by binge-eating, where massive amounts of food are consumed and then purged from the body to avoid weight gain.

Morley *et al.* first proposed NPY and/or PYY as candidates in the pathogenesis of human eating disorders such as bulimia. This was based on observations of a huge increase in daily food intake following central administration of these peptides in rodents (Morley *et al.*, 1985). Stanley *et al.* showed that animals given PFH injections of high-dose NPY consumed a huge meal similar to that observed in bulimics (Stanley *et al.*, 1993).

Evidence also exists to implicate other members of the pancreatic polypeptide family in bulimia. Levels of PYY are raised in the cerebrospinal fluid (CSF) of bulimic patients prevented from binge-eating, and are normalized when bingeing resumed (Berrettini *et al.*, 1988). Thus it was suggested that the binge-eating was aided by excessive hypothalamic PYY and that food consumption reversed this. To date, this is the clearest evidence implicating endogenous PYY in human eating disorders. Underweight anorexic patients have elevated levels of NPY in their CSF, and treatment to regain near normal body weight led to a fall in these levels (Kaye *et al.*, 1990).

These data suggest that both NPY and PYY may be sensitive to factors regulating body weight in humans. The evidence provided by these studies, however, is not conclusive of the involvement of NPY or PYY in the pathology of such eating disorders, and is regarded by many as a simplistic view of what are highly complex diseases. Further research is needed to assess the role of these peptides in bulimia and anorexia nervosa.

2.9 NPY and diabetes

Hypothalamic NPY has been implicated in the pathophysiology of diabetes. A relationship between NPY and circulating levels of insulin has been proposed, which may account for the characteristic hyperphagia observed in diabetic animals. As discussed earlier in this chapter, an ICV or intrahypothalamic injection of NPY raises levels of circulating insulin independent of the availability of food (Moltz and McDonald, 1985; van Dijk *et al.*, 1994). This is accompanied by a small increase in plasma glucose levels, but more frequently no change is observed. As a rise in insulin levels promotes cellular utilization of glucose, it appears that NPY has counter regulatory effects to the action of insulin. This is supported by its increasing of plasma glucagon and corticosterone (Pettersson *et al.*, 1987; Wahlestedt *et al.*, 1987; McKibbin *et al.*, 1991a), which promote a rise in glucose levels mainly through gluconeogenesis and glycogenolysis. NPY also reduces growth hormone secretion (McDonald *et al.*, 1985; Härfstrand *et al.*, 1987), which may increase cellular utilization of glucose. NPY has a potent effect on carbohydrate ingestion and increases the respiratory quotient (Menendez *et al.*, 1990). Together these endocrine effects should collectively lead to a rise in plasma glucose, but this is not the case. NPY appears to be exclusive in this respect, since PVN injection of other stimulators of feeding such as the catecholamines NA and ADR lead to a rise in plasma glucose, while at the same time increasing circulating levels of insulin and corticosterone (Leibowitz *et al.*, 1988; Ionescu *et al.*, 1989). Thus, stimulators of feeding appear to have their own definitive pattern of endocrine response.

Manipulation of circulating levels of insulin has been shown to cause profound changes in the levels of hypothalamic NPY. For example, rats made insulin deficient by the beta-cell toxin streptozotocin have been shown to have raised levels of both NPY mRNA and peptide within the hypothalamus (Williams *et al.*, 1988b; Sahu *et al.*, 1990; White *et al.*, 1990; Jones *et al.*, 1992). On closer examination this was found to be specific to certain hypothalamic nuclei, namely the paraventricular and ventromedial nuclei, and the lateral hypothalamic area (Williams *et al.*, 1989a). Indeed NPY is the only hypothalamic peptide to be consistently altered in diabetic animals (Williams *et al.*, 1988b). This increase in NPY mRNA is suggestive of increased NPYergic activity. This is consistent with the observation that secretion of NPY from the area of the PVN is increased in the streptozotocin diabetic rat (Sahu *et al.*, 1992b; Lambert *et al.*, 1994). Genetic models of diabetes have also been shown to have disturbances in their hypothalamic NPY system. The spontaneously diabetic BB/E Wistar rat has elevated levels of NPY within the central hypothalamus (Williams *et al.*, 1989b), whereas the spontaneously diabetic Chinese hamster displays a reduction in hypothalamic NPY concentration (Williams *et al.*, 1988a). By giving insulin replacement to such animals, the disturbance in NPY activity can be partially reversed (Williams *et al.*, 1989b; Sahu *et al.*, 1990; White *et al.*, 1990). It is likely that insulin alters the levels of NPY by a direct effect on NPY gene transcription within the brain. This is based on the fact that ICV insulin reduces the elevated levels of NPY mRNA induced by food deprivation in the arcuate nucleus of the hypothalamus (Schwartz *et al.*, 1991, 1992), whereas peripheral injections of insulin are ineffective (Corrin *et al.*, 1991). These findings of disturbances in the hypothalmic NPY system in diabetic rats suggest that increased hypothalamic NPY may be responsible for the hyperphagia characteristic of these animals.

2.10 Conclusion

NPY is one of the most potent central physiological regulators of feeding behaviour and metabolism yet discovered. It stimulates feeding in a variety of mammals and has marked effects on peripheral metabolism, such as decreasing brown adipose tissue thermogenesis and stimulating lipoprotein lipase activity. NPY also has profound effects on sexual function and the growth hormone axis.

Chronic central administration of NPY causes hyperphagia and weight gain disproportionate to the amount of food consumed. This led to the suggestion that NPY may be involved in the development of obesity and its associated metabolic disorders. Indeed the effects of NPY on feeding and metabolism in non-obese rodents are similar to certain characteristics of genetically obese rodents, such as hyperphagia, dyslipidaemia and decreased thermogenic activity. Dysfunctions in the hypothalamic NPY system are present in genetically obese animals at an early age and may contribute to the disturbances in their feeding behaviour and metabolism.

The feeding receptor has been characterized. A further rat hypothalamic NPY receptor (termed Y5) has now been cloned that is proposed to be the feeding receptor. Binding data of several NPY analogues correlates well with their effects on feeding behaviour. However central administration of NPY(13–36), an agonist at the Y5 receptor, has no effect on food intake. This finding opposes the proposed role of the Y5 receptor as the feeding receptor. The development of specific antagonists to this receptor will allow investigation of its precise role. It is not known if an NPY receptor type exists that solely affects feeding. In view of NPYs diverse and potent effects on other systems, namely sexual function, the HPA and growth hormone axes, the identification of such a receptor is obviously of great importance for the development of specific antagonists to the NPY feeding receptor, with the ultimate aim of providing a new generation of anti-obesity agents.

References

Adams, E.F., Venetikou, M.S., Woods, C.A., Lacoumenta, S. & Burrin, J.M. (1987) Neuropeptide Y directly inhibits growth hormone secretion by human pituitary somatotropic tumours. *Acta Endocrinol. Copenh.* **115**, 149–154.

Akabayashi, A., Watanabe, Y., Wahlestedt, C., McEwen, B.S., Paez, X. & Leibowitz, S.F. (1994) Hypothalamic neuropeptide Y, its gene expression and receptor activity: Relation to circulating corticosterone in adrenalectomized rats. *Brain Res.* **665**, 201–212.

Albers, H.E., Ottenweller, J.E., Liou, S.Y., Lumpkin, M.D. & Anderson, E.R. (1990) Neuropeptide Y in the hypothalamus: Effect on corticosterone and single-unit activity. *Am. J. Physiol.* **258**, R376–382.

Allen, Y.S., Adrian, T.E., Allen, J.M., Tatemoto, K., Crow, T.J., Bloom, S.R. & Polak, J.M. (1983) Neuropeptide Y distribution in the rat brain. *Science* **221**, 877–879.

Bai, F.L., Yamano, M., Shiotani, Y., Emson, P.C., Smith, A.D., Powell, J.F. & Tohyama, M. (1985) An arcuato-paraventricular and -dorsomedial hypothalamic neuropeptide Y-containing system which lacks noradrenaline in the rat. *Brain Res.* **331**, 172–175.

Barnea, A., Cho, G., Hajibeigi, A., Aguila, M.C. & Magni, P. (1991) Dexamethasone-induced accumulation of neuropeptide-Y by aggregating fetal brain cells in culture: A process dependent on the developmental age of aggregates. *Endocrinology* **129**, 931–938.

Bauer Dantoin, A.C., McDonald, J.K. & Levine, J.E. (1992) Neuropeptide Y potentiates luteinizing hormone (LH)-releasing hormone-induced LH secretion only under conditions leading to preovulatory LH surges. *Endocrinology* **131**, 2946–2952.

Beck, B., Stricker Krongrad, A., Nicolas, J.P. & Burlet, C. (1992) Chronic and continuous intracerebroventricular infusion of neuropeptide Y in Long–Evans rats mimics the feeding behaviour of obese Zucker rats. *Int. J. Obes. Relat. Metab. Disord.* **16**, 295–302.

Beck, B., Burlet, A., Nicolas, J.P. & Burlet, C. (1990) Hypothalamic neuropeptide Y (NPY) in obese Zucker rats: Implications in feeding and sexual behaviours. *Physiol. Behav.* **47**, 449–453.

Beck, B., Burlet, A., Bazin, R., Nicolas, J.P. & Burlet, C. (1993) Elevated neuropeptide Y in the arcuate nucleus of young obese Zucker rats may contribute to the development of their overeating. *J. Nutr.* **123**, 1168–1172.

Beck Sickinger, A.G. & Jung, G. (1995) Structure–activity relationships of neuropeptide Y analogues with respect to Y1 and Y2 receptors. *Biopolymers* **37**, 123–142.

Benotti, P.N. & Forse, R.A. (1995) The role of gastric surgery in the multidisciplinary management of severe obesity. *Am. J. Surg.* **169**, 361–367.

Berrettini, W.H., Kaye, W.H., Gwirtsman, H. & Allbright, A. (1988) Cerebrospinal fluid peptide YY immunoreactivity in eating disorders. *Neuropsychobiology* **19**, 121–124.

Billington, C.J., Briggs, J.E., Grace, M. & Levine, A.S. (1991) Effects of intracerebroventricular injection of neuropeptide Y on energy metabolism. *Am. J. Physiol.* **260**, R321–327.

Billington, C.J., Briggs, J.E., Harker, S., Grace, M. & Levine, A.S. (1994) Neuropeptide Y in hypothalamic paraventricular nucleus: a center coordinating energy metabolism. *Am. J. Physiol.* **266**, R1765–1770.

Bouali, S.M., Fournier, A., St Pierre, S. & Jolicoeur, F.B. (1994) In vivo central actions of NPY(1–30), an N-terminal fragment of neuropeptide Y. *Peptides* **15**, 799–802.

Bouali, S.M., Fournier, A., St Pierre, S. & Jolicoeur, F.B. (1995) Effects of NPY and NPY2–36 on body temperature and food intake following administration into hypothalamic nuclei. *Brain Res. Bull.* **36**, 131–135.

Brady, L.S., Smith, M.A., Gold, P.W. & Herkenham, M. (1990) Altered expression of hypothalamic neuropeptide mRNAs in food-restricted and food-deprived rats. *Neuroendocrinology* **52**, 441–447.

Brief, D.J., Sipols, A.J. & Woods, S.C. (1992) Intraventricular neuropeptide Y injections stimulate food intake in lean, but not obese Zucker rats. *Physiol. Behav.* **51**, 1105–1110.

Brindley, D.N. & Russell, J.C. (1995) Metabolic abnormalities linked to obesity: effects of dexfenfluramine in the corpulent rat. *Metabolism* **44**, 23–27.

Brownell, K.D., Greenwood, M.R., Stellar, E. & Shrager, E.E. (1986) The effects of repeated cycles of weight loss and regain in rats. *Physiol. Behav.* **38**, 459–464.

Bruno, J.F., Olchovsky, D., White, J.D., Leidy, J.W., Song, J. & Berelowitz, M. (1990) Influence of food deprivation on the rat on hypothalamic expression of growth hormone-releasing factor and somatostatin. *Endocrinology* **127**, 2111–2116.

Chronwall, B.M., DiMaggio, D.A., Massari, V.J., Pickel, V.M., Ruggiero, D.A. & O'Donohue,

T.L. (1985) The anatomy of neuropeptide-Y-containing neurons in rat brain. *Neuroscience* **15**, 1159–1181.

Chua, S.C., Jr, Brown, A.W., Kim, J., Hennessey, K.L., Leibel, R.L. & Hirsch, J. (1991) Food deprivation and hypothalamic neuropeptide gene expression: effects of strain background and the diabetes mutation. *Brain Res. Mol. Brain Res.* **11**, 291–299.

Clark, J.T., Kalra, P.S., Crowley, W.R. & Kalra, S.P. (1984) Neuropeptide Y and human pancreatic polypeptide stimulate feeding behavior in rats. *Endocrinology* **115**, 427–429.

Clark, J.T., Kalra, P.S. & Kalra, S.P. (1985) Neuropeptide Y stimulates feeding but inhibits sexual behavior in rats. *Endocrinology* **117**, 2435–2442.

Corder, R., Pralong, F., Turnill, D., Saudan, P., Muller, A.F. & Gaillard, R.C. (1988) Dexamethasone treatment increases neuropeptide Y levels in rat hypothalamic neurones. *Life Sci.* **43**, 1879–1886.

Corrin, S.E., McCarthy, H.D., McKibbin, P.E. & Williams, G. (1991) Unchanged hypothalamic neuropeptide Y concentrations in hyperphagic, hypoglycemic rats: evidence for specific metabolic regulation of hypothalamic NPY. *Peptides* **12**, 425–430.

De Quidt, M.E. & Emson, P.C. (1986) Distribution of neuropeptide Y-like immunoreactivity in the rat central nervous system – II. Immunohistochemical analysis. *Neuroscience* **18**, 545–618.

Dryden, S., Pickavance, L., Frankish, H.M. & Williams, G. (1995) Increased neuropeptide Y secretion in the hypothalamic paraventricular nucleus of obese *(fa/fa)* Zucker rats. *Brain Res.* **690**, 185–188.

Dube, M.G., Xu, B., Crowley, W.R., Kalra, P.S. & Kalra, S.P. (1994) Evidence that neuropeptide Y is a physiological signal for normal food intake. *Brain Res.* **646**, 341–344.

Dunbar, J.C., Ergene, E. & Barraco, R.A. (1992) Neuropeptide-Y stimulation of insulin secretion is mediated via the nucleus tractus solitarius. *Horm. Metab. Res.* **24**, 103–105.

Egawa, M., Yoshimatsu, H. & Bray, G.A. (1991) Neuropeptide Y suppresses sympathetic activity to interscapular brown adipose tissue in rats. *Am. J. Physiol.* **260**, R328–R334.

Erickson, J.C., Clegg, K.E. & Palmiter, R.D. (1996) Sensitivity to leptin and susceptibility to seizures of mice lacking neuropeptide Y. *Nature* **381**, 415–418.

Ferini Strambi, L., Franceschi, M., Cattaneo, A.G., Smirne, S., Calori, G. & Caviezel, F. (1991) Sleep-related growth hormone secretion in human obesity: effect of dietary treatment. *Neuroendocrinology* **54**, 412–415.

Fletcher, J.M., Haggarty, P., Wahle, K.W. & Reeds, P.J. (1986) Hormonal studies of young lean and obese Zucker rats. *Horm. Metab Res.* **18**, 290–295.

Garlind, A., Fowler, C.J., Alafuzoff, I., Winblad, B. & Cowburn, R.F. (1992) Neurotransmitter-mediated inhibition of post-mortem human brain adenylyl cyclase. *J. Neural Transm. Gen. Sect.* **87**, 113–124.

Gehlert, D.R., Chronwall, B.M., Schafer, M.P. & O'Donohue, T.L. (1987) Localization of neuropeptide Y messenger ribonucleic acid in rat and mouse brain by in situ hybridization. *Synapse* **1**, 25–31.

Gerald, C., Walker, M.W., Criscione, L., *et al.* (1996) A receptor subtype involved in neuropeptide Y-induced food intake. *Nature* **382**, 168–171.

Glick, Z., Teague, R.J. & Bray, G.A. (1981) Brown adipose tissue: thermic response increased by a single low protein, high carbohydrate meal. *Science* **213**, 1125–1127.

Gold, R.M., Jones, A.P. & Sawchenko, P.E. (1977) Paraventricular area: Critical focus of a longitudinal neurocircuitry mediating food intake. *Physiol. Behav.* **18**, 1111–1119.

Grandison, L. & Guidotti, A. (1977) Stimulation of food intake by muscimol and beta endorphin. *Neuropharmacology* **16**, 533–536.

Grundemar, L., Mörner, S.E.J.N., Högestätt, E.D., Wahlestedt, C. & Håkanson, R. (1992) Characterization of vascular neuropeptide Y receptors. *Br. J. Pharmacol.* **105**, 45–50.

Haas, D.A. & George, S.R. (1989) Neuropeptide Y-induced effects on hypothalamic corticotropin-releasing factor content and release are dependent on noradrenergic/adrenergic neurotransmission. *Brain Res.* **498**, 333–338.

Hamann, A., Flier, J.S. & Lowell, B.B. (1996) Decreased brown fat markedly enhances susceptibility to diet-induced obesity, diabetes, and hyperlipidemia. *Endocrinology* **137**, 21–29.

Härfstrand, A., Eneroth, P., Agnati, L. & Fuxe, K. (1987) Further studies on the effects of central administration of neuropeptide Y on neuroendocrine function in the male rat: relationship to hypothalamic catecholamines [published erratum appears in *Regul. Pept.* 1987 **17**, 300]. *Regul. Pept.* **17**, 167–179.

Heilig, M., McLeod, S., Brot, M., Heinrichs, S.C., Menzaghi, F., Koob, G.F. & Britton, K.T. (1993) Anxiolytic-like action of neuropeptide Y: mediation by Y1 receptors in amygdala, and dissociation from food intake effects. *Neuropsychopharmacology* **8**, 357–363.

Higuchi, H., Yang, H.Y. & Sabol, S.L. (1988) Rat neuropeptide Y precursor gene expression. mRNA structure, tissue distribution, and regulation by glucocorticoids, cyclic AMP, and phorbol ester. *J. Biol. Chem.* **263**, 6288–6295.

Himms Hagen, J. & Desautels, M. (1978) A mitochondrial defect in brown adipose tissue of the obese (*ob/ob*) mouse: reduced binding of purine nucleotides and a failure to respond to cold by an increase in binding. *Biochem. Biophys. Res. Commun.* **83**, 628–634.

Hisano, S., Tsuruo, Y., Kagotani, Y., Daikoku, S. & Chihara, K. (1990) Immunohistochemical evidence for synaptic connections between neuropeptide Y-containing axons and periventricular somatostatin neurons in the anterior hypothalamus in rats. *Brain Res.* **520**, 170–177.

Holt, S., York, D.A. & Fitzsimons, J.T. (1983) The effects of corticosterone, cold exposure and overfeeding with sucrose on brown adipose tissue of obese Zucker rats (*fa/fa*). *Biochem. J.* **214**, 215–223.

Horwitz, B.A., Inokuchi, T., Wickler, S.J. & Stern, J.S. (1984) Lipoprotein lipase activity and cellularity in brown and white adipose tissue in Zucker obese rats. *Metabolism* **33**, 354–357.

Inui, Z., Morioka, H., Okita, M., Inoue, T., Sakatani, N., Oya, M., Hatanaka, H., Mizuno, N., Oimomi, M. & Baba, S. (1989) Physiological antagonism between prostaglandin E2 and neuropeptide Y on thermoregulation in the dog. *Peptides* **10**, 869–871.

Ionescu, E., Coimbra, C.C., Walker, C.D. & Jeanrenaud, B. (1989) Paraventricular nucleus modulation of glycemia and insulinemia in freely moving lean rats. *Am. J. Physiol.* **257**, R1370–6.

Jhanwar Uniyal, M., Beck, B., Burlet, C. & Leibowitz, S.F. (1990) Diurnal rhythm of neuropeptide Y-like immunoreactivity in the suprachiasmatic, arcuate and paraventricular nuclei and other hypothalamic sites. *Brain Res.* **536**, 331–334.

Jolicoeur, F.B., Michaud, J.N., Menard, D. & Fournier, A. (1991a) In vivo structure activity study supports the existence of heterogeneous neuropeptide Y receptors. *Brain Res. Bull.* **26**, 309–311.

Jolicoeur, F.B., Michaud, J.N., Rivest, R., Menard, D., Gaudin, D., Fournier, A. & St Pierre, S. (1991b) Neurobehavioral profile of neuropeptide Y. *Brain Res. Bull.* **26**, 265–268.

Jolicoeur, F.B., Bouali, S.M., Fournier, A. & St Pierre, S. (1995) Mapping of hypothalamic sites involved in the effects of NPY on body temperature and food intake. *Brain Res. Bull.* **36**, 125–129.

Jones, P.M., Pierson, A.M., Williams, G., Ghatei, M.A. & Bloom, S.R. (1992) Increased hypothalamic neuropeptide Y messenger RNA levels in two rat models of diabetes. *Diabet. Med.* **9**, 76–80.

Kagotani, Y., Hashimoto, T., Tsuruo, Y., Kawano, H., Daikoku, S. & Chihara, K. (1989) Development of the neuronal system containing neuropeptide Y in the rat hypothalamus. *Int. J. Dev. Neurosci.* **7**, 359–374.

Kalra, S.P. (1993) Mandatory neuropeptide-steroid signaling for the preovulatory luteinizing hormone-releasing hormone discharge. *Endocr. Rev.* **14**, 507–538.

Kalra, S.P. & Crowley, W.R. (1984) Norepinephrine-like effects of neuropeptide Y on LH release in the rat. *Life Sci.* **35**, 1173–1176.

Kalra, S.P. & Crowley, W.R. (1992) Neuropeptide Y: A novel neuroendocrine peptide in the control of pituitary hormone secretion, and its relation to luteinizing hormone. *Front. Neuroendocrinol.* **13**, 1–46.

Kalra, S.P., Dube, M.G., Fournier, A. & Kalra, P.S. (1991a) Structure–function analysis of stimulation of food intake by neuropeptide Y: effects of receptor agonists. *Physiol. Behav.* **50**, 5–9.

Kalra, S.P., Dube, M.G., Sahu, A., Phelps, C.P. & Kalra, P.S. (1991b) Neuropeptide Y secretion increases in the paraventricular nucleus in association with increased appetite for food. *Proc. Natl Acad. Sci. USA* **88**, 10 931–10 935.

Kaye, W.H., Berrettini, W., Gwirtsman, H. & George, D.T. (1990) Altered cerebrospinal fluid neuropeptide Y and peptide YY immunoreactivity in anorexia and bulimia nervosa. *Arch. Gen. Psychiatry* **47**, 548–556.

Kelly, J., Alheid, G.F., Newberg, A. & Grossman, S.P. (1977) GABA stimulation and blockade in the hypothalamus and midbrain: effects on feeding and locomotor activity. *Pharmacol. Biochem. Behav.* **7**, 537–541.

Kerkerian, L. & Pelletier, G. (1986) Effects of monosodium L-glutamate administration on neuropeptide Y-containing neurons in the rat hypothalamus. *Brain Res.* **369**, 388–390.

Kirby, D.A., Koerber, S.C., May, J.M., Hagaman, C., Cullen, M.J., Pelleymounter, M.A. & Rivier, J.E. (1995) Y-1 and Y-2 receptor-selective neuropeptide-Y analogs – evidence for a Y-1 receptor subclass. *J. Medicinal Chem.* **38**, 4579–4586.

Koenig, J.I. (1990) Regulation of the hypothalamo-pituitary axis by neuropeptide Y. *Ann. N. York Acad. Sci.* **611**, 317–328.

Kyrkouli, S.E., Stanley, B.G. & Leibowitz, S.F. (1986) Galanin: stimulation of feeding induced by medial hypothalamic injection of this novel peptide. *Eur. J. Pharmacol.* **122**, 159–160.

Lambert, P.D., Wilding, J.P., Al Dokhayel, A.A., Bohuon, C., Comoy, E., Gilbey, S.G. & Bloom, S.R. (1993) A role for neuropeptide-Y, dynorphin, and noradrenaline in the central control of food intake after food deprivation. *Endocrinology* **133**, 29–32.

Lambert, P.D., Wilding, J.P., Turton, M.D., Ghatei, M.A. & Bloom, S.R. (1994) Effect of food deprivation and streptozotocin-induced diabetes on hypothalamic neuropeptide Y release as measured by a radioimmunoassay-linked microdialysis procedure. *Brain Res.* **656**, 135–140.

Lambert, P.D., Phillips, P.J., Wilding, J.P., Bloom, S.R. & Herbert, J. (1995) c-fos expression in the paraventricular nucleus of the hypothalamus following intracerebroventricular infusions of neuropeptide Y. *Brain Res.* **670**, 59–65.

Larsen, P.J., Sheikh, S.P., Jakobsen, C.R., Schwartz, T.W. & Mikkelsen, J.D. (1993) Regional distribution of putative NPY Y1 receptors and neurons expressing Y1 mRNA in forebrain areas of the rat central nervous system. *Eur. J. Neurosci.* **5**, 1622–1637.

Larsen, P.J., Jessop, D.S., Chowdrey, H.S., Lightman, S.L. & Mikkelsen, J.D. (1994) Chronic administration of glucocorticoids directly upregulates prepro-neuropeptide Y and Y1-receptor mRNA levels in the arcuate nucleus of the rat. *J. Neuroendocrinol.* **6**, 153–159.

Lee, G.H., Proenca, R., Montez, J.M., Carroll, K.M., Darvishzadeh, J.G., Lee, J.I. & Friedman, J.M. (1996) Abnormal splicing of the leptin receptor in diabetic mice. *Nature* **379**, 632–635.

Leibel, R.L., Rosenbaum, M. & Hirsch, J. (1995) Changes in energy expenditure resulting from altered body weight [see comments]. *N. Engl. J. Med.* **332**, 621–628.

Leibowitz, S.F. (1978) Paraventricular nucleus: a primary site mediating adrenergic stimulation of feeding and drinking. *Pharmacol. Biochem. Behav.* **8**, 163–175.

Leibowitz, S.F. (1990) Hypothalamic neuropeptide Y in relation to energy balance. *Ann. N. York Acad. Sci.* **611**, 284–301.

Leibowitz, S.F. (1991) Brain neuropeptide Y: an integrator of endocrine, metabolic and behavioural processes. *Brain Res. Bull.* **27**, 333–337.

Leibowitz, S.F. (1988) Hypothalamic paraventricular nucleus: interaction between alpha 2-noradrenergic system and circulating hormones and nutrients in relation to energy balance. *Neurosci. Biobehav. Rev.* **12**, 101–109.

Leibowitz, S.F., Hammer, N.J. & Chang, K. (1981) Hypothalamic paraventricular nucleus lesions produce overeating and obesity in the rat. *Physiol. Behav.* **27**, 1031–1040.

Leibowitz, S.F., Sladek, C., Spencer, L. & Tempel, D. (1988) Neuropeptide Y, epinephrine and norepinephrine in the paraventricular nucleus: stimulation of feeding and the release of corticosterone, vasopressin and glucose. *Brain Res. Bull.* **21**, 905–912.

Levine, A.S. & Morley, J.E. (1984) Neuropeptide Y: a potent inducer of consummatory behaviour in rats. *Peptides* **5**, 1025–1029.

Li, B.H., Xu, B., Rowland, N.E. & Kalra, S.P. (1994). c-fos expression in the rat brain following central administration of neuropeptide Y and effects of food consumption. *Brain Res.* **665**, 277–284.

Liposits, Z., Sievers, L. & Paull, W.K. (1988) Neuropeptide-Y and ACTH-immunoreactive innervation of corticotropin releasing factor (CRF)-synthesizing neurons in the hypothalamus of the rat. An immunocytochemical analysis at the light and electron microscopic levels. *Histochemistry* **88**, 227–234.

Lundberg, J.M., Terenius, L., Hokfelt, T. & Tatemoto, K. (1984) Comparative immunohistochemical and biochemical analysis of pancreatic polypeptide-like peptides with special reference to presence of neuropeptide Y in central and peripheral neurons. *J. Neurosci.* **4**, 2376–2386.

Matthews, J.W., Booth, D.A. & Stolerman, I.P. (1978) Factors influencing feeding elicited by intracranial noradrenaline in rats. *Brain Res.* **141**, 119–128.

McDonald, J.K., Lumpkin, M.D., Samson, W.K. & McCann, S.M. (1985) Neuropeptide Y affects secretion of luteinizing hormone and growth hormone in ovariectomized rats. *Proc. Natl Acad. Sci USA* **82**, 561–564.

McKibbin, P.E., Cotton, S.J. McMillan, S., Holloway, B., Mayers, R., McCarthy, H.D. & Williams, G. (1991a) Altered neuropeptide Y concentrations in specific hypothalamic regions of obese (*fa/fa*) Zucker rats. Possible relationship to obesity and neuroendocrine disturbances. *Diabetes* **40**, 1423–1429.

McKibbin, P.E., Rogers, P. & Williams, G. (1991b) Increased neuropeptide Y concentrations in the lateral hypothalamic area of the rat after the onset of darkness: possible relevance to the circadian periodicity of feeding behaviour. *Life Sci.* **48**, 2527–2533.

Menendez, J.A., McGregor, I.S., Healey, P.A., Atrens, D.M. & Leibowitz, S.F. (1990) Metabolic effects of neuropeptide Y injections into the paraventricular nucleus of the hypothalamus. *Brain Res.* **516**, 8–14.

Michel, M.C. (1991) Receptors for neuropeptide Y: multiple subtypes and multiple second messengers [published erratum appears in *Trends Pharmacol. Sci.* 1991, **12**, 448]. *Trends. Pharmacol. Sci.* **12**, 389–394.

Miura, M., Inui, A., Teranishi, A., Hirosue, Y., Nakajima, M., Okita, M., Inoue, T., Baba, S. & Kasuga, M. (1992) Structural requirements for the effects of neuropeptide Y on the hypothalamic–pituitary–adrenal axis in the dog. *Neuropeptides* **23**, 15–18.

Miyachi, Y., Jitsuishi, W., Miyoshi, A., Fujita, S., Mizuchi, A. & Tatemoto, K. (1986) The distribution of polypeptide YY-like immunoreactivity in rat tissues. *Endocrinology* **118**, 2163–2167.

Moltz, J.H. & McDonald, J.K. (1985) Neuropeptide Y: direct and indirect action on insulin secretion in the rat. *Peptides* **6**, 1155–1159.

Morley, J.E., Levine, A.S., Grace, M. & Kneip, J. (1982) Dynorphin-(1–13), dopamine and feeding in rats. *Pharmacol. Biochem. Behav.* **16**, 701–705.

Morley, J.E., Levine, A.S., Grace, M. & Kneip, J. (1985) Peptide YY (PYY), a potent orexigenic agent. *Brain Res.* **341**, 200–203.

Morley, J.E., Levine, A.S., Gosnell, B.A., Kneip, J. & Grace, M. (1987) Effect of neuropeptide Y on ingestive behaviors in the rat. *Am. J. Physiol.* **252**, R599–609.

Morris, B.J. (1989) Neuronal localisation of neuropeptide Y gene expression in rat brain. *J. Comp. Neurol.* **290**, 358–368.

Okada, K., Sugihara, H., Minami, S. & Wakabayashi, I. (1993) Effect of parenteral administration of selected nutrients and central injection of gamma-globulin from antiserum to neuropeptide Y on growth hormone secretory pattern in food-deprived rats. *Neuroendocrinology* **57**, 678–686.

Olchovsky, D., Bruno, J.F., Wood, T.L., Gelato, M.C., Leidy, J.W., Jr, Gilbert, J.M., Jr & Berelowitz, M. (1990) Altered pituitary growth hormone (GH) regulation in streptozotocin-diabetic rats: a combined defect of hypothalamic somatostatin and GH-releasing factor. *Endocrinology* **126**, 53–61.

O'Shea, D., Morgan, D.G., Meeran, K., *et al.* (1996) Neuropeptide Y induced feeding in the rat is mediated by a novel receptor. *Endocrinology* (in press).

Peng, C., Huang, Y.P. & Peter, R.E. (1990) Neuropeptide Y stimulates growth hormone and gonadotropin release from the goldfish pituitary in vitro. *Neuroendocrinology* **52**, 28–34.

Peng, C., Humphries, S., Peter, R.E., Rivier, J.E., Blomqvist, A.G. & Larhammar, D. (1993) Actions of goldfish neuropeptide Y on the secretion of growth hormone and gonadotropin-II in female goldfish. *Gen. Comp. Endocrinol.* **90**, 306–317.

Pesonen, U., Rouru, J., Huupponen, R. & Koulu, M. (1991) Effects of repeated administration of mifepristone and 8-OH-DPAT on expression of preproneuropeptide Y mRNA in the arcuate nucleus of obese Zucker rats. *Brain Res. Mol. Brain Res.* **10**, 267–272.

Pettersson, M., Lundquist, I. & Ahren, B. (1987) Neuropeptide Y and calcitonin gene-related peptide: effects on glucagon and insulin secretion in the mouse. *Endocr. Res.* **13**, 407–417.

Pierroz, D.D., Catzeflis, C., Aebi, A.C., Rivier, J.E. & Aubert, M.L. (1996) Chronic administration of neuropeptide-Y into the lateral ventricle inhibits both the pituitary-testicular axis and growth-hormone and insulin-like growth-factor-1 secretion in intact adult male rats. *Endocrinology* **137**, 3–12.

Quirion, R., Martel, J.C., Dumont, Y., Cadieux, A., Jolicoeur, F., St Pierre, S. & Fournier, A. (1990) Neuropeptide Y receptors: autoradiographic distribution in the brain and structure–activity relationships. *Ann. N. York Acad. Sci.* **611**, 58–72.

Rettori, V., Milenkovic, L., Aguila, M.C. & McCann, S.M. (1990a) Physiologically significant effect of neuropeptide Y to suppress growth hormone release by stimulating somatostatin discharge. *Endocrinology* **126**, 2296–2301.

Rettori, V., Milenkovic, L., Riedel, M. & McCann, S.M. (1990b) Physiological role of neuropeptide Y (NPY) in control of anterior pituitary hormone release in the rat. *Endocrinol. Exp.* **24**, 37–45.

Rink, T.J. (1994) Genetics. In search of a satiety factor [news; comment]. *Nature* **372**, 406–407.

Rothwell, N.J. & Stock, M.J. (1979) A role for brown adipose tissue in diet-induced thermogenesis. *Nature* **281**, 31–35.

Rothwell, N.J. & Stock, M.J. (1981) A role for insulin in the diet-induced thermogenesis of cafeteria-fed rats. *Metabolism* **30**, 673–678.

Rothwell, N.J., Saville, M.E. & Stock, M.J. (1982) Effects of feeding a 'cafeteria' diet on energy balance and diet-induced thermogenesis in four strains of rat. *J. Nutr.* **112**, 1515–1524.

Ruiz de Elvira, M.C. & Coen, C.W. (1990) Centrally administered neuropeptide Y enhances the hypothermia induced by peripheral administration of adrenoceptor antagonists. *Peptides* **11**, 963–967.

Sagar, S.M., Sharp, F.R. & Curran, T. (1988) Expression of c-fos protein in brain: metabolic mapping at the cellular level. *Science* **240**, 1328–1331.

Sahu, A., Kalra, P.S. & Kalra, S.P. (1988a) Food deprivation and ingestion induce reciprocal changes in neuropeptide Y concentrations in the paraventricular nucleus. *Peptides* **9**, 83–86.

Sahu, A., Kalra, S.P., Crowley, W.R. & Kalra, P.S. (1988b) Evidence that NPY-containing neurons in the brainstem project into selected hypothalamic nuclei: implication in feeding behaviour. *Brain Res.* **457**, 376–378.

Sahu, A., Kalra, S.P., Crowley, W.R. & Kalra, P.S. (1989) Testosterone raises neuropeptide-Y concentration in selected hypothalamic sites and in vitro release from the medial basal hypothalamus of castrated male rats. *Endocrinology* **124**, 410–414.

Sahu, A., Sninsky, C.A., Kalra, P.S. & Kalra, S.P. (1990) Neuropeptide-Y concentration in microdissected hypothalamic regions and in vitro release from the medial basal hypothalamus-preoptic area of streptozotocin-diabetic rats with and without insulin substitution therapy. *Endocrinology* **126**, 192–198.

Sahu, A., Phelps, C.P., White, J.D., Crowley, W.R., Kalra, S.P. & Kalra, P.S. (1992a) Steroidal regulation of hypothalamic neuropeptide Y release and gene expression. *Endocrinology* **130**, 3331–3336.

Sahu, A., Sninsky, C.A., Phelps, C.P., Dube, M.G., Kalra, P.S. & Kalra, S.P. (1992b) Neuropeptide Y release from the paraventricular nucleus increases in association with hyperphagia in streptozotocin-induced diabetic rats. *Endocrinology* **131**, 2979–2985.

Sanacora, G., Kershaw, M., Finkelstein, J.A. & White, J.D. (1990) Increased hypothalamic content of preproneuropeptide Y messenger ribonucleic acid in genetically obese Zucker rats and its regulation by food deprivation. *Endocrinology* **127**, 730–737.

Sawchenko, P.E., Swanson, L.W., Grzanna, R., Howe, P.R., Bloom, S.R. & Polak, J.M. (1985) Colocalization of neuropeptide Y immunoreactivity in brainstem catecholaminergic neurons that project to the paraventricular nucleus of the hypothalamus. *J. Comp. Neurol.* **241**, 138–153.

Scallet, A.C. & Olney, J.W. (1986) Components of hypothalmic obesity: bipiperidyl-mustard lesions add hyperphagia to monosodium glutamate-induced hyperinsulinemia. *Brain Res.* **374**, 380–384.

Schwartz, M.W., Marks, J.L., Sipols, A.J., Baskin, D.G., Woods, S.C., Kahn, S.E. & Porte, D., Jr (1991) Central insulin administration reduces neuropeptide Y mRNA expression in the arcuate nucleus of food-deprived lean (*Fa/Fa*) but not obese (*fa/fa*) Zucker rats. *Endocrinology* **128**, 2645–2647.

Schwartz, M.W., Sipols, A.J., Marks, J.L., Sanacora, G., White, J.D., Scheurink, A., Kahn, S.E., Baskin, D.G., Woods, S.C., Figlewicz, D.P. *et al.* (1992) Inhibition of hypothalamic neuropeptide Y gene expression by insulin. *Endocrinology* **130**, 3608–3616.

Schwartz, M.W., Figlewicz, D.P., Woods, S.C., Porte, D., Jr & Baskin, D.G. (1993) Insulin, neuropeptide Y, and food intake. *Ann. N. York Acad. Sci.* **692**, 60–71.

Schwartz, M.W., Baskin, D.G., Bukowski, T.R., Kuijper, J.L., Foster, D., Lasser, G., Prunkard, D.E., Porte, D., Jr., Woods, S.C., Seeley, R.J. & Weigle, D.S. (1996) Specificity of leptin action on elevated blood glucose levels and hypothalamic neuropeptide Y expression in *ob/ob* mice. *Diabetes* **45**, 531–535.

Scott, J. (1996) New chapter for the fat controller. *Nature* **379**, 113–114.

Sipols, A.J., Baskin, D.G. & Schwartz, M.W. (1995) Effect of intracerebroventricular insulin infusion on diabetic hyperphagia and hypothalamic neuropeptide gene expression. *Diabetes* **44**, 147–151.

Smith, B.K., York, D.A. & Bray, G.A. (1994) Chronic cerebroventricular galanin does not induce sustained hyperphagia or obesity. *Peptides* **15**, 1267–1272.

Stanley, B.G. & Leibowitz, S.F. (1984) Neuropeptide Y: stimulation of feeding and drinking by injection into the paraventricular nucleus. *Life Sci.* **35**, 2635–2642.

Stanley, B.G. & Leibowitz, S.F. (1985) Neuropeptide Y injected in the paraventricular hypothalamus: a powerful stimulant of feeding behaviour. *Proc. Natl Acad. Sci. USA* **82**, 3940–3943.

Stanley, B.G., Chin, A.S. & Leibowitz, S.F. (1985a) Feeding and drinking elictied by central injection of neuropeptide Y: evidence for a hypothalamic site(s) of action. *Brain Res. Bull.* **14**, 521–524.

Stanley, B.G., Daniel, D.R., Chin, A.S. & Leibowitz, S.F. (1985b) Paraventricular nucleus injections of peptide YY and neuropeptide Y preferentially enhance carbohydrate ingestion. *Peptides* **6**, 1205–1211.

Stanley, B.G., Kyrkouli, S.E., Lampert, S. & Leibowitz, S.F. (1986) Neuropeptide Y chronically injected into the hypothalmus: a powerful neurochemical inducer of hyperphagia and obesity. *Peptides* **7**, 1189–1192.

Stanley, B.G., Anderson, K.C., Grayson, M.H. & Leibowitz, S.F. (1989) Repeated hypothalamic stimulation with neuropeptide Y increases daily carbohydrate and fat intake and body weight gain in female rats. *Physiol. Behav.* **46**, 173–177.

Stanley, B.G., Magdalin, W., Seirafi, A., Nguyen, M.M. & Leibowitz, S.F. (1992) Evidence for neuropeptide Y mediation of eating produced by food deprivation and for a variant of the Y1 receptor mediating this peptide's effect. *Peptides* **13**, 581–587.

Stanley, B.G., Magdalin, W., Seirafi, A., Thomas, W.J. & Leibowitz, S.F. (1993) The periforni-cal area: the major focus of (a) patchily distributed hypothalamic neuropeptide Y-sensitive feeding system(s). *Brain Res.* **604**, 304–317.

Stephens, T.W., Basinski, M., Bristow, P.K., Bue-Valleskey, J.M., Burgett, S.G., Craft, L., Hale, J., Hoffmann, J., Hsiung, H.M., Kriauciunas, A., Mackellar, W., Rosteck, P.R., Schoner, B., Smith, D., Tinsley, F.C., Zhang, X-Y. & Heiman, M. (1995) The role of neuropeptide Y in the antiobesity action of the obese gene product. *Nature* **377**, 530–532.

Tannenbaum, G.S. (1981) Growth hormone secretory dynamics in streptozotocin diabetes: evidence of a role for endogenous circulating somatostatin. *Endocrinology* **108**, 76–82.

Tannenbaum, G.S., Rorstad, O. & Brazeau, P. (1979) Effects of prolonged food deprivation on the ultradian growth hormone rhythm and immunoreactive somatostatin tissue levels in the rat. *Endocrinology* **104**, 1733–1738.

Tatemoto, K., Carlquist, M. & Mutt, V. (1982) Neuropeptide Y – a novel brain peptide with structural similarities to peptide YY and pancreatic polypeptide. *Nature* **296**, 659–660.

Tempel, D.L. & Leibowitz, S.F. (1990) Diurnal variations in the feeding responses to norepinephrine, neuropeptide Y and galanin in the PVN. *Brain Res. Bull.* **25**, 821–825.

Tempel, D.L., Leibowitz, K.J. & Leibowitz, S.F. (1988). Effects of PVN galanin on macronutient selection. *Peptides* **9**, 309–314.

Tempel, D.L., Shor Posner, G., Dwyer, D. & Leibowitz, S.F. (1989). Nocturnal patterns of macronutrient intake in freely feeding and food-deprived rats. *Am. J. Physiol*, **256**, R541–548.

Tsagarakis, S., Rees, L.H., Besser, G.M. & Grossman, A. (1989) Neuropeptide-Y stimulates CRF-41 release from rat hypothalami in vitro. *Brain Res.* **502**, 167–170.

Tulp, O.L., Gregory, M.H. & Danforth, E., Jr (1982) Characteristics of diet-induced brown adipose tissue growth and thermogenesis in rats. *Life Sci.* **30**, 1525–1530.

Turton, M.D., O'Shea, D., Gunn, I., Beak, S.A., Edwards, C.M., Meeran, K., Choi, S.J., Taylor, G.M., Heath, M.M., Lambert, P.D., Wilding, J.P., Smith, D.M., Ghatei, M.A., Herbert, J. & Bloom, S.R. (1996) A role for glucagon-like peptide-1 in the central regulation of feeding. *Nature* **379**, 69–72.

Vaccarino, F.J., Bloom, F.E., Rivier, J., Vale, W. & Koob, G.F. (1985) Stimulation of food intake in rats by centrally administered hypothalamic growth hormone-releasing factor. *Nature* **314**, 167–168.

Van Dijk, G., Bottone, A.E., Strubbe, J.H. & Steffens, A.B. (1994) Hormonal and metabolic effects of paraventricular hypothalamic administration of neuropeptide Y during rest and feeding. *Brain Res.* **660**, 96–103.

Vettor, R., Zarjevski, N., Cusin, I., Rohner Jeanrenaud, F. & Jeanrenaud, B. (1994) Induction and reversibility of an obesity syndrome by intracerebroventricular neuropeptide Y administration to normal rats. *Diabetologia* **37**, 1202–1208.

Wahlestedt, C., Skagerberg, G., Ekman, R., Heilig, M., Sundler, F. & Hakanson, R. (1987) Neuropeptide Y (NPY) in the area of the hypothalamic paraventricular nucleus activates the pituitary-adrenocortical axis in the rat. *Brain Res.* **417**, 33–38.

Wahlestedt, C., Pich, E.M., Koob, G.F., Yee, F. & Heilig, M. (1993) Modulation of anxiety and neuropeptide Y-Y1 receptors by antisense oligodeoxynucleotides. *Science* **259**, 528–531.

Weinberg, D.H., Sirinathsinghji, D.J.S., Tan, C.P. *et al.* (1996) Cloning and functional expression of a novel neuropeptide Y receptor. *J. Biol. Chem.* **271**, 16435–16438.

White, J.D., Olchovsky, D., Kershaw, M. & Berelowitz, M. (1990) Increased hypothalamic content of preproneuropeptide-Y messenger ribonucleic acid in streptozotocin-diabetic rats. *Endocrinology* **126**, 765–772.

Wilding, J.P., Gilbey, S.G., Mannan, M., Aslam, N., Ghatei, M.A. & Bloom, S.R. (1992) Increased neuropeptide Y content in individual hypothalamic nuclei, but not neuropeptide Y mRNA, in diet-induced obesity in rats. *J. Endocrinol.* **132**, 299–304.

Wilding, J.P., Gilbey, S.G., Bailey, C.J., Batt, R.A., Williams, G., Ghatei, M.A. & Bloom, S.R. (1993a) Increased neuropeptide-Y messenger ribonucleic acid (mRNA) and decreased neurotensin mRNA in the hypothalamus of the obese (*ob/ob*) mouse. *Endocrinology* **132**, 1939–1944.

Wilding, J.P., Gilbey, S.G., Lambert, P.D., Ghatei, M.A. & Bloom, S.R. (1993b) Increases in neuropeptide Y content and gene expression in the hypothalamus of rats treated with dexamethasone are prevented by insulin. *Neuroendocrinology* **57**, 581–587.

Wilding, J.P.H., Kruszynska, Y.T., Lambert, P.D. & Bloom, S.R. (1995) Acute effects of central neuropeptide-y injection on glucose-metabolism in fasted rats. *Clin. Sci.* **89**, 543–548.

Williams, G., Ghatei, M.A., Diani, A.R., Gerritsen, G.C. & Bloom, S.R. (1988a) Reduced hypothalamic somatostatin and neuropeptide Y concentrations in the spontaneously-diabetic Chinese hamster. *Horm. Metab. Res.* **20**, 668–670.

Williams, G., Steel, J.H., Cardoso, H., Ghatei, M.A., Lee, Y.C., Gill, J.S., Burrin, J.M., Polak, J.M. & Bloom, S.R. (1988b) Increased hypothalamic neuropeptide Y concentrations in diabetic rats. *Diabetes* **37**, 763–772.

Williams, G., Gill, J.S., Lee, Y.C., Cardoso, H.M., Okpere, B.E. & Bloom, S.R. (1989a) Increased neuropeptide Y concentrations in specific hypothalamic regions of streptozocin-induced diabetic rats. *Diabetes* **38**, 321–327.

Williams, G., Lee, Y.C., Ghatei, M.A., Cardoso, H.M., Ball, J.A., Bone, A.J., Baird, J.D. & Bloom, S.R. (1989b) Elevated neuropeptide Y concentrations in the central hypothalamus of the spontaneously diabetic BB/E Wistar rat. *Diabet. Med.* **6**, 601–607.

Williams, G., Cardoso, H.M., Lee, Y.C., Ball, J.M., Ghatei, M.A., Stock, M.J. & Bloom, S.R. (1991) Hypothalamic regulatory peptides in obese and lean Zucker rats. *Clin. Sci. Colch.* **80**, 419–426.

Williams, G. & Bloom, S.R. (1989) Regulatory peptides, the hypothalamus and diabetes. *Diabet. Med.* **6**, 472–485.

Xu, B., Li, B.H., Rowland, N.E. & Kalra, S.P. (1995) Neuropeptide Y injection into the fourth cerebroventricle stimulates c-Fos expression in the paraventricular nucleus and other nuclei in the forebrain: effect of food consumption. *Brain Res.* **698**, 227–231.

Zarjevski, N., Cusin, I., Vettor, R., Rohner Jeanrenaud, F. & Jeanrenaud, B. (1993) Chronic intracerebroventricular neuropeptide-Y administration to normal rats mimics hormonal and metabolic changes of obesity. *Endocrinology* **133**, 1753–1758.

Zarjevski, N., Cusin, I., Vettor, R., Rohner Jeanrenaud, F. & Jeanrenaud, B. (1994) Intracerebroventricular administration of neuropeptide Y to normal rats has divergent effects on glucose utilization by adipose tissue and skeletal muscle. *Diabetes* **43**, 764–769.

Zhang, Y., Proenca, R., Maffei, M., Barone, M., Leopold, L. & Friedman, J.M. (1994) Positional cloning of the mouse obese gene and its human homologue. *Nature* **372**, 425–432.

Zucker, L.M. & Antoniades, H.N. (1972) Insulin and obesity in the Zucker genetically obese rat 'fatty'. *Endocrinology* **90**, 1320–1330.

CHAPTER 3

NEUROPEPTIDE Y IN SYMPATHETIC NERVES – EVIDENCE FOR Y1 RECEPTOR MEDIATED VASCULAR CONTROL

Rickard E. Malmström and Jan M. Lundberg

Table of Contents

3.1 Introduction

The 36-amino-acid peptide neuropeptide Y (NPY) is the neuronal counterpart to peptide YY (PYY), which is mainly present in intestinal endocrine cells (Lundberg *et al.*, 1982a). NPY is widely distributed in the central (Gray and Morely, 1986) and peripheral (Lundberg *et al.*, 1982b) nervous system, and exogenous NPY can evoke various functional responses. The co-localization of NPY with noradrenaline (NA) in sympathetic nerves was demonstrated (Lundberg *et al.*, 1982b, 1983) in accordance with earlier data from studies using antibodies to the related avian pancreatic polypeptide. NPY is co-released with NA from sympathetic nerves, preferentially on high-frequency stimulation or strong reflex activation (see Lundberg *et al.*, 1990). Nerve activity seems to be crucial for NPY synthesis. Thus, elevated levels of mRNA for NPY and axonal transport of the peptide (Schalling *et al.*, 1991) are seen after reserpine treatment, when the firing rate of sympathetic neurons is increased. Conversely, the expression of NPY mRNA in sympathetic ganglion cells decreases after blockade of ganglionic nicotinic receptors or surgical preganglionic denervation (Schalling *et al.*, 1991). Hence, the importance of this peptide in sympathetic transmission may change with the degree of environmental stress.

Neuropeptide Y and Drug Development
ISBN 0-12-304990-3

3.2 Prejunctional regulation of sympathetic transmitter release

The release of transmitters – adenosine triphosphate (ATP), NA, NPY – from sympathetic nerves is influenced by autoinhibition, mainly via endogenous NA acting on prejunctional α_2-adrenoceptors. Thus, α_2-adrenoceptor agonists like clonidine and UK 14304 inhibit and α_2-adrenoceptor antagonists like phenoxybenzamine and phentolamine increase nerve stimulation evoked transmitter release. This prejunctional α_2-adrenoceptor-mediated regulation of NPY release may be the decisive factor in suppression of NPY release on low-frequency stimulation. It can also explain why it is difficult to deplete the tissues of NPY and eliminate NPY release on prolonged stimulation under control conditions (Modin *et al.*, 1993a). With single nerve impulses there is no autoinhibition of release, but available data suggest that NPY is not released under these conditions, probably because it is stored exclusively in large dense-cored vesicles (see Lundberg, 1996). NA is not the only factor that modulates transmitter release, however. Prejunctional NPY receptors can also depress sympathetic neurotransmitter release, acting via different receptor subtypes in various tissues (see below). Thus, PYY has been shown to suppress overflow of endogenous NPY evoked by sympathetic nerve stimulation (Pernow and Lundberg, 1989a). In rat vas deferens the prejunctional NPY receptor inhibiting transmitter release is of the Y2 type (Wahlestedt *et al.*, 1986), while in rabbit vas deferens it is of the Y1 type (Doods and Krause, 1991). Enhancement of release of NPY-like immunoreactivity (NPY-LI) has been demonstrated upon stimulation of angiotensin II receptors (Pernow and Lundberg, 1989a) and β-adrenoceptors (Dahlöf *et al.*, 1991). However, these effects are much less significant than those mediated via prejunctional α_2-adrenoceptors.

3.3 NPY in plasma and its clearance

With the exception of rats, where the NPY found in plasma seems to emanate primarily from platelets (see Lundberg *et al.*, 1990), plasma NPY in most species is derived mainly from sympathetic nerves and reaches the circulation by spillover after release. Thus, in healthy people under a variety of conditions, NPY levels in plasma correlate with those of NA rather than those of adrenaline (Lundberg *et al.*, 1990). Actually, peptide washout is an important mechanism by which NPY released from sympathetic nerve terminals is "inactivated'. Washout is likely to be more prominent in tissue with fenestrated endothelium like kidney and spleen. In accordance with this, only little and delayed overflow of NPY can be detected in venous effluent from, for example, skeletal muscle or nasal mucosa after sympathetic nerve activation (see Lundberg *et al.*, 1990). Release of NPY into plasma effluent is detected by radioimmunoassay and local overflow can be evoked from various vascular beds by electrical nerve stimulation (Lundberg *et al.*, 1984b, 1990; Rudehill *et al.*, 1986) or reflexogenous sympathetic nerve activation as by endotoxin shock, haemorrhagic hypovolemia or during physical exercise in man (Lundberg *et al.*, 1985; Pernow *et al.*,

1986b, 1988c, 1990; Rudehill *et al.*, 1987). However, strong sympathetic activation is required to release enough NPY to raise systemic plasma NPY levels in man (Lundberg *et al.*, 1985; Pernow *et al.*, 1986a).

The adrenals of many species co-store NPY and NA but, as indicated above, the physiological role of adrenal NPY remains unclear. Thus, like NA, plasma NPY can be used as an indicator of high sympathetic tone rather than documenting NPY concentration at its site of receptor activation.

NPY has a slow clearance from plasma with a long half-life of about 5 min in pig (Rudehill *et al.*, 1987) and man (Pernow *et al.*, 1987a). Recently, the enzymes involved in NPY degradation were characterized. NPY is initially cleaved into NPY3–36, which thus also circulates in plasma. This cleavage is catalysed by dipeptidyl peptidase IV (Mentlein *et al.*, 1993). Interestingly, NPY3–36 is a selective agonist at Y2 receptors. NPY3–36 then may be further degraded by neuroendopeptidases to biologically inactive forms (Medeiros and Turner, 1994).

3.4 NPY in sympathetic neurotransmission

3.4.1 Localization of NPY receptor types

NPY receptors exist in many central and peripheral tissues crucial for cardiovascular control. Peripheral NPY receptor-types have been identified by various methods. Radioligand binding has demonstrated Y1 receptors in pig renal artery and dog spleen (Lundberg and Modin, 1995), while Y2 receptors have been identified in pig spleen (Lundberg and Modin, 1995) and rabbit kidney (Sheikh *et al.*, 1989). In blood vessels of human kidney, Y1 receptor mRNA has been detected with *in situ* hybridization (Wharton *et al.*, 1993). Mainly Y1 receptors have been demonstrated in cultured vascular smooth muscle cells from porcine and rat arteries and veins (Mihara *et al.*, 1990; Shigeri *et al.*, 1991; Grundemar *et al.*, 1992). Autoradiographic studies have labelled mainly Y1 receptors in small arteries in, for example, rabbit kidney (Leys *et al.*, 1987) and rat pancreas (Sheikh *et al.*, 1991), and intracardiac arterioles (Allen *et al.*, 1993). On the other hand Y3-like receptors may be present in rat heart (Balasubramaniam *et al.*, 1990).

3.4.2 NPY in sympathetic vasoconstriction

In vivo, exogenous NPY evokes long-lasting vasoconstriction, which mimics the non-adrenergic vascular response to sympathetic nerve stimulation (Lundberg and Tatemoto, 1982). NPY has been shown to reduce local blood flow in a variety of vascular beds (Rudehill *et al.*, 1987) and species, including man. Thus, NPY-evoked vasoconstriction in man has been demonstrated in skeletal muscle (Pernow *et al.*, 1987a), heart (Clarke *et al.*, 1987), kidney and splanchnic circulation (Ahlborg *et al.*, 1992). *In vitro*, NPY evokes contraction in small human vessels, for example, cerebral (Mejia *et al.*, 1988), coronary (Franco-Cereceda and Lundberg, 1987), renal (Pernow *et al.*, 1987b) and skeletal muscle arteries (Pernow and Lundberg, 1986). The NPY-evoked contraction is independent of the endothelium (Pernow, 1989). In contrast, most isolated large blood vessels with the exception of guinea-pig vena cava, do not respond to NPY with contractions *in vitro*.

Involvement of NPY in non-adrenergic sympathetic vascular control can be studied using a combined α- and β-adrenoceptor blockade. However, because of the risk of incomplete receptor blockade, NA depletion by reserpine treatment may provide more favourable conditions for these studies. When combined with transection of sympathetic nerves (at a preganglionic level) to interrupt nerve activity, reserpinization creates a situation in which tissue levels of NPY are maintained, but the levels of NA are reduced by over 90%. This in turn leads to an up to five-fold increase of NPY release upon nerve stimulation owing to the lack of prejunctional inhibition via α_2-adrenoceptors. Initially it was shown that NPY mimicked the prolonged vasoconstriction evoked by high-frequency stimulation in the presence of α- and β-adrenoceptor blockade in cat submandibular gland (Lundberg and Tatemoto, 1982). Subsequently, such long-lasting vasoconstriction was demonstrated *in vivo* in many other vascular beds, for example, skeletal muscle (Pernow *et al.*, 1988a; Modin *et al.*, 1993b), kidney (Pernow and Lundberg, 1989b) and nasal mucosa (Lundblad *et al.*, 1987; Lacroix *et al.*, 1988). These vasoconstrictor effects were also shown to be resistant to reserpine treatment (Lundblad *et al.*, 1987; Lacroix *et al.*, 1988; Pernow *et al.*, 1988b; Pernow and Lundberg, 1989b). Several other findings have supported NPY as a sympathetic mediator of non-adrenergic vasoconstriction. Thus, (1) NPY overflow is highly correlated to non-adrenergic vascular responses, including the decline seen upon repeated stimulation (Lundberg *et al.*, 1989b; Modin *et al.*, 1993a); (2) plasma NPY levels in pig splenic venous effluent upon nerve stimulation are within the vasoconstrictor range (Rudehill *et al.*, 1987; Lundberg *et al.*, 1989a); (3) sympathetic denervation in pig nasal mucosa (Lacroix and Lundberg, 1989) and rat tail artery (Neild, 1987) results in supersensitivity to NPY-evoked vasoconstriction; (4) tachyphylaxis to NPY or Y1 receptor agonists inhibits non-adrenergic sympathetic nerve responses (Öhlén *et al.*, 1990; Morris, 1991).

3.4.3 Final evidence for Y1 receptor mechanisms in sympathetic vasoconstriction

The introduction of the non-peptide Y1 receptor antagonists BIBP 3226 (Rudolf *et al.*, 1994) and SR 120107A (Serradeil-Le Gal *et al.*, 1994) has made it possible to establish finally that endogenous NPY acting on the Y1 receptor mediates long-lasting vasoconstriction in guinea-pig caval vein on transmural sympathetic nerve stimulation (Malmström and Lundberg, 1995a,b) (Figure 1). Thus, both of these Y1 receptor antagonists were shown to have potent inhibitory effects on the prolonged contraction of guinea-pig vena cava on high-frequency sympathetic nerve stimulation. In the presence of BIBP 3226 or SR 120107A only the initial rapid peak of contraction remained, which in turn was adrenergic, since it was abolished by subsequent addi-

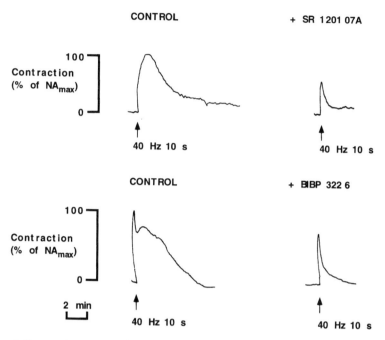

Figure 1 Contractions evoked in guinea-pig vena cava by electrical field stimulation at 40 Hz for 10 s (arrows), shown before and after pretreatment with SR 120107A (1 μM) (top panel) or BIBP 3226 (1 μM) (lower panel). Note that it is mainly the prolonged contraction that is reduced in the presence of the Y1-receptor antagonists.

tion of the α-adrenoceptor antagonist phentolamine (Malmström and Lundberg, 1995b). This further strengthens the theory of 'NPY-ergic' and adrenergic co-transmission. Selectivity was demonstrated, as the S-enantiomer to BIBP 3226, BIBP 3435, which has virtually no activity at Y1 receptors (Rudolf et al., 1994), did not affect the sympathetic contraction of the caval vein (Malmström and Lundberg, 1995b). SR120107A and BIBP 3226 were also equally potent inhibitors of the contraction response to exogenously administered NPY, and neither antagonist affected contractions evoked by exogenous NA.

The satisfactory results obtained in vitro were supported when BIBP 3226 and SR 120107A were used in pigs in vivo. In the presence of either of these Y1 receptor antagonists the long-lasting component of reserpine-resistant vasoconstriction on high-frequency sympathetic nerve stimulation in hind limb (skeletal muscle) and nasal mucosa was nearly abolished, revealing the crucial importance of Y1 receptors in this mechanism (Lundberg and Modin, 1995; Malmström et al., 1996) (Figure 2). Furthermore, the peak vasoconstrictor responses were also attenuated, especially in kidney (where Y1 receptors predominate) but also in spleen (Lundberg and Modin, 1995; Malmström et al., 1996) (Figure 2). In contrast, neither BIBP 3226 or SR 120107A had no effect on the vasoconstrictor response to single impulse stimulation

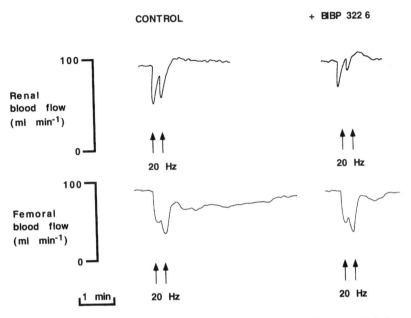

Figure 2 Vascular responses to sympathetic nerve stimulation with two bursts at 20 Hz (arrows) in reserpinized pigs *in vivo*. Vascular responses are shown in the absence and presence of BIBP 3226 (1 mg kg^{-1}). Note the inhibition of the prolonged vasoconstriction in the femoral artery and the attentuation of the peak vascular response in the kidney.

(which is only observed in nasal mucosa and hind limb). These small vascular responses are more prominent in control pigs than in reserpinized and mainly sensitive to α- and β-adrenergic blockade, leaving a small component that may be mediated by other (P$_{2x}$ purinergic?) mechanisms. The release of NA (control pigs) or NPY (reserpinized pigs) upon sympathetic nerve stimulation of spleen and kidney was not influenced by either BIBP 3226 or SR 120107A, excluding prejunctional Y1 receptor action at least in these vascular beds. Taken together, these findings confirm that endogenous NPY acting on the Y1 receptor is crucial for the long-lasting non-adrenergic vasoconstrictor response to high-frequency stimulation. In the kidney the non-adrenergic vasoconstriction seems to be mainly Y1 receptor mediated even though this response is of short duration (Figure 2), presumably owing to efficient autoregulation and/or clearance of NPY by diffusion. One of the consistent differences between vascular beds with short and long-lasting vascular responses is the permeability of the endothelium. Thus, neurotransmitter washout from the tissue through the fenestrated endothelium in kidney (and spleen) could be of crucial importance in explaining the short duration of vascular responses despite the long half-life of NPY. The inhibitory effects of BIBP 3226 and SR 120107A upon sympathetic vasoconstriction in spleen indicate that endogenously released NPY mainly activates Y1 receptors, which are presumably located near the neuronal release sites, while circulating NPY preferably activates the Y2 receptor, situated at sites easy accessible via the circulation. This is shown, for example, by the observation that vascular responses to intravenously administered exogenous NPY in spleen are not influenced by BIBP 3226 (Lundberg and Modin, 1995). In control pigs, with normal NA levels, BIBP 3226 has much smaller inhibitory effects on sympathetic vasoconstriction (Lundberg and Modin, 1995). Hence, the role of NPY in control pigs is less clear.

It is well known that NPY can serve as a regulating factor and enhance the effects of other vasoconstrictor agents, including NA (Ekblad et al., 1984; Pernow et al., 1986b). This potentiation is most pronounced in large vessels, where NPY evokes a minor contraction or no contraction by itself. However, the relevance of this remains to be established in vivo.

3.4.4 NPY in prejunctional sympathetic regulation

Another prominent action of NPY is prejunctional inhibition of release of sympathetic transmitters (NA, NPY and ATP). Thus, NPY inhibits the ATP-mediated response to single impulse stimulation of the sympathetic nerves in rat vas deferens (Lundberg et al., 1982b), and the inhibitory effect parallels inhibition of NA release in this tissue (Lundberg and Stjärne, 1984). This inhibitory effect of NPY was suggested to be prejunctional, and the notion was supported by studies monitoring NA release from perivascular nerves in vitro (Pernow et al., 1987b) and sympathetic nerves in pig kidney in vivo (Pernow and Lundberg, 1989a). The prejunctional inhibitory effect of NPY on sympathetic transmitter release is usually Y2-receptor mediated according to in vitro experiments performed mainly on rat vas deferens (Wahlestedt et al., 1986; Grundemar and Håkanson, 1990) and it occurs independently of α_2-adrenoceptors (Lundberg and Stjärne, 1984; Stjärne et al., 1986). However, in mouse vas deferens NPY also potentiates the contractile effects of α,β-methylene ATP and NA, indicating a dual role for NPY in this tissue (Stjärne et al., 1986). Y1 receptors can also be prejunctional and inhibit sympathetic transmitter release, as in rabbit vas deferens where Y1 receptor agonists inhibit responses to sympathetic nerve stimulation (Doods and Krause, 1991). This was confirmed when SR 120819A as well as BIBP 3226 were shown to reverse the inhibition of rabbit vas deferens contractions evoked by the Y1 receptor agonist [Leu^{31}Pro^{34}] NPY and NPY (Serradeil-Le Gal et al., 1995; Doods et al., 1995) in a potent and competitive manner.

NPY can also inhibit the release of acetylcholine from vagal cholinergic nerves in the heart (Lundberg et al., 1984a; Potter, 1985, 1987, 1988). It has also been suggested that NPY released from cardiac sympathetic nerves on high-frequency stimulation can cause long-lasting depression of cardiac vagal tone in dogs in vivo (Warner and Levy, 1989; Hall et al., 1990; Warner et al., 1991). Similar inhibitory actions remain after adrenoceptor blockade (Potter, 1988; Warner and Levy, 1989) and reserpine treatment (Moriarty et al., 1993) but disappear after guanethidine (Potter, 1988), clearly suggesting NPY as the mediator of this effect. The inhibitory effect of NPY on vagal function in the heart is probably mediated via Y2 receptors (Potter et al., 1989). Indirect evidence also suggests that Y2 receptors can mediate the inhibition of parasympathetic vasodilatation seen after sympathetic nerve stimulation (Lacroix et al., 1994).

3.4.5 NPY actions on cardiac muscle

It is well known that systemic administration of NPY reduces cardiac output, but the effects of NPY in the heart are complex: NPY acts at many sites both within the heart and outside it, to regulate cardiovascular function. Thus, NPY can alter cardiac function indirectly via central effects or by causing alterations in afterload directly by its own vasoconstrictory effects or by potentiating those of other vasoconstrictors. Furthermore, NPY can enhance preload via venous vasoconstriction or reduce it owing to secondary histamine release. NPY might also act directly to cause coronary vasoconstriction and alter the release of autonomous neurotransmitters in the heart via prejunctional inhibition (see above). Possibly, NPY may also affect inotropy, chronotropy and dromotropy. However, the results have been somewhat divergent and the effects of NPY on inotropy thus vary in different species and tissue preparations. Thus, NPY has been shown to exert negative, positive and no effects on cardiac muscle strips. Inotropy was not affected by NPY in human atrial strips (Franco-Cereceda et al., 1987; Michel et al., 1989). Negative inotropic effects of NPY were demonstrated in adult rat cardiomyocytes and the opposite in those of adult guinea-pig (Millar et al., 1991).

3.5 NPY and cardiovascular disorders

It has been suggested that altered tissue content or release of neurotransmitters parallels various cardiovascular diseases. NPY content in various peripheral tissues has been studied in this regard, and the results seem to depend on the tissue or animal model used. Thus, cardiac NPY content seems to be unchanged in all forms of hypertensive rats (Allen et al., 1986; Ballesta et al., 1987; Kong et al., 1991; Zukowska-Grojec et al., 1993a), while renal NPY content may be decreased in some forms of acquired hypertension in rats (Allen et al., 1986; Ballesta et al., 1987). Data on arterial NPY content have not been conclusive. However, at an early prehypertensive stage, spontaneously hypertensive rats (SHR) have a more dense perivascular innervation with NPY-containing fibres compared to control rats (Dhital et al., 1988; Lee et al., 1988). Furthermore, pressor responsiveness to NPY increased in parallel with the development of hypertension in SHR (Miller and Tessel, 1991). However, Y1 antagonists ought to be used to test the relevance of NPY in this model. Recent data suggest that BIBP 3226 does not influence basal blood pressure in SHR (Doods et al., 1995). In contrast, BIBP 3226 reduce the long-lasting meseuteric vasoconstriction seen in conscious rats subjected to cold stress, suggesting an involvement of Y1 receptor mechanisms (Zukowska-Grojec et al., 1996). It has been shown that NPY-mediated prejunctional inhibition of NA release is less potent in SHR rats than in control rats (Westfall et al., 1987), a finding that is true also of other mediators in states of chronic hypertension (Tsuda and Masuyama, 1991).

Plasma levels of NPY are elevated in several cardiovascular diseases in which vasoconstriction plays an important role in pathogenesis, such as acute myocardial infarction and angina pectoris (Ullman *et al.*, 1990), heart failure (Hulting *et al.*, 1990) and hypertension (Chalmers *et al.*, 1989; Solt *et al.*, 1990; Lettgen *et al.*, 1994). The highest circulating levels of NPY were found in patients with phaeochromocytoma (Corder *et al.*, 1985; Lundberg *et al.*, 1986; Grouzman *et al.*, 1989), but there are no studies that have shown correlations between plasma NPY levels with changes in blood pressure. However, manipulation of the tumour, as in surgery, triggers the release of NPY to the circulation (Lundberg *et al.*, 1986; Connell *et al.*, 1987) and surgical situations are known to evoke dangerous rises in arterial blood pressure.

Exercise-induced elevation of plasma NPY seems to be attenuated in patients with moderate heart failure (Ullman *et al.*, 1994), and depletion of NA and NPY from human heart tissue has been reported in patients with severe and long-lasting heart failure associated with prolonged sympathetic activation (Andersson *et al.*, 1992). This indicates that synthesis may be insufficient to maintain NPY levels during conditions of prolonged increase of nerve activity. Circulating plasma levels of NPY in patients with severe cardiac failure (Hulting *et al.*, 1990) are clearly within the range that evokes vasoconstriction in man *in vivo* (Pernow *et al.*, 1987a).

Furthermore, intracoronary injection of NPY in patients with angina pectoris causes symptoms and ECG changes typical of cardiac ischaemia (Clarke *et al.*, 1987). Thus, it would be interesting to study the effects of Y1 receptor antagonists on stress-evoked myocardial ischaemia and hypertension. Since NPY inhibits vagal activity in the heart (see above), a Y2 antagonist could be relevant in the treatment of stress-evoked cardiac arrhythmias. NPY antagonists could be advantageous compared to drugs that influence other transmitters involved in sympathetic vasoconstriction, given that basal vascular tone or mild reflex adjustments are less likely to be influenced by NPY antagonists. Chronic NPY receptor stimulation enhances DNA synthesis in vascular smooth muscle cells (Shigeri and Fujimoto, 1993; Zukowska-Grojec *et al.*, 1993b), cardiomyocytes (Millar *et al.*, 1994) and renal cells (Voisin *et al.*, 1993). Hence, NPY can possibly play a role in the development of hypertrophy and hyperplasia under pathophysiological conditions.

To conclude, the presently available Y1 antagonists have at last made it possible to establish that endogenous NPY can act as a sympathetic vasoconstrictor. The next task is to study the relevance of NPY in cardiovascular pathophysiology in various animal models. With the development of more potent and selective NPY antagonists, these studies should ultimately be extended to include man.

References

Ahlborg, G., Weitzberg, E., Sollevi, A. & Lundberg, J.M. (1992) Splanchnic and renal vasoconstrictor and metabolic responses to neuropeptide Y in resting and exercising man. *Acta Physiol. Scand.* **145**, 139–149.

Allen, J.M., Godfrey, N.P., Yeats, J.C., Bing, R.F. & Bloom, S.R. (1986) Neuropeptide Y in renovascular models of hypertension in the rat. *Clin. Sci. Colch.* **70**, 485–488.

Allen, C.J., Ghilardi, J.R., Vigna, S.R., Mannon, P.J., Taylor, I.L., McVey, D.C. *et al.* (1993) Neuropeptide Y/peptide YY receptor binding sites in the heart: Localization and pharmacological characterization. *Neuroscience* **53**, 889–898.

Andersson, F.L., Port, J.D., Reid, B.B., Larrabee, P., Hanson, G. & Bristow, M.R. (1992) Myocardial catecholamine and neuropeptide Y depletion in failing ventricles of patients with idiopathic dilated cardiomyopathy. Correlation with β-adrenergic receptor downregulation. *Circulation* **85**, 45–53.

Balasubramaniam, A., Sheriff, S., Rigel, D.F. & Fischer, J.E. (1990) Characterization of neuropeptide Y binding sites in rat cardiac ventricular membranes. *Peptides* **11**, 545–550.

Ballesta, J., Lawson, J.A., Pals, D.T., Ludens, J.H., Lee, Y.C., Bloom, S.R. *et al.* (1987) Significant depletion of NPY in the innervation of the rat mesenteric, renal arteries and kidneys in experimentally (aorta coarctation) induced hypertension. *Histochemistry* **87**, 273–278.

Chalmers, J., Morris, M., Kapoor, V., Cain, M., Elliot, J., Russel, A. *et al.* (1989) Neuropeptide Y in the sympathetic control of blood pressure in hypertensive patients. *J. Clin. Exp. Hypertens.* **A11** (Suppl. 1), 59–66.

Clarke, J.G., Kerwin, R., Larkin, S., Lee, Y., Yacoub, M., Davies, G.J. *et al.* (1987) Coronary artery infusion of neuropeptide Y in patients with angina pectoris. *Lancet* **I**(8541), 1057–1059.

Connell, J.M.C., Corder, R., Asbury, J., Macpherson, S., Inglis, G.C., Lowry, P. *et al.* (1987) Neuropeptide Y in multiple endocrine neoplasia: release during surgery for pheochromocytoma. *Clin. Endocrinol.* **26**, 75–84.

Corder, R., Lowry, P.J., Emson, P.C. & Gaillard, R.C. (1985) Chromatographic characterization of the circulating neuropeptide Y immunoreactivity from patients with phaeochromocytoma. *Regul. Pept.* **10**, 91–97.

Dahlöf, P., Tarizzo, V.I., Lundberg, J.M. & Dahlöf, C. (1991) α- and β-adrenoceptor-mediated effects on nerve stimulation-evoked release of neuropeptide Y (NPY)-like immunoreactivity in the pithed guinea-pig. *J. Auton. Nerv. Syst.* **35**, 199–210.

Dhital, K.K., Gerli, R., Lincoln, J., Milner, P., Tanganelli, P., Weber, G. *et al.* (1988) Increased density of perivascular nerves to the major cerebral vessels of the spontaneously hypertensive rat: differential changes in noradrenaline and neuropeptide Y during development. *Brain Res.* **444**, 33–45.

Doods, H.N. & Krause, J. (1991) Different neuropeptide Y receptor subtypes in rat and rabbit vas deferens. *Eur. J. Pharmacol.* **204**, 101–103.

Doods, H.N., Wienen, W., Entzeroth, M., Rudolf, K., Eberlein, W., Engel, W. *et al.* (1995) Pharmacological characterization of the selective nonpeptide neuropeptide Y Y1 receptor antagonist BIBP 3226. *J. Pharm. Exp. Ther.* **275**, 136–142.

Ekblad, E., Edvinsson, L., Wahlestedt, C., Uddman, R., Håkanson, R. & Sundler, F. (1984) Neuropeptide Y co-exists and co-operates with noradrenaline in perivascular nerve fibers. *Regul. Pept.* **8**, 225–235.

Franco-Cereceda, A. & Lundberg, J.M. (1987) Potent effects of neuropeptide Y and calcitonin gene-related peptide on human coronary vascular tone in vitro. *Acta Physiol. Scand.* **131**, 159–160.

Franco-Cereceda, A., Bengtsson, L. & Lundberg, J.M. (1987) Inotropic effects of calcitonin-gene related peptide, vasoactive intestinal peptide and somatostatin on the human right atrium in vitro. *Eur. J. Pharmacol.* **134**, 69–76.

Gray, T.S. & Morely, J.E. (1986) Neuropeptide Y: anatomical distribution and possible function in mammalian nervous system. *Nature* **38**, 389–401.

Grouzman, E., Comoy, E. & Bouhon, C. (1989) Plasma neuropeptide Y concentrations in patients with neuroendocrine tumours. *J. Clin. Endocr. Metab.* **68**, 808–813.

Grundemar, L. & Håkanson, R. (1990) Effects of various neuropeptide Y/peptide YY fragments on electrically-evoked contractions of rat vas deferens. *Br. J. Pharmacol.* **100**, 190–192.

Grundemar, L., Jonas, S.E., Mörner, N., Högestätt, E.D., Wahlestedt, C. & Håkanson, R. (1992) Characterization of vascular neuropeptide Y receptors. *Br. J. Pharmacol.* **105**, 45–50.

Hall, G.T., Gardner, T.D. & Potter, E.K. (1990) Attenuation of long-lasting effects of sympathetic stimulation after repeated stimulation. *Circ. Res.* **67**, 193–198.

Hulting, J., Sollevi, A., Ullman, B., Franco-Cereceda, A. & Lundberg, J.M. (1990) Plasma neuropeptide Y on admission to a coronary care unit: raised in patients with left heart failure. *Cardiovasc. Res.* **24**, 102–108.

Kong, J.Q., Curto, K.A., Fleming, W.W., Kotchen, T.A. & Taylor, D. (1991) Catecholamine and neuropeptide Y levels in tissues from young Dahl rats following 5 days low- or high-salt diet. *Blood Vessels* **28**, 442–451.

Lacroix, J.S. & Lundberg, J.M. (1989) Adrenergic and neuropeptide Y supersensitivity in denervated nasal mucosa vasculature of the pig. *Eur. J. Pharmacol.* **169**, 125–136.

Lacroix, J.S., Stjärne, P., Änggård, A. & Lundberg, J.M. (1988) Sympathetic vascular control of the pig nasal mucosa. (2): reserpine-resistant, non-adrenergic nervous responses in relation to neuropeptide Y and ATP. *Acta Physiol. Scand.* **133**, 183–197.

Lacroix, J.S., Ulman, L.G. & Potter, E.K. (1994) Modulation by neuropeptide Y of parasympathetic nerve-evoked nasal vasodilatation via Y2 prejunctional receptor. *Br. J. Pharmacol.* **113**, 479–484.

Lee, R.M.K., Nagahama, M., McKenzie, R. & Daniel, E.E. (1988) Peptide-containing nerves around blood vessels of stroke-prone spontaneously hypertensive rats. *Hypertension* **11** (Suppl. 1), I117–I120.

Lettgen, B., Wagner, S., Hänze, J., Lang, R.E. & Rascher, W. (1994) Elevated plasma concentration of neuropeptide Y in adolescents with primary hypertension. *J. Hum. Hypertens.* **8**, 345–349.

Leys, K., Schachter, M. & Sever, P. (1987) Autoradiographic localization of NPY receptors in rabbit kidney: comparison with rat, guinea-pig and human. *Eur. J. Pharmacol.* **134**, 233–237.

Lundberg, J.M. (1996) Pharmacology of cotransmission in the autonomic nervous system: Integrative aspects on amines, neuropeptides, ATP, amino acids and nitric oxide. *Pharm. Rev.* **48**, 113–178.

Lundberg, J.M. & Modin, A. (1995) Inhibition of sympathetic vasoconstriction in pigs in vivo by the neuropeptide Y–Y1 receptor antagonist BIBP 3226. *Br. J. Pharmacol.* **116**, 2971–2982.

Lundberg, J.M. & Stjärne, L. (1984) Neuropeptide Y (NPY) depresses the secretion of 3H-noradrenaline and the contractile response evoked by field stimulation, in rat vas deferens. *Acta Physiol. Scand.* **120**, 477–479.

Lundberg, J.M. & Tatemoto, K. (1982) Pancreatic polypeptide family (APP, BPP, NPY, PYY) in relation to sympathetic vasoconstriction resistant to α-adrenoceptor blockade. *Acta Physiol. Scand.* **116**, 393–402.

Lundberg, J.M., Tatemoto, K., Terenius, L., Hellström, P.M., Mutt, V., Hökfelt, T. *et al.* (1982a) Localization of the peptide YY (PYY) in gastrointestinal endocrine cells and effects on intestinal blood flow and motility. *Proc. Natl Acad. Sci. USA* **79**, 4471–4475.

Lundberg, J.M., Terenius, L., Hökfelt, T., Martling, C.-R., Tatemoto, K., Mutt, V. *et al.* (1982b) Neuropeptide Y (NPY)-like immunoreactivity in peripheral noradrenergic neurons and effects of NPY on sympathetic function. *Acta Physiol. Scand.* **116**, 477–480.

Lundberg, J.M., Terenius, L., Hökfelt, T. & Goldstein, M. (1983) High levels of neuropeptide Y in peripheral noradrenergic neurons in various mammals including man. *Neurosci. Lett.* **42**, 167–172.

Lundberg, J.M., Hua, X.-Y. & Franco-Cereceda, A. (1984a) Effects of neuropeptide Y (NPY) on mechanical activity and neurotransmission in the heart, vas deferens and urinary bladder of the guinea-pig. *Acta Physiol. Scand.* **121**, 325–332.

Lundberg, J.M., Änggård, A., Theodorsson-Norheim, E. & Pernow, J. (1984b) Guanethidine-sensitive release of neuropeptide Y-like immunoreactivity in the cat spleen by sympathetic nerve stimulation. *Neurosci. Lett.* **52**, 175–180.

Lundberg, J.M., Martinson, A., Hemsén, A., Theodorsson-Norheim, A., Svedenhag, J., Ekblom, B. *et al.* (1985) Corelease of neuropeptide Y and catecholamines during physical exercise in man. *Biochem. Biophys. Res. Comm.* **133**, 30–36.

Lundberg, J.M., Hökfelt, T., Hemsén, A., Theodorsson-Norheim, E., Pernow, J., Hamberger, B. et al. (1986) Neuropeptide Y-like immunoreactivity in adrenaline cells of adrenal medulla and in tumours and plasma of pheochromocytoma patients. Regul. Pept. **13**, 169–182.

Lundberg, J.M., Rudehill, A. & Sollevi, A. (1989a) Pharmacological characterization of neuropeptide Y and noradrenaline mechanisms in sympathetic control of pig spleen. Eur. J. Pharmacol. **163**, 103–113.

Lundberg, J.M., Rudehill, A., Sollevi, A. & Hamberger, B. (1989b) Evidence for co-transmitter role of neuropeptide Y in the pig spleen. Br. J. Pharmacol. **96**, 675–687.

Lundberg, J.M., Franco-Cereceda, A., Hemsén, A., Lacroix, J.S. & Pernow, J. (1990) Pharmacology of noradrenaline and neuropeptide tyrosine (NPY)-mediated sympathetic cotransmission. Fundam. Clin. Pharmacol. **4**, 373–391.

Lundblad, L., Änggård, A., Saria, A. & Lundberg, J.M. (1987) Neuropeptide Y and non-adrenergic sympathetic vascular control of the cat nasal mucosa. J. Auton. Nerv. Syst. **20**, 189–197.

Malmström, R.E. and Lundberg, J.M. (1995a) Endogenous NPY acting on the Y1 receptor accounts for the long lasting part of the sympathetic contraction in guinea-pig vena cava: evidence using SR 120107A. Acta Physiol. Scand. **155**, 329–330.

Malmström, R.E. & Lundberg, J.M. (1995b) Neuropeptide Y accounts for sympathetic vasoconstriction in guinea-pig vena cava: evidence using BIBP 3226 and 3435. Eur. J. Pharmacol. **294**, 661–668.

Malmström, R.E., Modin, A. & Lundberg, J.M. (1996) SR 120107A antagonizes neuropeptide Y Y1 receptor mediated sympathetic vasoconstriction in pigs in vivo. Eur. J. Pharmacol. **305**, 145–154.

Medeiros, M.S. & Turner, A.J. (1994) Post-secretory processing of regulatory peptides: the pancreatic polypeptide family as a model example. Biochimie **76**, 283–287.

Mejia, J.A., Pernow, J., Holst, H.V., Rudehill, A. & Lundberg, J.M. (1988) Effects of neuropeptide Y, calcitonin gene-related peptide, substance P and capsaicin on cerebral arteries in man and animals. J. Neurosurg. **69**, 913–918.

Mentlein, R., Dahms, P., Grandt, D. & Kruger, R. (1993) Proteolytic processing of neuropeptide Y and peptide YY by dipeptidyl peptidase IV. Regul. Pept. **49**, 133–144.

Michel, M.C., Wirth, C., Zerkowski, H.-R., Maisel, A.S. & Motulsky, H.J. (1989) Lack of inotropic effects of neuropeptide Y in human myocardium. J. Cardiovasc. Pharmacol. **14**, 919–922.

Mihara, S.-I., Shigeri, Y. & Fujimoto, M. (1990) Neuropeptide Y receptor in cultured vascular smooth muscle cells: ligand binding and increase in cytosolic free Ca^{2+}. Biochem. Int. **22**, 205–212.

Millar, B.C., Weis, T., Piper, H.M., Weber, M., Borchard, U., McDermott, B.J. et al. (1991) Positive and negative contractile effects of neuropeptide Y on ventricular cardiomyocytes. Am. J. Physiol. **261**, H1727–H1733.

Millar, B.C., Schlüter, K.-D., Zhou, X.-J., McDermott, B.J. & Piper, H.M. (1994) Neuropeptide Y stimulates hypertrophy of adult ventricular cardiomyocytes. Am. J. Physiol. **266**, C1271–C1277.

Miller, D.W. & Tessel, R. (1991) Age-dependent hyperresponsiveness of spontaneously hypertensive rats (SHR) to the pressor effects of intravenous neuropeptide Y (NPY): The role of mode of peptide administration and plasma NPY-like immunoreactivity. J. Cardiovasc. Pharmacol. **18**, 647–656.

Modin, A., Pernow, J. & Lundberg, J.M. (1993a) Repeated renal and splenic sympathetic nerve stimulation in anaesthetized pigs: maintained overflow of neuropeptide Y in controls but not after reserpine. J. Auton. Nerv. Syst. **49**, 123–134.

Modin, A., Pernow, J. & Lundberg, J.M. (1993b) Sympathetic regulation of skeletal muscle blood flow in the pig: a non-adrenergic component likely to be mediated by neuropeptide Y. Acta Physiol. Scand. **148**, 1–11.

Moriarty, M., Potter, E.K. & McCloskey, D.I. (1993) Pharmacological separation of cardioacceleration and vagal inhibitory capacities of sympathetic nerves. *J. Auton. Nerv. Syst.* **43**, 7–16.

Morris, J.L. (1991) Roles of neuropeptide Y and noradrenaline in sympathetic neurotransmission to the thoracic vena cava and aorta of guinea-pigs. *Regul. Pept.* **32**, 297–310.

Neild, T.O. (1987) Actions of neuropeptide Y on innervated and denervated rat tail arteries. *J. Physiol.* (Lond.) **386**, 19–30.

Öhlén, A., Persson, M., Lindbom, L., Gustafsson, L.E. & Hedqvist, P. (1990) Nerve-induced nonadrenergic vasoconstriction and vasodilatation in skeletal muscle. *Am. J. Physiol.* **258**, H1334–H1338.

Pernow, J. (1989) Actions of constrictor (NPY and endothelin) and dilator (substance P, CGRP and VIP) peptides on pig splenic and human skeletal muscle arteries: involvement of the endothelium. *Br. J. Pharmacol.* **97**, 983–989.

Pernow, J. & Lundberg, J.M. (1986) Neuropeptide Y constricts human skeletal muscle arteries via a nifedipine-sensitive mechanism independent of extracellular calcium? *Acta Physiol. Scand.* **128**, 655–656.

Pernow, J. & Lundberg, J.M. (1989a) Modulation of noradrenaline and neuropeptide Y (NPY) release in the pig kidney in vivo: involvement of alpha2, NPY and angiotensin II receptors. *Naunyn-Schmiedeberg's Arch. Pharmacol.* **340**, 379–385.

Pernow, J. & Lundberg, J.M. (1989b) Release and vasoconstrictor effects of neuropeptide Y in relation to non-adrenergic sympathetic control of renal blood flow in the pig. *Acta Physiol. Scand.* **136**, 507–517.

Pernow, J., Lundberg, J.M., Kaijser, L., Hjemdahl, P., Theodorsson-Norheim, E., Martinsson, E. *et al.* (1986a) Plasma neuropeptide Y-like immunoreactivity and catecholamines during various degrees of sympathetc activation in man. *Clin. Physiol.* **6**, 561–578.

Pernow, J., Saria, A. & Lundberg, J.M. (1986b) Mechanisms underlying pre- and postjunctional effects of neuropeptide Y in sympathetic vascular control. *Acta Physiol. Scand.* **126**, 239–249.

Pernow, J., Lundberg, J.M. & Kaijser, L. (1987a) Vasoconstrictor effects in vivo and plasma disappearance rate of neuropeptide Y in man. *Life Sci.* **40**, 47–54.

Pernow, J., Svenberg, T. & Lundberg, J.M. (1987b) Actions of calcium antagonists on pre- and postjunctional effects of neuropeptide Y on human peripheral blood vessels in vitro. *Eur. J. Pharmacol.* **136**, 207–218.

Pernow, J., Kahan, T., Hjemdahl, P. & Lundberg, J.M. (1988a) Possible involvement of neuropeptide Y in sympathetic vascular control of canine skeletal muscle. *Acta Physiol. Scand.* **132**, 43–50.

Pernow, J., Kahan, T. & Lundberg, J.M. (1988b) Neuropeptide Y and reserpine-resistant vasoconstriction evoked by sympathetic nerve stimulation in dog skeletal muscle. *Br. J. Pharmacol.* **94**, 952–960.

Pernow, J., Lundberg, J.M. & Kaijser, L. (1988c) α-Adrenoceptor influence on plasma levels of neuropeptide Y-like immunoreactivity and catecholamines during rest and sympathoadrenal activation in humans. *J. Cardiovasc. Pharmacol.* **12**, 593–599.

Pernow, J., Hemsén, A., Hallén, A. & Lundberg, J.M. (1990) Release of endothelin-like immunoreactivity in relation to neuropeptide Y and catecholamines during endotoxin shock and asphyxia in the pig. *Acta Physiol. Scand.* **140**, 311–322.

Potter, E.K. (1985) Prolonged non-adrenergic inhibition of cardiac vagal action following sympathetic stimulation: Neuromodulation by neuropeptide Y? *Neurosci. Lett.* **54**, 117–121.

Potter, E.K. (1987) Presynaptic inhibition of cardiac vagal postganglionic nerves by neuropeptide Y. *Neurosci. Lett.* **83**, 101–106.

Potter, E.K. (1988) Neuropeptide Y as an autonomic neurotransmitter. *Pharmacol. Ther.* **37**, 251–273.

Potter, E.K., Michell, L., McCloskey, M.J.D., Tseng, A., Goodman, A.E., Shine, J. *et al.* (1989) Pre- and postjunctional actions of neuropeptide Y and related peptides. *Regul. Pept.* **25**, 167–177.

Rudehill, A., Sollevi, A., Franco-Cereceda, A. & Lundberg, J.M. (1986) Neuropeptide Y (NPY) and the pig heart: release and coronary vasoconstrictor effects. *Peptides* **7**, 821–826.

Rudehill, A., Olcen, M., Sollevi, A., Hamberger, B. & Lundberg, J.M. (1987) Release of neuropeptide Y upon haemorrhagic hypovolemia in relation to vasoconstrictor effects in the pig. *Acta Physiol. Scand.* **131**, 517–523.

Rudolf, K., Eberlein, W., Engel, W., Wieland, H.A., Willim, K.D., Entzeroth, M. *et al.* (1994) The first highly potent and selective non-peptide neuropeptide Y Y1 receptor antagonist: BIBP3226. *Eur. J. Pharmacol.* **271**, R11–R13.

Schalling, M., Franco-Cereceda, A., Hemsén, A., Dagerlind, Å., Seroogy, K., Persson, H. *et al.* (1991) Neuropeptide Y and catecholamine synthesizing enzymes and their mRNAs in rat sympathetic neurons and adrenal glands: studies on expression, synthesis and axonal transport after pharmacological and experimental manipulations using hybridization techniques and radioimmunoassay. *Neuroscience* **41**, 753–766.

Serradeil-Le Gal, C., Valette, G., Rouby, P.E., Pellet, A., Villanova, G., Foulon, L. *et al.* (1994) SR 120107A and SR 120819A: two potent and selective orally-effective antagonists for NPY Y1 receptors. *Soc. Neurosci. Abstr.* **20**, 907.

Serradeil-Le Gal, C., Valette, G., Rouby, P.-E., Pellet, A., Oury-Donat, F., Brossard, G. *et al.* (1995) SR120819A, an orally-active and selective neuropeptide Y Y1 receptor antagonist. *FEBS Lett.* **362**, 192–196.

Sheikh, S.P., Sheikh, M.I. & Schwartz, T.W. (1989) Y2-type receptors for peptide YY on renal proximal tubular cells in the rabbit. *Am. J. Physiol.* **257**, F978–F984.

Sheikh, S.P., Roach, E., Fuhlendorff, J. & Williams, J.A. (1991) Localization of Y1 receptors for NPY and PYY on vascular smooth muscle cells in rat pancreas. *Am. J. Physiol.* **260**, G250–G257.

Shigeri, Y. & Fujimoto, M. (1993) Neuropeptide Y stimulates DNA synthesis in vascular smooth muscle cells. *Neurosci, Lett.* **149**, 19–22.

Shigeri, Y., Mihara, S.-I. & Fujimoto, M. (1991) Neuropeptide Y receptor in vascular smooth muscle. *J. Neurochem.* **56**, 852–859.

Solt, V.B., Brown, M.R., Kennedy, B., Kolterman, O.G. & Ziegler, M.G. (1990) Elevated insulin, norepinephrine and neuropeptide Y in hypertension. *Am. J. Hypertens.* **3**, 823–828.

Stjärne, L., Lundberg, J.M. & Åstrand, P. (1986) Neuropeptide Y – a co-transmitter with noradrenaline and adenosine-5'-triphosphate in the sympathetic nerves of the mouse vas deferens? A biochemical, physical and electropharmacological study. *Neuroscience* **18**, 151–166.

Tsuda, K. & Masuyama, Y. (1991) Presynaptic regulation of neurotransmitter release in hypertension. *Clin. Exp. Pharmacol. Physiol.* **18**, 455–467.

Ullman, B., Franco-Cereceda, A., Hulting, J., Lundberg, J.M. & Sollevi, A. (1990) Elevation of plasma neuropeptide Y-like immunoreactivity and noradrenaline during myocardial ischemia in man. *J. Intern. Med.* **228**, 583–589.

Ullman, B., Lindvall, K., Lundberg, J.M., Sigurdsson, A. & Swedberg, K. (1994) Response of plasma neuropeptide Y and noradrenaline to dynamic exercise and ramipril treatment in patients with congestive heart failure. *Clin. Physiol.* **14**, 123–134.

Voisin, T., Bens, M., Cluzeaud, F., Vandewalle, A. & Laburthe, M. (1993) Peptide YY receptors in the proximal tubule PKCSV-PCT cell line derived from transgenic mice. Relation with cell growth. *J. Biol. Chem.* **268**, 20 547–20 554.

Wahlestedt, C., Yanaihara, N. & Håkanson, R. (1986) Evidence for different pre- and postjunctional receptors for neuropeptide Y and related peptides. *Regul. Pept.* **13**, 307–318.

Warner, M.R. & Levy, M.N. (1989) Inhibition of cardiac vagal effects by neurally released and exogenous neuropeptide Y. *Circ. Res.* **65**, 1536–1546.

Warner, M.R., Desilva-Senanayake, P., Ferrario, C.M. & Levy, M.N. (1991) Sympathetic stimulation-evoked overflow of norepinephrine and neuropeptide Y from the heart. *Circ. Res.* **69**, 455–465.

Westfall, T.C., Qualy, J.M., Meldrum, M.J., Zhang, S.-Q., Carpentier, S. & Naes, L. (1987)

Central and peripheral alterations in noradrenergic transmission in experimental hypertension: modulation by prejunctional receptors. *J. Cardiovasc. Pharmacol.* **10** (Suppl. 4), S62–S67.
Wharton, J., Gordon, L., Byrne, J., Herzog, H., Selbie, L.A., Moore, K. *et al.* (1993) Expression of the human neuropeptide tyrosine Y1 receptor. *Proc. Natl Acad. Sci. USA* **90**, 687–691.
Zukowska-Grojec, Z., Golczynska, M., Shen, G.H., Torres-Duarte, A., Haass, M., Wahlestedt, C. *et al.* (1993a) Modulation of vascular function by neuropeptide Y during development of hypertension in spontaneously hypertensive rats. *Pediatr. Nephrol.* **7**, 845–852.
Zukowska-Grojec, Z., Pruszczyk, P., Colton, C., Yao, J., Shen, G.H., Mayers, A.K. *et al.* (1993b) Mitogenic effect of neuropeptide Y in rat vascular smooth muscle cells. *Peptides* **14**, 263–268.
Zukowska-Grojec, Z., Dayao, E.K., Karwatowska-Prokopczuk, E., *et al.* (1996) Stress-induced meseuteric vasoconstriction in rats is mediated by neuropeptide Y-Y1 receptors. *Am. J. Physiol.* **270**, H796–800.

_____ CHAPTER 4 _____

NEUROPEPTIDE Y RECEPTOR TYPES IN THE MAMMALIAN BRAIN: SPECIES DIFFERENCES AND STATUS IN THE HUMAN CENTRAL NERVOUS SYSTEM

Yvan Dumont, Danielle Jacques, Jacques-André St-Pierre and
Rémi Quirion

Table of Contents

4.1 Introduction

Neuropeptide Y (NPY) is one of the most abundant peptides found in mammalian brain (Chronwall *et al.*, 1985; O'Donohue *et al.*, 1985; DeQuidt and Emson, 1986a,b). NPY-like immunoreactivity is widely distributed and especially concentrated in brain structures associated with the limbic system, including cortical areas and the hippocampal formation, as well as in the hypothalamus and various brainstem nuclei (Chronwall *et al.*, 1985; O'Donohue *et al.*, 1985; DeQuidt and Emson, 1986a,b; Hendry, 1993). This distribution confers several potential physiological roles to NPY in the regulation of CNS functions.

Intracerebroventricular (ICV) injections of NPY or its congener peptide YY (PYY) as well as direct administration into specific hypothalamic nuclei, such as the paraventricular hypothalamic nucleus and the prefornical nucleus, have revealed that these peptides induce a robust increase in food intake in several species including rat, mouse, sheep and pig (for reviews, see Chapter 1, this volume; Dumont *et al.*, 1992; Stanley, 1993, Wahlestedt and Reis, 1993). Moreover, they increase respiratory

Neuropeptide Y and Drug Development
ISBN 0-12-304990-3

quotient indicating an increase of carbohydrate utilization as energy substrate (Menéndez et al., 1990).

It has also been reported that NPY and PYY can facilitate learning and memory processes (Flood et al., 1987), modulate locomotor behaviours (Heilig and Murison, 1987; Jolicoeur et al., 1991a), produce hypothermia (Esteban et al., 1989; Jolicoeur et al., 1991b), inhibit sexual behavior (Clark et al., 1985), shift circadian rhythms (Albers et al., 1984; Calzá et al., 1990), modulate cardiorespiratory parameters (McAuley et al., 1993) and generate anxiolytic-like effects (Heilig et al., 1993). Neuroendocrine hormones are also altered by NPY-like peptides. For example, NPY and PYY modulate the release (depending on the hormonal status) of luteinizing hormone releasing hormone (LHRH) (Kalra and Crowley, 1992), induce the release of corticotrophin-releasing factor (CRF) (Tsagarakis et al., 1989) and affect those of growth hormone, prolactin and thyrotropin (Härfstrand et al., 1986, 1987). Furthermore, the central administration of NPY increases plasma levels of vasopressin (Leibowitz et al., 1988), adrenocorticotrophic hormone (ACTH) and consequently, of corticosterone and aldosterone (Härfstrand et al., 1986, 1987). Insulin secretion is also altered following the ICV injection of NPY and derivatives (Kuenzel and McMurty, 1988), while gastric acid secretion is inhibited (Humphreys et al., 1988).

Several of these effects appear to be physiologically relevant based on studies involving NPY antibody or NPY antisense oligonucleotides. Following passive immunization using NPY antibody into the central nervous system (CNS), it has been demonstrated that endogenous NPY had a tonic inhibitory effect on baroreceptor reflexes (Shih et al., 1992). Additionally, neutralizing endogenous NPY effects by the administration of NPY antibody into the brain resulted in the development of amnesia (Flood et al., 1989) and a decrease of food intake (Walter et al., 1994). Similarly, blocking the synthesis of NPY by ICV administration of NPY antisense oligonucleotides resulted in a decrease in food intake (Akabayashi et al., 1994; Husley et al., 1995) and an attentuation of the progesterone-induced LH surge by suppressing NPY levels in hypothalamic areas that are involved in this behavior (Kalra et al., 1995).

It is also well accepted that these effects of NPY and related peptides are mediated by the activation of NPY/PYY receptors located on cell plasma membranes. Over the last decade, a variety of radiolabelled probes have been used to characterize brain NPY receptor sites including [^{3}H]NPY (Martel et al., 1986, 1990a; Chang et al., 1988; Widdowson and Halaris, 1990), [^{125}I]NPY (Walker and Miller, 1988; Sheikh et al., 1989a,b), [^{125}I]Bolton–Hunter(BH)-NPY (Chang et al., 1985; Lynch et al., 1989; Martel et al., 1987, 1990b; Ohkubo et al., 1990), [^{125}I]PYY (Walker and Miller, 1988; Lynch et al., 1989; Martel et al., 1990b), [^{125}I]NPY13–36 (Sheikh et al., 1989a), [^{125}I][Leu^{31},Pro^{34}]NPY (Larsen et al., 1993), [^{125}I]NPY2–36 (Scohber and Gehlert 1993), and more recently, [^{125}I][Leu^{31},Pro^{34}]PYY and [^{125}I]PYY3–36 (Dumont et al., 1995a). All bind with high affinity to brain tissues. While most investigators detected a single class of high-affinity sites, others clearly demonstrated the existence of multiple receptor affinity sites or states (see Dumont et al., 1992; Quirion and Martel, 1992, for more details).

Anatomical studies have shown that NPY binding sites are mostly concentrated in the hippocampal formation, cortical areas, anterior olfactory nuclei and the lateral septum in the rat brain, while lower but still significant amounts of binding sites were detected in the striatum and thalamic, hypothalamic and brainstem nuclei, as well as in the cerebellum (Inui *et al.*, 1988, 1989; Lynch *et al.*, 1989; Martel *et al.*, 1986, 1987, 1990b; Ohkubo *et al.*, 1990; Rosier *et al.*, 1990). Most radiolabeled probes demonstrated similar distributional profiles. However, few differences were observed between the localization of specific $[^{125}I]$BH-NPY and $[^{125}I]$PYY sites (Lynch *et al.*, 1989; Martel *et al.*, 1990b), especially at the levels of the hypothalamus and the cerebellum suggesting the possible heterogeneity of NPY receptor sites.

4.2 Comparative distribution of NPY receptor types

At least four classes of NPY receptors are present in various tissues, designated Y1, Y2 and Y3 (Dumont *et al.*, 1992; Gehlert 1994, Grundemar *et al.*, 1993; Wahlestedt *et al.*, 1992; Wahlestedt and Reis, 1993) with the most recent three cloned receptors referred to the Y4 (Bard *et al.*, 1995) or PP1 (Lundell *et al.*, 1995), Y5 (Gerald *et al.*, 1996) and Y6 (Weinberg *et al.*, 1996) receptor types. The profile of each of these receptors has been well established by the rank order of potency of various NPY/PYY derivatives and pancreatic polypeptides (PPs). NPY, PYY, $[Leu^{31},Pro^{34}]$NPY and $[Leu^{31},Pro^{34}]$PYY are highly potent, while the C-terminal fragments of NPY and PYY, and the PPs are active only in the micromolar range at the Y1 receptor type (Dumont *et al.*, 1994, 1995; Gehlert, 1994; Grundemar *et al.*, 1993; Wahlestedt and Reis, 1993). On the other hand, the Y2 receptor type is activated by NPY, PYY and their C-terminal fragments, whereas the $[Leu^{31},Pro^{34}]$-substituted analogues and the PPs demonstrate much lower affinity (Grundemar *et al.*, 1993; Wahlestedt and Reis, 1993; Gehlert, 1994). In contrast to the Y1 and the Y2 receptors, the Y3 type has preferential affinity for NPY-related peptides (Grundemar *et al.*, 1993; Wahlestedt and Reis, 1993; Dumont *et al.*, 1994). One of the characteristics of the purported PP1/Y4 receptor class is its high affinity for PP-related peptides, such as human (h) PP, rat (r) PP, bovine (b) PP and salmon (s) PP (Bard *et al.*, 1995; Schober *et al.*, 1995), contrasting with low affinity of PPs for the other receptor types of this peptide family (Grundemar *et al.*, 1993, Wahlestedt and Reis, 1993). PYY and its derivatives also possess rather high affinity for the PP1/Y4 receptor type (Bard *et al.*, 1995; Gackenheimer *et al.*, 1995). The Y5 receptor type has high affinity for hPP, NPY, PYY, $[Leu^{31},Pro^{34}]$NPY, $[Leu^{31},Pro^{34}]$PYY, NPY2–36 and PYY3–36 but low affinity for short C-terminal fragments such as NPY13–36 and PYY13–36 as well as for rPP (Gerald *et al.*, 1996). The pharmacological profile of the Y6 receptor type is rather similar to the Y5 except that hPP is not potent on this receptor class (Weinberg *et al.*, 1996).

4.2.1 Rat brain

The first demonstration of a differential distribution of the Y1 and Y2 receptor types in the rat brain was reported 6 years ago using $[^{125}I]$PYY as radioligand in the presence of masking concentrations of [Pro^{34}]NPY or NPY13–36 (Dumont *et al.*, 1990). Most of the specific [^{125}I]PYY binding sites detected in cortical areas were potently inhibited by [Pro^{34}]NPY, a Y1 receptor agonist (Fuhlendorff *et al.*, 1990; Schwartz *et al.*, 1990) but not by NPY13–36, a Y2 receptor agonist (Wahlestedt *et al.*, 1986). In contrast, [^{125}I]PYY binding in the hippocampus was highly sensitive to the Y2 receptor agonist but more resistant to [Pro^{34}]NPY. These results were subsequently confirmed by other groups using similar approaches (Aicher *et al.*, 1991; Gehlert *et al.*, 1992).

In follow-up studies, the respective distribution of the Y1 and Y2 receptor types was evaluated in greater details. Membrane binding assays revealed that the Y1 receptor agonist, [Leu^{31},Pro^{34}]NPY competed for [^{125}I]PYY binding with a competition profile best fitted by a two-site model with high- and low-affinity components representing Y1 and Y2 sites, respectively (Dumont *et al.*, 1993, 1994). These studies clearly demonstrated that both receptor-types were present in various brain regions but their densities greatly varied as a function of the area. For example, 70% of [^{125}I]PYY binding in the frontoparietal cortex are of the Y1 type, while 90% of those found in the hippocampus are of the Y2 class (Dumont *et al.*, 1993, 1994). Autoradiographic studies confirmed these findings (Aicher *et al.*, 1991; Gehlert *et al.*, 1992; Dumont *et al.*, 1993; Larsen *et al.*, 1993). These studies were performed using concentrations of 10–300 nM of [Pro^{34}]NPY and 100–1000 nM of NPY13–36, to mask specifically the Y1 and Y2 receptor type, respectively. This approach is not optimal, as it is suggested from the competition curve that is difficult to establish the concentration precisely of the Y1 or Y2 agonist that will fully occupy one class of receptors without interfering at all with the other. This is especially evident here since they used Y1 and Y2 receptor blockers that are not fully selective for one class of site over the other. This issue has been discussed elsewhere for various classes of peptides and non-peptides receptors (Seeman, 1980; Quirion *et al.*, 1983; Quirion, 1985; Frazer *et al.*, 1990). Thus, the development of more selective agonists and antagonists and their use as radiolabeled probes is essential to precisely define the characteristics of each NPY receptor-type. In that regard, [^{125}I] [Leu^{31},Pro^{34}]NPY has been used to target the Y1 receptor-type in the rat brain (Larsen *et al.*, 1993). Additionally, [^{125}I]NPY2–36 (Schober and Gehlert, 1993) was developed in order to facilitate the characterization of the atypical Y1/Y2 receptor type believed to be responsible for the effect of NPY on food intake (Jolicoeur *et al.*, 1991a,b; Quirion *et al.*, 1990; Stanley *et al.*, 1992). However, NPY2–36 was unable to discriminate clearly between the typical Y1 and Y2 receptor types and failed to establish the existence of the atypical site (Schober and Gehlert, 1993). Additionally, NPY2–36 and [Leu^{31},Pro^{34}]NPY were shown to have relatively high affinity for the Y3 receptor type (Dumont *et al.*, 1994) and hence cannot be used in tissue possibly expressing this receptor class such as the CNS (see Grundemar *et al.*, 1991).

We have developed [Leu^{31},Pro^{34}]PYY and PYY3–36 as putative Y1 and Y2 receptor agonists, respectively (Dumont *et al.*, 1994). One major advantage of these PYY derivatives over their NPY counterpart, relates to their lack of affinity for the Y3 receptor (Dumont *et al.*, 1994). These peptides were subsequently radiolabelled (^{125}I) and the respective competition profile of various homologues including NPY, NPY13–36, [Leu^{31},Pro^{34}]NPY, PYY, PYY13–36, [Leu^{31},Pro^{34}]PYY and PPs was established (Dumont *et al.*, 1995). Hill coefficients lower than unity suggested further heterogeneity of both $[^{125}I][Leu^{31},Pro^{34}]PYY/Y1$-like and $[^{125}I]PYY3$–$36/Y2$-like binding sites in the rat brain (Dumont *et al.*, 1995; see below).

As shown in Plate 1, the autoradiographic distribution of $[^{125}I][Leu^{31},Pro^{34}]$ PYY/Y1-like binding revealed high levels of sites in the superficial layers of the cortex, olfactory bulb, islands of Calleja, tenia tecta, molecular layer of the dentate gyrus, several thalamic nuclei and the posterior part of the medial mammillary nucleus. $[^{125}I]PYY3$–$36/Y2$-like binding was found to be most abundant in several regions including the lateral septum, piriform cortex, triangular septal nucleus, bed nucleus of the stria terminalis, oriens and stratum radiatum layers of the dorsal hippocampus, ventral tegmental area, substantia nigra, dorsal raphe nucleus and granular cell layer of the cerebellum (Plate 2). Moreover, few areas contained significant levels of both $[^{125}I][Leu^{31},Pro^{34}]PYY$ and $[^{125}I]PYY3$–36 labeling such as the anterior olfactory nuclei, oriens layer and stratum radiatum of the ventral hippocampus, nucleus tractus solitarius, area postrema and inferior olive (Plates 1 and 2). This regional distribution of the putative Y1 and Y2 receptor-types using direct labeling conditions (Dumont *et al.*, 1996a) was largely consistent with other reports employing masking conditions (Dumont *et al.*, 1990, 1993; Aicher *et al.*, 1991; Gehlert *et al.*, 1992; Larsen *et al.*, 1993). However, higher levels of putative Y1 binding sites were detected in the anterior olfactory nucleus, ventral part of the hippocampal formation, amygdaloid body and various thalamic nuclei using a direct labeling technique (Dumont *et al.*, 1996a). Further, the distribution of the NPY Y1 receptor mRNA as shown by *in situ* hybridization (Eva *et al.*, 1990; Larsen *et al.*, 1993; Tong *et al.*, 1993) and the localization of $[^{125}I][Leu^{31},Pro^{34}]PYY$ binding sites (Dumont *et al.*, 1996a) are generally very similar supporting the local synthesis and expression of the Y1 receptor.

The newly developed non-peptide receptor antagonists, BIBP3226 (Rudolf *et al.*, 1994) and SR 12898A (Serradeil-Le Gal *et al.*, 1995) have been demonstrated to be highly selective for the Y1 receptor-type (for details, see Chapters 7 and 8). The selectivity and specificity of BIBP3226 for the Y1 versus Y2 and Y3 receptor types have been demonstrated in various binding assays and bioassays (Rudolf *et al.*, 1994; Jacques *et al.*, 1995). Moreover, its selectivity has further been confirmed in binding assays with Y1-, Y2-, Y4- and Y5-transfected cell lines (Gerald *et al.*, 1996). The tritiated form of BIBP3226 has also been used to characterize the Y1 receptor type expressed in neuroblastoma cell lines (Entzeroth *et al.*, 1995) and we compared the distribution of specific $[^{3}H]BIBP3226$ sites with that of $[^{125}I][Leu^{31},Pro^{34}]PYY$ sites and observed a rather similar pattern (Plate 3). However, few areas are more densely labeled with $[^{125}I]Leu^{31},Pro^{34}]PYY$ than $[^{3}H]BIBP3226$ binding (Dumont *et al.*, 1996b). As shown in Plate 3, intense labeling with $[^{125}I][Leu^{31},Pro^{34}]PYY$ was visualized in the external plexiform layer of the olfactory bulb, lateral septum, nucleus tractus solitarius and area postrema compared to levels detected using the Y1 receptor antagonist, $[^{3}H]BIBP3226$. It is unlikely that differences seen between the two Y1 receptor radioligands can be explained by the nature of the radioisotope used and their respective affinity for the Y1 receptor (Dumont *et al.*, 1996b). A more likely hypothesis is that previously used Y1 receptor radioligands, such as

[^{125}I] [Leu^{31},Pro^{34}]NPY (Larsen *et al.*, 1993) and [^{125}I] [Leu^{31},Pro^{34}]PYY (Dumont *et al.*, 1995) each recognize additional class(es) of sites. The low Hill coefficient observed in homogenates binding assays (Dumont *et al.*, 1995) and the significant potency of [Leu^{31},Pro^{34}]PYY (Dumont *et al.*, 1994) and [Leu^{31},Pro^{34}]NPY (Jørgensen *et al.*, 1990) to inhibit the rat vas deferens twitch response supports this contention. In fact, it would now appear that [Leu^{31},Pro^{34}]NPY also label the Y3 receptor (Grundemar *et al.*, 1991; Wahlestedt *et al.*, 1992), while [Leu^{31},Pro^{34}]PYY and [Leu^{31},Pro^{34}]NPY can recognize the newly cloned PP1/Y4 (Bard *et al.*, 1995; Gackenheimer *et al.*, 1995), Y5 (Gerald *et al.*, 1996) and Y6 (Weinberg *et al.*, 1996) receptor types.

An extensive competition binding study in rat brain membrane homogenates using [^{125}I] [Leu^{31},Pro^{34}]PYY as radioligand in the presence of either one of the following peptides NPY, NPY2–36, NPY13–36, NPY18–36, [Leu^{31},Pro^{34}]NPY, PYY, PYY3–36, PYY13–36, [Leu^{31},Pro^{34}]PYY, hPP, rPP and aPP or antagonists, BIBP3226 and BIBP3435 (S-enantiomer of BIBP3226) at concentrations ranging from 10^{-12} to 10^{-6} M confirmed that BIBP3226, in contrast to NPY, PYY and PP-related homologs was unable to compete for the totality of specific [^{125}I] [Leu^{31},Pro^{34}]PYY binding (Dumont and Quirion, 1995). It thus appears that sites recognized by [^{125}I] [Leu^{31},Pro^{34}]PYY also include a population of sites that are insensitive to BIBP3226. The later class of receptor has been characterized by blocking [^{125}I] [Leu^{31},Pro^{34}]PYY binding to the Y1 receptor-type with 2 μM BIBP3226. Under such experimental conditions, competition binding analysis revealed that hPP was the most potent competitor (IC$_{50}$: 2 nM) followed by PYY and NPY (IC$_{50}$: 4–6 nM) while rPP, aPP and C-terminal fragments of NPY and PYY (NPY13–36, NPY18–36 and PYY13–36) were much less potent (>300 nM) (Dumont and Quirion, 1995). Hence, the competition binding profile of this receptor type is clearly different from the Y1, Y2 and Y3 receptor class. As shown in Plate 4, this site is mostly concentrated in the external plexiform layer of the olfactory bulb, septal area, anteroventral thalamic nucleus, nucleus tractus solitarius and area postrema. Discriminating between effects induced by hPP but not rPP may prove useful in understanding the role of this new class of NPY-related sites. Relationship to the recently cloned PP1/Y4 receptor type also remains to be fully established, differences being in the rather low potency of rPP in our assay compared to its high affinity for the cloned receptor (Bard *et al.*, 1995). On the other hand, the pharmacological profile of [^{125}I] [Leu^{31},Pro^{34}]PYY/BIBP3226-insensitive binding site is rather similar to the Y5 receptor (Gerald *et al.*, 1996).

Preliminary evidence also suggests the possible heterogeneity of the Y2-like receptor population present in the rat brain. It is well known that Y1 (Herzog *et al.*, 1992; Larhammar *et al.*, 1992), Y2 (Gerald *et al.*, 1995) and PP1/Y4 (Bard *et al.*, 1995; Lundell *et al.*, 1995), Y5 (Gerald *et al.*, 1996) and Y6 (Weinberg *et al.*, 1996), all belong to the seven transmembrane domain G-protein-coupled receptor superfamily, and thus can be modulated by GTP and its stable analogue, GTPγS. In fact, 100 μM GTPγS decreased specific [^{125}I]PYY binding by 45% and 25% in Y1- and Y2-enriched preparations, respectively (Figure 1 and Table 1) suggesting that a proportion of high-affinity receptors had shifted to low-affinity states. Moreover, in the hippocampus (Y2-enriched preparation), the occlusion of the Y1 receptor class (20 nM

HIPPOCAMPUS

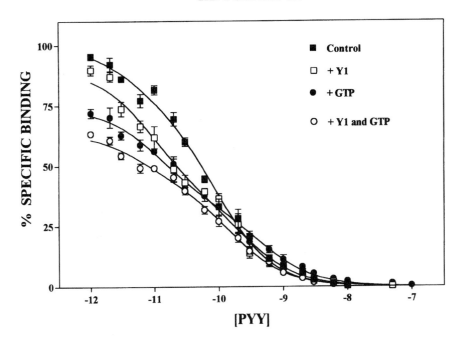

Figure 1 Effect of 100 μM GTPγS on [^{125}I]PYY in the presence of 20 nM [Leu^{31},Pro^{34}]NPY in rat hippocampal membrane preparations.

[Leu^{31},Pro^{34}]NPY) in the presence of 100 μM GTPγS resulted in a further 10–15% decrease of [^{125}I]PYY binding sites (Figure 1) and binding curves were best fitted to a two-site model with high- and low-affinity components (Table 1). Additionally, Hill coefficients lower than one were also noted for most NPY/PYY competitors against [^{125}I]PYY3–36/Y2-like binding (Dumont *et al.*, 1995). Taken together, these data suggest the possible heterogeneity of the Y2-like receptor family. However, in order to confirm this hypothesis fully, Y2 receptor antagonists will need to be developed that could discriminate between [^{125}I]PYY3–36/Y2 antagonist-sensitive and antagonist-insensitive binding sites as shown for BIBP3226 (Dumont *et al.*, 1996b).

Little is known on the putative distribution of the Y3 receptor type in the rat brain. It may be restricted to brainstem nuclei such as the nucleus tractus solitarius and area postrema (Grundemar *et al.*, 1991). Currently, the only means of investigating the brain distribution of the Y3 receptor type is to use [^{125}I]BH-NPY in the presence of PYY (to block Y1 and Y2 sites) or Y1 and Y2 blockers (1 μM [Leu^{31},Pro^{34}]PYY + 1 μM PYY3–36). As shown in Plate 5, [^{125}I]BH-NPY binding under these blocking conditions was almost identical to non-specific binding (in the presence of 1 μM pNPY). These results suggest that if the Y3 receptor type is in fact present in the rat brain, it is expressed only in very low concentrations.

Table 1 Binding parameters derived from [^{125}I]PYY competition curves in the presence and absence of 20 nM [Leu^{31},Pro^{34}]NPY plus 100 μM GTPγS in frontoparietal (Y1-enriched) and hippocampal (Y2-enriched) membrane preparations

Regions and conditions	PYY		
	K_{D1}(pM)	K_{D2}	%R1
Hippocampus (100%)	15±10	500±200	52±5
+Y1 (89±6%)	10±8	260±120	56±6
+GTPγS (74±6%)	30±15	1100±250	37±6
+Y1 and GTPγS (63±4%)	26±9	950±230	42±5
Frontoparietal cortex (100%)	85±20	1900±530	39±5
+Y1 (32±4%)	10±5	180±90	34±7
+GTPγS (44±3%)	75±15	2300±900	29±4

K_{D1} and K_{D2} represent the affinity of PYY for the high- and low-affinity sites, respectively. % R1 represents the percentage of sites in the high-affinity mode observed in the presence and absence of a 20 nM blocking concentration of [Leu^{31},Pro^{34}]NPY (Y1) and /or 100 μM GTPγS.
Numbers in parenthesis represents the percentage of specific binding that remains in the presence of Y1 agonist or the GTP analog.

Concerning the newly cloned PP1/Y4 receptor, its full autoradiographic distribution remains to be established but likely includes the interpendicular nucleus, nucleus tractus solitarius and the area postrema as defined using [^{125}I]bPP (Whitcomb *et al.*, 1990). Additional experiments are currently in progress to study, in detail, the discrete localization of this receptor class in the CNS, as well as for the Y5 and Y6 receptors.

4.2.2 Other species

Little is known with respect to the autoradiographic distribution of brain NPY receptor sites in other species. Few studies have reported the presence and distribution of NPY receptor sites in selected areas of the hamster (Martel *et al.*, 1987), guinea-pig (Martel *et al.*, 1987), monkey (Martel *et al.*, 1987; Rosier *et al.*, 1990), cat (Rosier *et al.*, 1990) and human (Martel *et al.*, 1990c; Widdowson and Halaris, 1990; Widdowson, 1993) brains. In all these species, very high densities of specific labeling were detected in the hippocampus and cortical areas. However, differences with respect to the distributional profile were seen in various subcortical areas. For example, striate nuclei are enriched with [^{125}I]BH-NPY or [^{125}I]PYY sites in the guinea-pig, monkey and human brains as compared to the rat and mouse (Martel *et al.*, 1987). Further, recent studies have shown that, in contrast to the rat brain, very low levels of the Y1 receptor-type are present in the human brain (Widdowson, 1993).

Using the Y1/[^{125}I][Leu^{31},Pro^{34}]PYY and Y2/[^{125}I]PYY3–36 receptor probes, we have demonstrated that the brain distribution of these two classes of sites varied between species. Rat and mouse brains have a similar distributional profile, while in the guinea-pig brain, the Y2 receptor type is expressed only in low concentrations, including within the hippocampus (Rouissi *et al.*, 1994). In contrast, in the monkey and human brains, only low levels of $[^{125}I][Leu^{31},Pro^{34}]PYY/Y1$ sites were detected in all regions, except in the dentate gyrus of the hippocampus (Rouissi *et al.*, 1994; see below).

4.2.2.1 Mouse

The distributional pattern of Y1-like/$[^{125}I][Leu^{31},Pro^{34}]PYY$ (Plate 6) and Y2-like/$[^{125}I]PYY3–36$ (Plate 7) binding sites is generally similar to those of the rat brain (Plates 1 and 2). $[^{125}I][Leu^{31},Pro^{34}]PYY$ binding sites were found in high concentrations in cortical areas, the dentate gyrus of the hippocampus, the olfactory tubercle and islands of Calleja (Plate 6), while $[^{125}I]PYY3–36$ labeling was mostly localized in the ependymal and subependymal layers of the olfactory bulb, the septal area, the hippocampal formation, the stria terminalis and the amygdaloid complex (Plate 7). Moreover, as in the rat brain, hypothalamic nuclei contained low to very low levels of $[^{125}I][Leu^{31},Pro^{34}]PYY$ (Plate 6) and $[^{125}I]PYY3–36$ (Plate 7) binding sites.

However, it is noteworthy that a few differences exist between the two species. In the mouse brain, the anterior olfactory nucleus contains considerably lower amounts of $[^{125}I]PYY3–36$ binding sites (Plate 7) compared to levels detected in the rat brain (Plate 2). Higher concentrations of $[^{125}I][Leu^{31},Pro^{34}]PYY$ binding sites were detected in the mouse caudate putamen, while all thalamic nuclei including the geniculate nuclei revealed considerably less labeling (Plate 6) as compared to the rat brain (Plate 1).

Up to date, the distributional pattern of $[^{125}I][Leu^{31},Pro^{34}]PYY/BIBP3226$-insensitive binding sites has not been evaluated in the mouse. Neither has the distribution of the Y3 and PP1/Y4, Y5 and Y6 receptor types.

4.2.2.2 Guinea-pig

The discrete distribution of the purported Y1 and Y2 receptor types have been evaluated using $[^{125}I][Leu^{31},Pro^{34}]PYY$ and $[^{125}I]PYY3–36$, respectively. Suprisingly, in contrast to the results obtained in the rat and mouse, very low levels of $[^{125}I]PYY3–36$ labelling were detected in various regions of the guinea-pig brain. Most of the NPY receptors that are expressed in the guinea-pig brain appears to be of the Y1 receptor type (Rouissi *et al.*, 1994; Plates 8 and 9). Intense Y1-like labeling was detected in all cortical areas and the hippocampal formation (Plate 8), while only low levels of Y2/$[^{125}I]PYY3–36$ binding sites were detected in these areas (Plate 9). Additionally, only low amounts of both $[^{125}I][Leu^{31},Pro^{34}]PYY$ (Plate 8) and $[^{125}I]PYY3–36$ (Plate 9) binding were observed in structures associated with the olfactory system including the olfactory bulb, anterior olfactory nuclei and olfactory tubercle. This is in contrast with data obtained in the rat (Plates 1 and 2) and mouse (Plates 6 and 7) brains. Higher levels of $[^{125}I][Leu^{31},Pro^{34}]PYY$ labeling (Plate 8) was observed in the striatum of the guinea-pig as compared to the signal detected in the rat brain (Plate 1). In contrast, the septal area of the guinea-pig contains much lower concentrations of $[^{125}I]\ PYY3–36$ binding sites (Plate 9) in comparison to the levels seen in rat (Plate 2) and mouse (Plate 7). Most thalamic nuclei are only poorly labeled with either radioligands in the guinea-pig (Plates 8 and 9). The substantia nigra was enriched with [^{125}I] PYY3–36 labeling (Plate 9) but displayed only low levels of [^{125}I] [Leu^{31},Pro^{34}]PYY binding sites (Plate 8).

Interestingly, [^{125}I] [Leu^{31},Pro^{34}]PYY binding expressed in various regions of the guinea-pig brain does not appear to correspond to an homogeneous population of sites. As seen in the rat, the guinea-pig brain also contained two populations of [^{125}I] [Leu^{31},Pro^{34}]PYY sites, one which is sensitive to BIBP3226, the other not. However, in the guinea-pig, the regions of the brain containing a population of [^{125}I] [Leu^{31},Pro^{34}]PYY/BIBP3226-insensitive sites are not similar to those observed in the rat brain. For example, [^{125}I] [Leu^{31},Pro^{34}]PYY binding sites in the external plexiform layer of the olfactory bulb are competed for by a low micromolar concentration of BIBP3226 (Plate 10). Moreover, the striatum, lateral septum, hippocampal formation and locus coeruleus contained a significantly greater proportion of [^{125}I] [Leu^{31},Pro^{34}]PYY binding, which is resistant to micromolar concentrations of BIBP3226, while in other structures like the medial mammillary nuclei, all specific [^{125}I] [Leu^{31},Pro^{34}]PYY labeling is fully inhibited by 1 μM BIBP3226 (Plate 10). It remains to be established whether BIBP3226-insensitive sites are identical in the rat and guinea-pig brains. The presence and distribution of the Y3 and PP1/Y4, Y5 and Y6 receptor types have yet to be examined in the guinea-pig brain.

4.2.2.3 Monkey

As shown in Plate 11, cortical areas of the monkey (vervet) brain contain only low levels of Y1/[^{125}I] [Leu^{31},Pro^{34}]PYY binding sites. These data contrast with the large amounts of specific [^{125}I] [Leu^{31},Pro^{34}]PYY labeling detected in the rat (Plate 1), mouse (Plate 6) and guinea-pig (Plate 8) cortex. In fact, the distribution of specific NPY binding reported earlier using non-selective ligands (Martel *et al.*, 1987; Rosier *et al.*, 1990) correspond rather well with that of the Y2/[^{125}I]PYY3–36 binding in most regions of the monkey brain including the cortex, the hippocampal formation and various hypothalamic nuclei (Plate 11). The only area that contains significant amounts of Y1/[^{125}I] [Leu^{31},Pro^{34}]PYY labeling is the dentate gyrus of the hippocampus in the monkey brain. Data are not available yet on the presence and distribution of [^{125}I] [Leu^{31},Pro^{34}]PYY/BIBP3226-insensitive, Y3 and PP1/Y4, Y5 and Y6 sites in the monkey brain.

4.2.2.4 Human

Few studies have been reported thus far on the existence of NPY receptors in the human brain. Early reports have shown that NPY receptors are present in the human brain (Martel *et al.*, 1990c; Widdowson and Halaris, 1990). Later on, using masking conditions, it was reported that human brain tissues expressed very limited amounts of the Y1 receptor type, with most of the specific [^{125}I]PYY binding being of Y2 receptor class (Widdowson, 1993). Most recently, we carried out an extensive analysis of the respective distribution of specific Y1-like/[^{125}I] [Leu^{31},Pro^{34}]PYY, [^{125}I] [Leu^{31},Pro^{34}]

[¹²⁵I][Leu³¹,Pro³⁴]PYY   [¹²⁵I]PYY₃₋₃₆

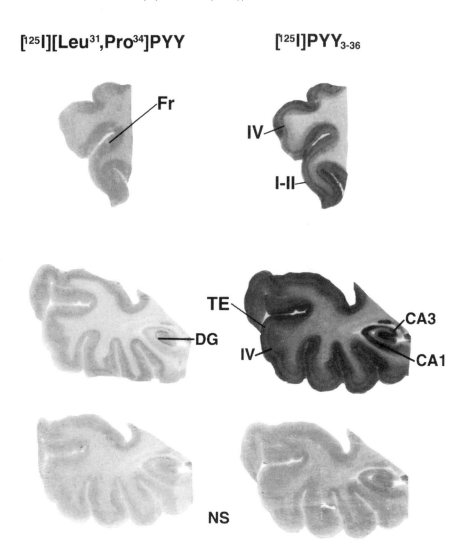

Figure 2 Photomicrographs of the comparative autoradiographic distribution of [¹²⁵I][Leu³¹,Pro³⁴]PYY/Y1-like and [¹²⁵I]PYY3–36/Y2-like binding sites at the level of the frontal cortex and the hippocampus of human brain. Adjacent coronal sections were incubated with 35 pM of either [¹²⁵I][Leu³¹,Pro³⁴]PYY or [¹²⁵I]PYY3–36 in the presence or absence of 1 μM pNPY in order to determine non-specific binding. See list of abbreviations for details of anatomical identification.

PYY/BIBP3226-insensitive and Y2-like/[¹²⁵I]PYY3–36 binding sites in various areas of the human brain. Very low levels of specific [¹²⁵I][Leu³¹,Pro³⁴]PYY were detected in frontal and temporal (Figure 2) cortices, while the dentate gyrus of the hippocampus was found to express significant amounts of Y1 binding sites (Figure 2). In con-

[¹²⁵I][Leu³¹,Pro³⁴]PYY   **BIBP3226 10⁻⁶M**

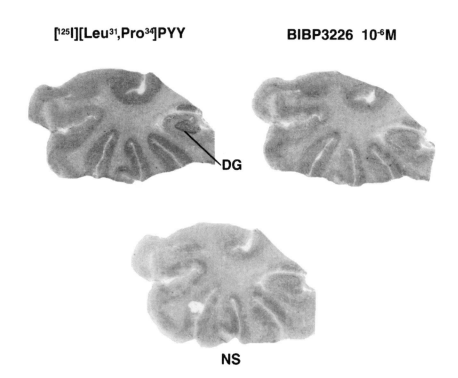

NS

Figure 3 Photomicrographs of the comparative autoradiographic distribution of [¹²⁵I] [Leu³¹,Pro³⁴]PYY in the presence or absence of 1 µM BIBP3226, a Y1 receptor antagonist at the level of the human brain hippocampus. Adjacent coronal sections were incubated with 35 pM [¹²⁵I] [Leu³¹,Pro³⁴]PYY in the presence or absence of 1 µM pNPY in order to determine non-specific binding. See list of abbreviations for details of anatomical identification.

trast, cortical areas and the hippocampus were enriched with specific [¹²⁵I] PYY3–36/Y2-like binding sites (Figure 2). These results have been confirmed using membrane binding assays. In human frontal cortex membrane homogenates, only the use of [¹²⁵I]PYY3–36 generates specific signals at reasonable protein concentration (Jacques *et al.*, 1994). Additionally, the Y1-like/[¹²⁵I] [Leu³¹,Pro³⁴]PYY binding sites expressed in the dentate gyrus were fully competed by the Y1 receptor antagonist, BIBP3226 (Figure 3). This suggest the absence (or very low level of expression) of the [¹²⁵I] [Leu³¹,Pro³⁴]PYY/BIBP3226-insensitive sites in the human brain.

Despite the paucity of Y1-like binding sites detected in most areas of the human brain (Widdowson, 1993; Jacques *et al.*, 1994; Figure 2), the Y1 receptor mRNA signal, as revealed by *in situ* hybridization, clearly showed a laminar distribution in frontal (Figure 4) and temporal (Figure 5) cortices. Moreover, the Y1 receptor mRNA appears to be more abundant than the translated protein in most brain structures including the claustrum, amygdaloid nuclei, and arcuate and paraventricular hypo-

[¹²⁵I][Leu³¹,Pro³⁴]PYY   **Y₁ R mRNA**

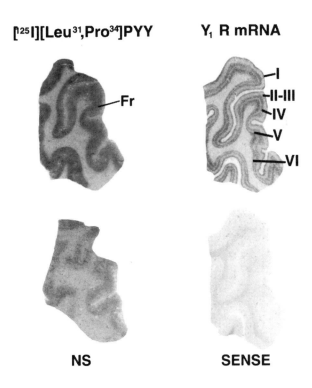

NS   **SENSE**

Figure 4 Photomicrographs of the comparative distribution of [¹²⁵I][Leu³¹,Pro³⁴]PYY binding sites and Y1 receptor mRNA in at the level of the frontal cortex of the human brain. Adjacent coronal sections were incubated with either 35 pM [¹²⁵I][Leu³¹,Pro³⁴]PYY in the presence or absence of 1 μM pNPY and ³⁵S-sense and ³⁵S-antisense of the NPY Y1 receptor mRNA. See list of abbreviations for details of anatomical identification.

thalamic nuclei (Jacques *et al.*, 1996). The dentate gyrus is the only area that contains significant amounts of both the Y1 receptor mRNA and its translated protein (Figure 5), suggesting the localization of the receptor on intrinsic neurons (Jacques *et al.*, 1996).

We have recently extended our study on the autoradiographic distribution of the purported Y1 and Y2 receptor types, as well as that of the NPY Y1 receptor mRNA, to include regions such as the basal ganglia, caudate and putamen, thalamus and hypothalamus, the brainstem, cerebellum and spinal cord (Jacques *et al.*, 1994, 1995, 1996). As shown in Table 2, only small numbers of Y1 binding sites are present in most brain regions, while the Y2 receptor type is more prominently distributed throughout the human brain. Surprisingly, Y1 receptor mRNA is relatively more abundant than the translated protein. The functional significance of this observation as well as the existence of the Y3 and PP1/Y4, Y5 and Y6 receptor classes in the human brain remain to be investigated.

Y. Dumont *et al.*

[¹²⁵I][Leu³¹,Pro³⁴]PYY   Y₁ R mRNA

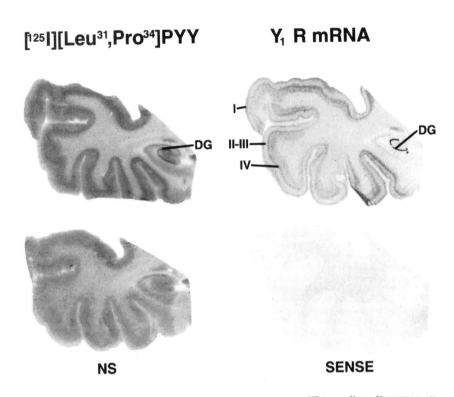

NS   SENSE

Figure 5 Photomicrographs of the comparative distribution of [¹²⁵I][Leu³¹,Pro³⁴]PYY binding sites and the Y1 receptor mRNA at the level of the human brain hippocampus. Adjacent coronal sections were incubated with either 35 pM [¹²⁵I][Leu³¹,Pro³⁴]PYY in the presence or absence of 1 µM pNPY and ³⁵S-sense and ³⁵S-antisense of the NPY Y1 receptor mRNA. See list of abbreviations for details of anatomical identification.

4.3 Functional significance of the various NPY receptor types

4.3.1 Rat brain

4.3.1.1 Striatum

Locomotor activity may be regulated by NPYergic neurons present in the striatum through the activation of the Y1 and Y2 receptor types. The activation of these two classes of receptors has been suggested to be responsible for the stimulation and inhibition of locomotor behavior, respectively (for review, see Heilig, 1993). NPY-like immunoreactive neurons in the rat striatum may represent a target for glutamatergic corticostriatal projections as well as nigrostriatal dopaminergic inputs and intrinsic GABA-ergic neurons (Aoki and Pickel, 1990). Studies suggested the existence of

70

Table 2 Quantitative autoradiographic distribution of [^{125}I][Leu^{31},Pro^{34}]PYY/Y1-like (Y1), [^{125}I]PYY3–36/Y2-like (Y2) binding sites and Y1 receptor mRNA (Y1 R mRNA) in normal human brain, post-mortem

Brain regions	Relative intensity of the signal detected		
	Y1	Y2	Y1 R mRNA
Frontal cortex			
Layer I–II	+	++++	+++
Layer III	+	++	++
Layer IV	+	+++	+++
Layer V–VI	+	++	++
Temporal cortex			
Layer I–II	+	+++	+++
Layer III	+	++	++
Layer IV	−	++	+++
Layer V–VI	+	++	++
Entorhinal cortex			
Layer I–II	+	++	ND
Layer III	+	++	ND
Layer IV	+	++	ND
Layer V–VI	+	+	ND
Hippocampus			
Stratum oriens	±	+	++
Stratum pyramidale			
CA1	±	+++	+
CA2	+	+++	+
CA3	±	+++	+
CA4	+	++++	+
Stratum radiatum	±	+++	ND
Stratum lacunosum	±	++	ND
Stratum moleculare	±	++	ND
Dentate gyrus			
Stratum moleculare	+++	±	++++
Stratum granulosum	++	±	++++
Polymorphic layer	++	±	++
Basal ganglia			
Septal nuclei	±	++	ND
Putamen	+	++	++
Bed nucleus of the stria terminalis	++	+	ND
Globus pallidus	+	+	—
Claustrum	+	+	+++

Table 2 (*cont.*)

Brain regions	Relative intensity of the signal detected		
	Y1	Y2	Y1 R mRNA
Paraolfactory gyrus	±	+	ND
Olfactory tubercle	±	+ +	—
Basal nucleus of Meynert	±	+ +	+ +
Hypothalamic nuclei			
Preoptic area	±	+ +	ND
Paraventricular	±	+	+ +
Periventricular	±	+	+ +
Arcuate	±	+	+ +
Dorsomedial	±	+	±
Ventromedial	±	+	+ +
Mammillary body	±	+	±
Posterior	±	+	ND
Thalamic nuclei			
Ventral lateral	±	±	±
Anterior	±	+	±
Dorsomedial	±	+	±
Midline	±	+	±
Lateral posterior	—	±	ND
Ventral posterolateral	±	±	ND
Centromedial	+	+	ND
Subthalamic	+	+	ND
Nucleus of medial geniculate body	+	+	+ + +
Amygdaloid nuclei	±	+ +	+ +
Substantia nigra	±	+ +	ND
Brainstem			
Red nucleus	+	+ +	—
Pontine nuclei	±	+	—
Nucleus of inferior colliculus	+ +	+ +	—
Superior colliculus	±	+ +	—
Dorsal raphe nucleus	±	+ +	—
Inferior olivary nucleus	—	+	—
Nucleus tractus solitarius	—	+ +	—
Interpeduncular nucleus	±	+ +	—
Decussation of superior cerebellar peduncle	—	±	—

Table 2 (*cont.*)

Brain regions	Relative intensity of the signal detected		
	Y1	Y2	Y1 R mRNA
Oculomotor nerve (III)	±	+	—
Reticular formation	—	+ +	—
Cerebellum			
Molecular layer	—	—	—
Granular layer	±	—	—
Medullary layer	±	±	—
Purkinje cell layer	±	ND	—

Values represent the mean from six brains using a concentration of 25–35 pM of either [^{125}I][Leu^{31},Pro^{34}]PYY or [^{125}I]PYY3–36. Non-specific labeling in the presence of 1 μM hNPY was digitally subtracted from all readings. For *in situ* hybridization, data are means obtained from four brains. ^{35}S-antisense NPY Y1 receptor mRNA was subtracted from value obtained with ^{35}S-sense NPY Y1 receptor mRNA. All results were expressed as follows: + + + +, very high levels; + + +, high amounts; + +, moderate concentrations; +, low signal; ±, very low density (at the limit of the detection); —, not detected; ND, not determined.

reciprocal regulatory mechanisms between dopaminergic and NPYergic neurons in the striatum. Intrastriatal or ICV injections of NPY-like peptides induced a dose-dependent increase in striatal dopamine turnover (Beal *et al.*, 1986a; Heilig *et al.*, 1990) by activating dopamine release (Goff *et al.*, 1992). It has also been shown that intra-striatal injections of low concentrations of NPY increased glutamate uptake while higher amounts decreased both glutamate and GABA uptake (Goff *et al.*, 1992). Additionally, biochemical and immunohistochemical data support the existence of a dual, direct interaction between dopaminergic and NPY systems in the striatum (Engber *et al.*, 1992; Goff *et al.*, 1992; Maeda *et al.*, 1993). However, the respective, distinctive contribution of each of the various NPY receptor-types present in the striatum will require further investigation using highly selective receptor antagonists such as BIBP3226 (Rudolf *et al.*, 1994) and SR120819A (Serradail-Le Gal *et al.*, 1995).

4.3.1.2 Cortical areas

The respective role(s) of the Y1, Y2 and [^{125}I][Leu^{31},Pro^{34}]PYY/BIBP3226-insensitive receptor-types in cortical areas are mostly unknown at this time. However, ICV injections of a Y1 receptor antisense was reported to decrease cortical Y1 binding by 60–70% without affecting the apparent density of the Y2 sites (Wahlestedt *et al.*, 1993). Interestingly, Y1 receptor antisense-treated rats showed a marked anxiogenic-like behaviour, without alterations in locomotor activity and food intake (Wehlestedt *et al.*, 1993). These results and others (Heilig, 1993; Heilig *et al.*, 1993) suggest that NPY, acting on Y1 receptors may have a role in anxiety-related behaviors (for reviews, see

Heilig, 1993; Wahlestedt and Reis, 1993). More recently, it has been confirmed that the administration of a Y1 receptor antisense, in addition of inducing an anxiogenic-like effect also attenuates the anxiolytic-like action of NPY in the amygdala (Heilig, 1995). However, the fact that the human brain is mostly devoid of Y1 receptors suggest that great care must be taken when extrapolating from data obtained in the rat (see below).

4.3.1.3 Hippocampal formation

In addition to the presence of high concentrations of NPY receptors in the rat hippocampus (mostly of the Y2 type), NPY-like immunoreactivity is also abundant in many hippocampal cell layers (except the pyramidal neurons) (Chronwall et al., 1985; O'Donohue et al., 1985; DeQuidt and Emson, 1986a,b). It has been shown that neurons containing NPY-like immunoreactivity in the hilus of the dentate gyrus and the CA1 and CA3 subfields of the stratum radiatum, frequently receive inputs from the septal area (Miettinen and Freund, 1992; Milner and Veznedaroglu, 1993), while CA1 NPY-like immunoreactive neurons are also targeted by afferents originating from the medium raphe nucleus (Meittiven and Freund, 1992). These anatomical data suggest that hippocampal NPY-like immunoreactive neurons are likely modulated by septal cholinergic/GABAergic and/or raphe serotonergic afferents. Regarding NPY itself, most electrophysiological data suggest that it inhibits glutamatergic excitatory synaptic transmission in the stratum radiatum of the hippocampus likely by acting on presynaptic Y2 receptors (for extensive reviews, see Bleakman et al., 1993; Colmers, 1990; Colmers and Bleakman, 1994). Behaviorally, the hippocampal Y2 receptor-type has been implicated in facilitating learning and memory processes with increases in memory retention induced by NPY (Flood et al., 1987). In further support of a physiological role for NPY in cognitive behaviours, it has been reported that a passive immunization by NPY antibodies injected into the hippocampus produced amnesia (Flood et al.., 1989).

Within the CA3 pyramidal cell layer, Monnet and co-workers (1992a,b) have reported that NPY can potentiate the electrophysiological response of these neurons to the well-known glutamate agonist, N-methyl-D-aspartate (NMDA). Interestingly, the potentiating effect of NPY is blocked by haloperidol, acting here as a sigma receptor antagonist (Monnet et al., 1992b). The pharmacological profile of this NPY-related effect does not correspond with any of the purported Y1, Y2 and Y3 receptor-types as PYY effectively antagonized the effects of NPY (Monnet et al., 1992a). We also reported that NPY can inhibit 25–30% of in vivo [^{3}H]SKF 10047/sigma labeling in the mouse hippocampus (Bouchard et al., 1993). While the precise mechanism(s) underlying these effects still remains largely unknown, it apparently does not involve a direct interaction between NPY and sigma receptors (Quirion et al., 1991; Tam and Mitchell, 1991).

The Y1 receptor-type may also be functionally important in the hippocampus as this site was found to be located in the dentate gyrus (and to a lesser extent in the ventral part of the hippocampus). Primary rat hippocampal cell cultures may be helpful in shedding light on this issue as they are highly enriched with this receptor class (St-Pierre *et al.*, 1994). The Y1 receptor-type may also be functioning as an autoreceptor modulating NPY release in the hippocampus. In support of this hypothesis, we observed specific [^{125}I][Leu^{31},Pro^{34}]PYY binding sites located on NPY-like immunoreactive neurons (St-Pierre *et al.*, 1995). Interestingly, these binding sites are fully sensitive to BIBP3226 confirming their Y1-like nature (St-Pierre *et al.*, unpublished results).

Very recently, it was shown that in freshly dissociated dentate granule cells, NPY, [Leu^{31},Pro^{34}]NPY and PYY reduced intracellular Ca^{2+} during depolarization (McQuiston *et al.*, 1996). It thus confirms that hippocampal Y1 receptors can regulate neuronal activity at least in the dentate gyrus. Moreover, since NPY13–36 was also effective in reducing intracellular Ca^{2+}, it suggests that the Y2 receptor type is also present in this preparation (McQuiston *et al.*, 1996). However, the number of cells that responded to [Leu^{31},Pro^{34}]NPY was more important than those affected by NPY13–36.

4.3.1.4 Thalamus and hypothalamus

Various thalamic nuclei expressed large amounts of specific Y1-like/[^{125}I] [Leu^{31},Pro^{34}]PYY binding sites, while only a few contain significant levels of [^{125}I]PYY3–36 labeling in the rat brain. The abundance of NPY receptors, especially of the Y1-type, contrasts with the rather low concentrations of NPY-like immunoreactivity found in most thalamic nuclei (Chronwall *et al.*, 1985; O'Donohue *et al.*, 1985; DeQuidt and Emson, 1986a,b). Little is currently known about the role of NPY and its receptors in the thalamus. It has been speculated that the modulation of locomotor behaviours observed following ICV injections of NPY-related peptides (for reviews, see Dumont *et al.*, 1992; Heilig, 1993) may at least partly be related to the activation of Y1 and/or Y2 receptors located in the thalamus. Discrete, intrathalamic injections of both Y1- and Y2-related molecules and their antagonists would be necessary to verify this hypothesis.

Even though it contains the largest amounts of NPY-like immunoreactivity in the rat brain (Chronwall *et al.*, 1985; O'Donohue *et al.*, 1985; DeQuidt and Emson, 1986a,b), only small to very small amounts of either Y1-like/[^{125}I][Leu^{31},Pro^{34}]PYY or Y2-like/[^{125}I]PYY3–36 binding sites are found in the rat hypothalamus. The Y2 binding sites are predominant over the Y1 sites in all hypothalamic nuclei, except in the suprachiasmatic nucleus. Despite the relative paucity of Y1 and Y2 receptor sites, the best characterized CNS effect of NPY-like peptides are related to actions at the level of the hypothalamus (for reviews, see Dumont *et al.*, 1992; Grundemar *et al.*, 1993; Kalra and Crowley, 1992; Leibowitz and Alexander, 1991; McAuley *et al.*, 1993; McDonald and Koenig, 1993; Stanley, 1993). For example, NPY is a potent stimulant of food intake, an effect apparently mediated by an atypical hypothalamic Y1 receptor subtype (Quirion *et al.*, 1990; Jolicoeur *et al.*, 1991a,b; Stanley *et al.*, 1992) now known as the Y5 receptor type (Gerald *et al.*, 1996). It is this action of NPY that stimulated most of the current interest on that peptide family, a suitable antagonist likely acting as a potent modulator of appetite (but see Erickson *et al.*, 1996). Additionally, Y1 receptors located in the hypothalamus are also likely to be involved in mediating the potent hypothermic effect (Jolicoeur *et al.*, 1991b) of NPY as well as the release of LHRH (Kalra and Crowley, 1992). Hypothalamic Y2 receptors are thought to be implicated in the release of corticotropin releasing factor, prolactin, thyrotropin and growth hormone (Härfstrand *et al.*, 1986, 1987). Hence, receptor functions are not necessarily associated with significant effects, since low levels of receptors are linked with similar potent actions of NPY and related peptides in the hypothalamus.

4.3.1.5 Brainstem

Among the highest densities of Y1-like/$[^{125}I]$$[Leu^{31},Pro^{34}]$PYY, Y2-like/$[^{125}I]$PYY3–36, $[^{125}I]$$[Leu^{31},Pro^{34}]$PYY/BIBP3226-insensitive (see Plates 1, 2 and 4) and $[^{125}I]$bPP (Whitcomb *et al.*, 1990) binding sites are expressed at the level of the nucleus tractus solitarius (NTS) and the area postrema in the rat brain. These receptors are likely to be involved in the CNS-mediated effects of NPY on various cardiovascular and respiratory parameters (for reviews, see Dumont *et al.*, 1992; McAuley *et al.*, 1993). For example, direct injections of NPY into the NTS produce vasodepressor effects, and supresses the baroreceptor reflex (Grundemar *et al.*, 1991; Shih *et al.*, 1992). The physiological role of NPY as a tonic inhibitor of baroreceptor reflexes was further supported by results obtained with NPY antibodies injected directly into the NTS (Shih *et al.*, 1992). The effects of NPY on this brainstem nucleus may be mediated by the Y2 receptor on the basis of the relative potency of NPY13–36 (Barraco *et al.*, 1990; Narvaez *et al.*, 1993). Furthermore, since PYY was apparently devoid of activity in modulating cardiorespiratory glutamate responses, Grundemar *et al.* (1991) proposed the existence of a unique receptor-type (Y3) with high affinity for NPY- but not PYY-derived molecules. Interestingly, Nakajima and co-workers (1986) reported that a significant proportion of $[^{125}I]$BH-NPY binding sites were insensitive to PYY in the NTS. Future studies will be required to delineate precisely the respective role of the Y1, Y2, and possibly Y3, Y4 and $[^{125}I]$$[Leu^{31},Pro^{34}]$ PYY/BIBP3226-insensitive receptors in various brainstem nuclei in the rat brain.

4.3.1.6 Glia

It is also worth mentioning that a few studies have suggested the existence of specific NPY receptors on cortical glial cells (Gimpl *et al.*, 1993; Hosli *et al.*, 1992; Hosli and Hosli, 1993). However, the receptor type involved remains to be established. Interestingly, NPY has been shown to modulate the intracellular concentrations of Ca^{2+} in astrocytes either inducing hyperpolarization or depolarization (Hosli *et al.*, 1992; Hosli and Hosli, 1993; Gimpl *et al.*, 1993). Hence, NPY and related peptides are likely to behave as potential modulators of glial cells in the rat brain.

4.3.2 Human brain

The distribution of NPY-like immunoreactivity in the human brain is rather similar to that observed in the rat. Substantial amounts of NPY-like immunoreactivity have been detected in various hypothalamic nuclei, caudate putamen, septal nuclei, hippocampus, amygdala and most cortical areas (Adrian et al., 1983; Pelletier E, 1984; Chan-Palay et al., 1985a,b). In humans, cortical, NPY-like immunoreactive neurons are small, aspiny bipolar or multipolar neurons, which are particularly abundant in deep cortical layers and subcortical white matter area (Chan-Palay et al., 1985a). Axonal plexuses are found throughout the cortex but are particularly abundant in the superficial layers (Chan-Palay et al., 1985a). The human hippocampus also expresses significant amounts of NPY-like immunoreactive neurons and fibers (Chan-Palay et al., 1986a) with densities of NPYergic neurons generally being greater in the human versus the rat hippocampi. The CA1 subfield demonstrated the highest amount of NPY-like immunoreactive neurons and fibers displaying a distinct laminar axonal organization. NPY-like immunoreactive fibers were also found in high densities within the strata moleculare and pyramidal cell layers, while small bipolar neurons are detected in the stratum oriens. In addition, the subiculum and entorhinal areas also showed high densities of small bipolar neurons enriched with NPY-like immunoreactivity. Moreover, these two areas and the parasubiculum were also densely innervated by NPY-like immunoreactive fibers. In situ hybridization revealed that the localization of NPY mRNA correlated well with the distribution of NPY-like immunoreactivity suggesting that NPY-like material is synthesized, processed and stored within these neurons (Terenghi et al., 1987; Chan-Palay et al., 1988).

Experiments in rodents have suggested that NPY-related peptides may play critical roles in the regulation of fluid and electrolyte balance, food intake, energy metabolism, thermoregulation, neuroendocrine secretion, cardiorespiratory function, locomotion and anxiety-related behaviours (see Section 4.3.1 for more details). However, the extent to which these effects apply to man is still largely unknown. Some evidence suggest that NPY may play similar roles in man. For example, higher cerebrospinal fluid (CSF) levels of NPY were measured in anorexic patients following the normalization of their body weight (Wahlestedt et al., 1993). However, the paucity of Y1-like receptor in the human brain suggests that data obtained in the rat brain with regard to the role of a given receptor type may not be fully applicable to the human situation. Accordingly, detailed study will have to be performed in humans to establish the NPY receptor type modulating appetite behaviours in man.

The hippocampal formation is associated with learning and memory processes in rodents and primates including man, and is one area severely affected in Alzheimer's disease (Terry and Davies, 1980). Moreover, several studies have reported significant decreases in NPY-like immunoreactivity in cortical, amygdaloid and hippocampal areas in Alzheimer's disease brains (Chan-Palay et al., 1985b, 1986b; Beal et al., 1986b). Similarly, [³H]NPY binding sites were reported to be reduced in temporal cortices and hippocampus of patients suffering from Alzheimer's disease (Martel et al., 1990c). Additionally, NPY-like immunoreactivity has been detected within neuritic plaques in the brains of patients with Alzheimer's disease (Chan-Palay et al., 1986b). This suggests that the degenerative processes occurring in this disease may also involve changes in NPY-related neurons. We are currently investigating the possible alterations of the Y1 and Y2 receptor types in Alzheimer's disease.

Temporal lobe epilepsy is another neurological disorder in which the hippocampal formation has been shown to be severely affected. In approximately two-thirds of cases, the hippocampus is often the only structure that shows pathological modifications (Amaral and Insausti, 1990). Considering that NPY-containing neurons degenerate in the hippocampus of patients with temporal lobe epilepsy (de Lanerolle *et al.*, 1989) and the NPY regulates neuronal excitability at least in the rat hippocampus (for extensive reviews, see Bleakman *et al.*, 1993; Colmers, 1990; Colmers and Bleakman, 1994), it may suggest that NPY may be involved in certain forms of epileptic seizures. Further studies in that regard are certainly warranted (see e.g., Sperk, 1994; Schwarzer *et al.*, 1995).

The levels of peptides and neurotransmitters in the CSF of patients suffering from neurological disorders may provide some indication of those likely affected/involved in a given disease. Interestingly, it has been shown that the concentration of NPY in the CSF of patients with major depression was reduced as compared to non-depressed patients (Widerlöv *et al.*, 1986, 1988). Similarly, cortical areas of tissues obtained from suicide victims having a medical history of depression revealed lower levels of NPY as compared to suicide victims with no reported depressive episodes (Widdowson *et al.*, 1992). Additionally, higher CSF NPY concentrations were found in depressed patients showing low symptoms of both psychological and somatic anxieties, while those who were anxious had lower levels of NPY in the CSF (Widerlöv *et al.*, 1989). These results and the reported changes in brain NPY contents following olfactory bulbectomy, electroconvulsive shocks and antidepressant drugs in rats (Heilig, 1993; Wahlestedt and Reis, 1993; see also Section 4.3.1), all argue in favor for a role of NPY in anxiety-related behaviors. While a Y1 receptor-type apparently mediates these effects in the rat (Heilig, 1993, 1995; Heilig *et al.*, 1993; Wahlestedt and Reis, 1993; Wahlestedt *et al.*, 1993), the paucity of this class of NPY receptor in the human brain does not permit extrapolation at this time.

4.4 Conclusion

In brief, it is clear from the data presented in this chapter that major species differences exist in the relative enrichment and distribution of a given NPY receptor-type. For example, while the mouse and rat brain cortices are enriched in Y1 receptor binding sites these same areas are mostly devoid of this class of sites in the monkey and human brain. The guinea-pig brain is particular enriched with the Y1 type. Hence, at least in regard to the two best studied classes of NPY receptors, the Y1 and Y2 types, great care must be taken when extrapolating to the human situation on the basis of results obtained in other species. It remains to be established whether similar consensus apply to Y3 and the newly characterized PP1/Y4, Y5 and Y6 receptor types, only very limited information currently being available on their expression in the mammalian brain. In any case it would appear that the use of human brain tissues is critical to establish clearly the relevance of data obtained in other species. Moreover, it is also clear that what has been designated as Y1- and Y2-mediated effects over the past few years, will have to be reevaluated in light of the recently cloned PP1/Y4, Y5 and Y6 receptors.

Acknowledgements

This study was supported by the Medical Research Council of Canada and Karl Thomae GmbH. Rémi Quirion is 'Chercheur-Boursier' of the 'Fonds de la Recherche en Santé du Québec'. Danielle Jacques holds a fellowship from the 'Fonds de la Recherche en Santé du Québec'. The authors would like to thank Drs Alain Fournier and Serge St-Pierre (INRS-Santé, Pointe-Claire, Québec, Canada) for NPY peptides. Mr Wayne Rowe for the critical review of this chapter and Mme Danielle Cecyre, Coordinator of the Douglas Hospital Research Center Brain Bank, for supplying us with human brain tissues.

References

Adrian, T.E., Allen, J.M., Bloom, S.R., Ghatei, M.A., Rossor, M.N., Roberts, G.W., Crow, T.J., Tatemoto, K. & Polak, J.M. (1983) Neuropeptide Y distribution in the human brain. *Nature* **306**, 584–586.
Aicher, S.A., Springston, M., Berger, S.B., Reis, D.J. & Wahlestedt, C. (1991) Receptor-selective analogs demonstrate NPY/PYY receptor heterogeneity in rat brain. *Neurosci. Lett.* **130**, 32–36.
Akabayashi, A., Wahlestedt, C., Alexander, J.T. & Leibowitz, S.F. (1994) Specific inhibition of endogenous neuropeptide Y synthesis in arcuate nucleus by antisense oligonucleotides suppresses feeding behaviour and insulin secretion. *Molec. Brain Res.* **21**, 55–61.
Albers, H.E., Ferris, C.F., Leeman, S.E. & Goldman, B.D. (1984) Avian pancreatic polypeptide phase shifts hamster circadian rhythms when microinjected into the suprachiasmatic region. *Science* **223**, 833–835.
Amaral, D.G. & Insausti, T. (1990) Hippocampal formation. In *The Human Nervous System* (ed. Paxinos, G.), pp. 711–755. London, Academic Press.
Aoki, C. & Pickel, V.M. (1990) Neuropeptide Y in cortex and striatum. *Ann. N. York Acad. Sci.* **611**, 186–205.
Bard, J.A., Walker, M.W., Branchek, T.A. & Weinshank, R.L. (1995) Cloning and functional expression of a human Y4 subtype receptor for pancreatic polypeptide, neuropeptide Y and peptide YY. *J. Biol. Chem.* **270**, 26762–26765.
Barraco, R.A., Ergene, E., Dunbar, J.C. & El-Ridi, M.R. (1990) Cardiorespiratory response patterns elicited by microinjections of neuropeptide Y in the nucleus tractus solitarius. *Brain Res. Bull.* **24**, 465–485.
Beal, M.F., Frank, R.C., Ellison, D.W. & Martin, J.B. (1986a) The effect of neuropeptide Y on striatal catecholamines. *Neurosci. Lett.* **71**, 118–123.
Beal, M.F., Mazurek, M.F., Chattha, G.K., Svendsen, C.N., Bird, E.D. & Martin, J.B. (1986b) Neuropeptide Y immunoreactivity is reduced in cerebral cortex in Alzheimer's disease. *Ann. Neurol.* **20**, 282–288.

Bleakman, D., Miller, R.J. & Colmers, W.F. (1993) Actions of neuropeptide Y on the electrophysiological properties of nerve cells. In *The Biology of Neuropeptide Y and Related Peptides* (eds Colmers, W.F. & Wahlestedt, C.), pp. 241–272. Totowa, NJ, Humana Press Inc.

Bouchard, P., Dumont, Y., Fournier, A., St-Pierre, S. & Quirion, R. (1993) Evidence for *in vivo* interactions between neuropeptide Y-related peptides and σ receptors in the mouse hippocampal formation. *J. Neurosci.* **13**, 3926–3931.

Calzá, L., Giardino, L., Zanni, M., Velardo, A., Parchi, P. & Marrama, P. (1990) Daily changes of neuropeptide Y-like immunoreactivity in the suprachiasmatic nucleus of the rat. *Regul. Pept.* **27**, 127–137.

Chang, R.S.L., Lotti, V.J., Chen, T.B., Cerino, D.J. & Kling, P.J. (1985) Neuropeptide Y (NPY) binding sites in rat brain labeled with ^{125}I-Bolton–Hunter NPY: Comparative potencies of various polypeptides on brain NPY binding and biological responses in the rat vas deferens. *Life Sci.* **37**, 2111–2122.

Chang, R.S.L., Lotti, V.J. & Chen, T.-B. (1988) Specific [3H] propionyl-neuropeptide Y (NPY) binding in rabbit aortic membranes: comparisons with binding in rat brain and biological response in rat vas deferens. *Biochem. Biophys. Res. Comm.* **151**, 1213–1219.

Chan-Palay, V., Lang, W., Allen, Y.S., Haesler, U. & Polak, J.M. (1985a) I Cytology and distribution in normal human cerebral cortex of neurons immunoreactive with antisera against neuropeptide Y. *J. Comp. Neurol.* **238**, 382–389.

Chan-Palay, V., Lang, W., Allen, Y.S., Haesler, U. & Polak, J.M. (1985b) II Cortical neurons immunoreactive with antisera against neuropeptide Y are altered in Alzheimer's-type dementia. *J. Comp. Neurol.* **238**, 390–400.

Chan-Palay, V., Kohler, C., Haesler, U., Lang, W. & Yasargil, G. (1986a) Distribution of neurons and axons immunoreactive with antisera against neuropeptide Y in the normal human hippocampus. *J. Comp. Neurol.* **248**, 360–375.

Chan-Palay, V., Lang, W., Haesler, U., Kohler, C. & Yasargil, G. (1986b) Distribution of altered hippocampal neurons and axons immunoreactive with antisera against neuropeptide Y in Alzheimer's-type dementia. *J. Comp. Neurol.* **248**, 376–394.

Chan-Palay, V., Vasargil, G., Hamid, Q., Polak, J.M. & Palay, S.L. (1988) Simultaneous demonstration of neuropeptide Y gene expression and peptide storage in single neurons of the human brain. *Proc. Natl Acad. Sci. USA* **85**, 3213–3215.

Chronwall, B.M., DiMaggio, D.A., Massari, V.J., Pickel, V.M., Ruggiero, D.A. & O'Donohue, T.L. (1985) The anatomy of neuropeptide Y containing neurons in rat brain. *Neuroscience* **15**, 1159–1181.

Clark, J.T., Kalra, P.S. & Kalra, S.P. (1985) Neuropeptide Y stimulates feeding but inhbits sexual behaviour in male rats. *Endocrinology* **117**, 2435–2442.

Colmers, W.F. (1990) Modulation of synaptic transmission in hippocampus by neuropeptide Y: presynaptic actions. *Ann. N. York Acad. Sci.* **611**, 206–218.

Colmers, W.F. & Bleakman, D. (1994) Effects of neuropeptide Y on the electrical properties of neurons. *Trends Neurosci.* **17**, 373–379.

De Lanerolle, N.C., Kim, J.H., Robbins, R.J. & Spencer, D.D. (1989) Hippocampal interneurons loss and plasticity in human temporal lobe epilepsy. *Brain Res.* **495**, 387–395.

DeQuidt, M.E. & Emson, P.C. (1986a) Distribution of neuropeptide Y-like immunoreactivity in the rat central nervous system I. radioimmunoassay and chromatographic characterization. *Neuroscience* **18**, 527–543.

DeQuidt, M.E. & Emson, P.C. (1986b) Distribution of neuropeptide Y-like immunoreactivity in the rat central nervous system II. immunohistochemical analysis. *Neuroscience* **18**, 545–618.

Dumont, Y., Fournier, A., St-Pierre, S., Schwartz, T.W. & Quirion, R. (1990) Differential distribution of neuropeptide Y1 and Y2 receptors in the rat brain. *Eur. J. Pharmacol.* **191**, 501–503.

Dumont, Y., Martel, J.C., Fournier, A., St-Pierre, S. & Quirion, R. (1992) Neuropeptide Y and neuropeptide Y receptor subtypes in brain and peripheral tissues. *Prog. Neurobiol.* **38**, 125–167.

Dumont, Y., Fournier, A., St-Pierre, S. & Quirion, R. (1993) Comparative characterization and autoradiographic distribution of neuropeptide Y receptor subtypes in rat brain. *J. Neurosci.* **13**, 73–86.

Dumont, Y., Cadieux, A., Pheng, L.H., Fournier, A., St-Pierre, S. & Quirion, R. (1994) Peptide YY derivatives as selective neuropeptide Y/peptide YY Y1 and Y2 agonists devoid of activity for the Y3 receptor subtype. *Molec, Brain Res.* **26**, 320–324.

Dumont, Y., Fournier, A., St-Pierre, S. & Quirion, R. (1995) Characterization of neuropeptide Y binding sites in rat brain membrane preparations using [^{125}I][Leu^{31},Pro^{34}]PYY and [^{125}I]PYY3–36 as selective Y1 and Y2 radioligands. *J. Pharmacol. Exp. Ther.* **272**, 673–680.

Dumont, Y. & Quirion, R. (1995) Possible Y1 receptor heterogeneity as revealed by using the newly developed non-peptide neuropeptide Y Y1 antagonist, BIBP3226. *The Physiologist* **38**, A253.

Dumont, Y., Fournier, A., St-Pierre, S. & Quirion, R. (1996a) Auroradiographic distribution of [^{125}I][Leu^{31},Pro^{34}]PYY and [^{125}I]PYY3–36 binding sites in the rat brain evaluated with two newly developed Y1 and Y2 receptor radioligands. *Synapse* **22**, 139–158.

Dumont, Y., St-Pierre, J.A. & Quirion, R. (1996b) Comparative autoradiographic distribution of neuropeptide Y Y1 receptors visualized with the Y1 receptor agonist [^{125}I][Leu^{31},Pro^{34}]PYY and the non-peptide antagonist [^{3}H]BIBP3226. *NeuroReport* **7**, 901–904.

Engber, T.M., Boldry, R.C., Kuo, S. & Chase, T.N. (1992) Dopaminergic modulation of striatal neuropeptides: differential effects of D1 and D2 receptor stimulation on somatostatin, neuropeptide Y, neurotensin, dynorphin and enkephalin. *Brain Res.* **581**, 261–268.

Entzeroth, M., Braunger, H., Eberlein, W., Engel, W., Rudolf, K., Wienen, W., Wieland, H.A., Willim, K.D. & Doods, H.N. (1995) Labeling of neuropeptide Y receptors in SK-N-MC cells using the novel nonpeptide Y1 receptor-selective antagonist [^{3}H]BIBP3226. *Eur. J. Pharmacol.* **278**, 239–242.

Erickson, J.C., Clegg, K.E. & Palmiter, R.D. (1996) Sensitivity to leptin and susceptibility to seizures of mice lacking neuropeptide Y. *Nature* **381**, 415–418.

Esteban, J., Chover, A.J., Sánchez, P.A., Micó, J.A. & Gibert-Rahola, J. (1989) Central administration of neuropeptide Y induces hypothermia in mice. Possible interaction with central noradrenergic systems. *Life Sci.* **45**, 2395–2400.

Eva, C., Keinanen, K., Monyer, H., Seeburg, P. & Sprengel, R. (1990) Molecular cloning of a novel G protein-coupled receptor that may belong to the neuropeptide receptor family. *FEBS Lett.* **271**, 81–84.

Flood, J.F., Hernandez, E.N. & Morley, J.E. (1987) Modulation of memory processing by neuropeptide Y. *Brain Res.* **421**, 280–290.

Flood, J.F., Baker, M.L., Hernandez, E.N. & Morley, J.E. (1989) Modulation of memory processing by neuropeptide Y varies with brain injection site. *Brain Res.* **503**, 73–82.

Frazer, A., Maayani, S. & Wolfe, B.B. (1990) Subtype of receptors for serotonin. *Ann. Rev. Pharmacol. Toxicol.* **30**, 307–348.

Fuhlendorff, J., Gether, U., Aakerlund, L., Langeland-Johansen, N., Thogersen, H., Melberg, S.G., Olsen, U.B., Thastrup, O. & Schwartz, T.W. (1990) [Leu^{31},Pro^{34}]Neuropeptide Y: a specific Y1 receptor agonist. *Proc. Natl Acad. Sci. USA* **87**, 182–186.

Gackenheimer, SlL., Lundell, I., Schimdt, R., Beavers, L., Gadski, R.A., Berglund, M., Schober, D.A., Mayne, N.L., Burnett, J.P., Larhammar, D. & Gehlert, D.R. (1995) Binding of [^{125}I][Leu^{31},Pro^{34}]PYY (LP-PYY) to receptors for neuropeptide Y (Y-1) and pancreatic polypeptide (PP1). *The Physiologist* **38**, A249.

Gehlert, D.R. (1994) Subtypes of receptors for NPY: Implications for the targeting of therapeutics. *Life Sci.*, **55**, 551–562.

Gehlert, D.R., Gackenheimer, S.L. & Schober, D.A. (1992) [Leu^{31},Pro^{34}] neuropeptide Y identifies a subtype of ^{125}I-labelled peptide YY binding sites in the rat brain. *Neurochem. Int.* **21**, 45–67.

Gerald, C., Walker, M.W., Vaysse, P.J.J., Branchek, T.A. & Weinshank, R.L. (1995) Expression, cloning and pharmacological characterization of a human hippocampal neuropeptide Y/peptide YY Y2 receptor subtype. *J. Biol. Chem.* **270**, 26758–26761.

Gerald, G., Walker, M.W., Criscione, L., *et al.* (1996) A receptor subtype involved in neuropeptide-Y-induced food intake. *Nature* **382**, 168–172.

Gimpl, G., Kirchhoff, F., Lang, R.E. & Kettenmann, H. (1993) Identification of neuropeptide Y receptors in cultured astrocytes from neonatal rat brain. *J. Neurosci. Res.* **34**, 198–205.

Goff, L.K., Forni, C., Samuel, D., Bloc, A., Dusticier, N. & Nieoullon, A. (1992) Intracerebroventricular administration of neuropeptide Y affects parameters of dopamine, glutamate, GABA activities in the rat striatum. *Brain Res. Bull.* **28**, 187–193.

Grundemar, L., Wahlestedt, C. & Reis, D.J. (1991) Neuropeptide Y acts at an atypical receptor to evoke cardiovascular depression and to inhibit glutamate responsiveness in the brainstem. *J. Pharmacol. Exp. Ther.* **258**, 633–638.

Grundemar, L., Sheikh, S.P. & Wahlestedt, C. (1993) Characterization of receptor types for neuropeptide Y and related peptides. In *The Biology of Neuropeptide Y and Related Peptides* (eds Colmers, W.F. & Wahlestedt, C.), pp. 197–240. Totowa, NJ, Humana Press Inc.

Härfstrand, A., Fuxe, K., Agnati, L.F., Eneroth, P., Zini, I., Zoli, M., Andersson, K., von Euler, G., Terenius, L., Mutt, V. & Goldstein, M. (1986) Studies on neuropeptide Y-catecholamine interactions in the hypothalamus and in the forebrain of the male rat. Relationship to neuroendocrine function. *Neurochem. Int.* **8**, 355–376.

Härfstrand, A., Eneroth, P., Agnati, L. & Fuxe, K. (1987) Further studies on the effects of central administration of neuropeptide Y on neuroendocrine function in the male rat: relationship to hypothalamic catecholamines. *Regul. Pept.* **17**, 167–179.

Heilig, M. (1993) Neuropeptide Y in relation to behaviour and psychiatric disorders: some animal and clinical observations. In *The Biology of Neuropeptide Y and Related Peptides* (eds Colmers, W.F. & Wahlestedt, C.), pp. 511–555. Totowa, NJ, Humana Press Inc.

Heilig, M. (1995) Antisense inhibition of neuropeptide Y (NPY)-Y1 receptor expression blocks the anxiolytic-like action of NPY in amygdala and paradoxically increases feeding. *Regul. Pept.* **59**, 201–205.

Heilig, M. & Murison, R. (1987) Intracerebroventricular neuropeptide Y (NPY) suppresses home cage and open field activity in the rat. *Regul. Pept.* **19**, 221–231.

Heilig, M., Vecsei, L., Wahlestedt, C., Alling, C.H. & Widerlöv, E. (1990) Effects of centrally administered neuropeptide Y (NPY) and NPY13–36 on the brain monoaminergic system of the rat. *J. Neural Transm.* **79**, 193–208.

Heilig, M., McLeod, S., Brot, M., Koob, G.F. & Briton, K.T. (1993) Anxiolytic-like action of neuropeptide Y: mediation by Y1 receptors in amygdala and dissociation from food intake effects. *Psychopharmacology* **8**, 357–363.

Hendry, S.H.C. (1993) Organization of neuropeptide Y neurons in the mammalian central nervous system. In *The Biology of Neuropeptide Y and Related Peptides* (eds Colmers, W.F. & Wahlestedt, C.), pp. 65–156. Totowa, NJ, Humana Press Inc.

Herzog, H., Hort, Y.J., Ball, H.J., Hayes, G., Shine, J. & Selbie, L.A. (1992) Cloned human neuropeptide Y receptor couples to two different second messenger systems. *Proc. Natl Acad. Sci. USA* **89**, 5794–5798.

Hosli, E. & Hosli, L. (1993) Autoradiographic localization of binding sites for neuropeptide Y and bradykinin on astrocytes. *NeuroReport* **4**, 159–162.

Hosli, L., Hosli, E., Kaeser, H. & Lefkovits, M. (1992) Colocalization of receptors for vasoactive peptides on astrocytes of cultured rat spinal cord and brain stem: electrophysiological effects of atrial and brain natriuretic peptide, neuropeptide Y and bradykinin. *Neurosci. Lett.* **148**, 114–116.

Humphreys, G.A., Davison, J.S. & Veale, W.L. (1988) Injection of neuropeptide Y into the paraventricular nucleus of the hypothalamus inhibits gastric acid secretion in the rat. *Brain Res.* **456**, 241–248.

Husley, M.G., Pless, C.M., White, B.D. & Martin, R.J. (1995) ICV administration of anti-NPY antisense oligonucleotide: Effects on feeding behavior, body weight, peptide content and peptide release. *Regul. Pept.* **59**, 207–214.

Inui, A., Oya, M., Okita, M., Inoue, T., Sakatani, N., Morioka, H., Shii, K., Yokono, K., Mizuno, N. & Baba, S. (1988) Peptide YY receptors in the brain. *Biochem. Biophys. Res. Commun.* **150**, 25–32.

Inui, A., Okita, M., Inoue, T., Sakatani, N., Oya, M., Morioka, H., Shii, K., Yokono, K., Mizuno, N. & Baba, S. (1989) Characterization of peptide YY receptors in the brain. *Endocrinology* **124**, 402–409.

Jacques, D., Dumont, Y., Rouissi, N., St-Pierre, S., Fournier, A. & Quirion, R. (1994) Characterization of neuropeptide Y receptor subtypes in the normal human brain. *Soc. Neurosci. Abst.* **20**, 85.

Jacques, D., Cadieux, A., Dumont, Y. & Quirion, R. (1995) Apparent affinity and potency of BIBP3226, a non-peptide neuropeptide Y receptor antagonist, on purported Y1, Y2 and Y3 receptors. *Eur. J. Pharmacol.* **278**, R3–R5.

Jacques, D., Tong, Y., Dumont, Y., Shen, S.H. & Quirion, R. (1996) Expression of the neuro-peptide Y Y1 mRNA in the human brain: an in situ hybridization study. *NeuroReport*, **7**(7), 1053–1056.

Jolicoeur, F.B., Michaud, J.N., Rivest, R., Menard, D., Gaudin, D., Fournier, A. & St-Pierre, S. (1991a) Neurobehavioural profile of neuropeptide Y. *Brain Res. Bull.* **26**, 265–268.

Jolicoeur, F.B., Michaud, J.N., Menard, D., Fournier, A. & St-Pierre, S. (1991b) In vivo struc-ture activity study supports the existence of heterogeneous neuropeptide Y receptors. *Brain Res. Bull.* **26**, 309–311.

Jørgensen, J.C., Fuhlendorff, J. & Schwartz, T.W. (1990) Structure function studies on neuro-peptide Y and pancreatic polypeptide evidence for two fold receptors in vas deferens. *Eur. J. Pharmacol.* **186**, 105–114.

Kalra, S.P. & Crowley, W.R. (1992) Neuropeptide Y: a noval neuroendocrine peptide in the control of pituitary hormone secretion with emphasis on luteinizing hormone. *Front. Neuroendocrinol,* **13**, 1–46.

Kalra, P.S., Bonavera, J.J. & Kalra, S.P. (1995) Central administration of antisense oligodeoxynucleotides to neuropeptide Y (NPY) mRNA reveals the critical role of newly syn-thesized NPY in regulation of LHRH release. *Regul. Pept.* **59**, 215–220.

Kuenzel, W.J. & McMurtry, J. (1988) Neuropeptide Y: Brain localization and central effects on plasma insulin in chicks. *Physiol. Behav.* **44**, 669–678.

Larhammar, D., Blomqvist, A.G., Yee, F., Jazin, E., Yoo, H. & Wahlestedt, C. (1992) Cloning and functional expression of a human neuropeptide Y/peptide YY receptor of Y1 type. *J. Biol. Chem.* **267**, 10 935–10 938.

Larsen, P.J., Sheikh, S.P., Jakobsen, C.R., Schwartz, T.W. & Mikkelsen, J.D. (1993) Regional dis-tribution of putative NPY Y1 receptors and neurons expressing Y1 mRNA in forebrain areas of the rat central nervous system. *Eur. J. Neurosci.* **5**, 1622–1637.

Leibowitz, S.F. & Alexander, J.T. (1991) Analysis of neuropeptide Y-induced feeding: dissocia-tion of Y1 and Y2 receptor effects on natural meal patterns. *Peptides* **12**, 1251–1260.

Leibowitz, S.F., Sladek, C., Spencer, L. & Tempel, D. (1988) Neuropeptide Y, epinephrine and norepinephrine in the paraventricular nucleus: stimulation of feeding and the release of cor-ticosterone, vasopressin and glucose. *Brain Res. Bull.* **21**, 905–912.

Lundell, I., Schober, D.A., Johnson, D., Statnick, M., Starback, P., Berglund, D.R., Gerlert, D.R. & Larhammar, D. (1995) Cloning of a rat receptor of the NPY receptor family with high affinity for pancreatic polypeptide. *The Physiologist*, **38**, A242.

Lynch, D.R., Walker, M.W., Miller, R.J. & Snyder, S.H. (1989) Neuropeptide Y receptor binding sites in rat brain: Differential localization with [^{125}I] peptide YY and [^{125}I] neuropep-tide Y imply receptor heterogenity. *J. Neurosci.* **9**, 2607–2619.

Maeda, K., Kawata, E., Sakai, K. & Chihara, K. (1993) Effects of putative cognitive function-enhancing drugs and dopaminergic agents on somatostatin and neuropeptide Y in rat brain. *Eur. J. Pharmacol.* **233**, 227–235.

Martel, J.C., St-Pierre, S. & Quirion, R. (1986) Neuropeptide Y receptors in rat brain: Autoradiographic localization. *Peptides* **7**, 55–60.

Martel, J.C., St-Pierre, S., Bédard, P.J. & Quirion, R. (1987) Comparison of [^{125}I]Bolton–Hunter neuropeptide Y binding sites in the forebrain of various mammalian species. *Brain Res.* **419**, 403–407.

Martel, J.C., Fournier, A., St-Pierre, S., Dumont, Y., Forest, M. & Quirion, R. (1990a) Comparative structural requirements of brain neuropeptide Y binding sites and vas deferens neuropeptide Y receptors. *Molec. Pharmacol.* **38**, 494–502.

Martel, J.C., Fournier, A., St-Pierre, S. & Quirion, R. (1990b) Quantitative autoradiographic distribution of [^{125}I]Bolton–Hunter neuropeptide Y receptor binding sites in rat brain. Comparison with [^{125}I]peptide YY receptor sites. *Neuroscience* **36**, 255–283.

Martel, J.C., Alagar, R., Robitaille, Y. & Quirion, R. (1990c) Neuropeptide Y receptor binding sites in human brain. Possible alteration in Alzheimer's disease. *Brain Res.* **456**, 228–235.

McAuley, M.A., Chen, X. & Westfall, T.C. (1993) Central cardiovascular actions of neuropeptide Y. In *The Biology of Neuropeptide Y and Related Peptides* (eds Colmers, W.F. & Wahlestedt, C.), p. 389–418. Totowa, NJ, Humana Press Inc.

McDonald, J.K. & Koenig, J.I. (1993) Neuropeptide Y actions on reproductive and endocrine functions. In *The Biology of Neuropeptide Y and Related Peptides* (eds Colmers, W.F. & Wahlestedt, C.) pp. 419–456. Totowa, NJ, Humana Press Inc.

McQuiston, A.R., Petrozzino, J.J., Connor, J.A. & Colmers, W.F. (1996) Neuropeptide Y1 receptors inhibit N-type calcium currents and reduce transient calcium increases in rat dentate granule cells. *J. Neurosci.* **16**, 1422–1429.

Menéndez, J.A., McGregor, I.S., Healey, P.A., Atrens, D.M. & Leibowitz, S.F. (1990) Metabolic effects of neuropeptide Y injections into the paraventricular nucleus of the hypothalamus. *Brain Res.* **516**, 8–14.

Miettinen, R. & Freund, T.F. (1992) Neuropeptide Y-containing interneurons in the hippocampus receive synaptic input from median raphe and gabaergic septal afferents. *Neuropeptides* **22**, 185–193.

Milner, T.A. & Veznedaroglu, E. (1993) Septal efferent axon terminals identified by anterograde degeneration show multiple sites of modulation of neuropeptide Y-containing neurons in the rat dentate gyrus. *Synapse,* **14**, 101–112.

Monnet, F.P., Fornier, A., Debonnel, G. & deMontigny, C. (1992a) Neuropeptide potentiates selectively the *N*-methyl-D-aspartate response in the rat CA3 dorsal hippocampus.1. Involvement of an atypical neuropeptide Y receptor. *J. Pharmacol. Exp. Ther.* **263**, 1212–1218.

Monnet, F.P., Debonnel, G., Fournier, A. & deMontigny, C. (1992b) Neuropeptide Y potentiates the *N*-methyl-D-aspartate response in the CA3 dorsal hippocampus. involvement of a subtype of sigma receptor. *J. Pharmacol. Exp. Ther.* **263**, 1219–1225.

Nakajima, T., Yashima, Y. & Nakamura, K. (1986) Quantitative autoradiographic localization of neuropeptide Y receptors in the rat lower brainstem. *Brain Res.* **380**, 144–150.

Narvaez, J.A., Aguire, J.A. & Fuxe, K. (1993) Subpicomolar amounts of NPY(13–36) injected into the nucleus tractus solitarius of rat counteract the cardiovascular response to l-glutamate. *Neurosci. Lett.* **151**, 182–186.

O'Donohue, T.L., Chronwall, B.M., Pruss, R.M., Mezey, E., Kiss, J.Z., Eiden, L.E., Massari, V.J., Tessel, R.E., Pickel, V.M., DiMaggio, D.A., Hotchkiss, A.J., Crowley, W.R. & Zukowska-Grojec, Z. (1985) Neuropeptide Y and peptide YY neuronal and endocrine systems. *Peptides* **6**, 755–768.

Ohkubo, T., Niwa, M., Yamashita, K., Kataoka, Y., Shigematsu, K. (1990) Neuropeptide Y (NPY) and peptide YY (PYY) receptors in rat brain. *Cell. Molec. Neurobiol.* **10**, 539–552.

Pelletier, G., Desy, L., Kerkerian, L. & Cote, J. (1984) Immunocytochemical localization of neuropeptide Y (NPY) in the human hypothalamus. *Cell Tissue Res.* **238**, 203–205.

Quirion, R. (1985) Multiple tachykinin receptors. *Trends NeuroSci.* **8**, 83–185.

Quirion, R. & Martel, J.C. (1992) Neuropeptide Y receptors in mammalian brains. In *Handbook of Chemical Neuroanatomy*, Vol. 11: *Neuropeptide Receptors in the CNS* (eds Bjorklund, A., Hökfelt, T.H. & Kuhar, M.J.), pp. 247–287. Amsterdam, Elsevier.

Quirion, R., Zajac, J.M., Morgat, J.L. & Roques, B.P. (1983) Autoradiographic distribution of mu and delta opiate receptors in rat brain using highly selective ligands. *Life Sci.* **33**, 227–230.

Quirion, R., Martel, J.C., Dumont, Y., Cadieux, A., Jolicoeur, F., St-Pierre, S. & Fournier, A. (1990) Neuropeptide Y receptors: autoradiographic distribution in the brain and structure–activity relationships. *Ann. N. York Acad. Sci.* **611**, 58–72.

Quirion, R., Mount, H., Chaudieu, I., Dumont, Y. & Boksa, P. (1991) Neuropeptide Y, polypeptide YY, phencyclidine and sigma related agents. Any relationships? In *NMDA and Related Agents: Biochemistry, Pharmacology and Behaviour* (eds Kameyama, T., Nabeshima, T. & Domino, E.F.), pp. 203–210. Ann Arbor, MI, NPP Press.

Rosier, A.M., Orban, G.A. & Vandesande, F. (1990) Regional distribution of binding sites for neuropeptide Y in cat and monkey visual cortex determined by in vitro receptor autoradiography. *J. Comp. Neurol.* **293**, 486–498.

Rouissi, N., Bouchard, P., Dumont, Y., Jacques, D. & Quirion, R. (1994) Comparative autoradiograhic distribution of the Y1 and Y2 receptor subtypes in the mammalian brain using selective radioligands: Differences between primates and other species. *Can. J. Physiol.* **72**, 412.

Rudolf, K., Eberlein, W., Engel, W., Wieland, H.A., Willim, K.D., Entzeroth, M., Wienen, W., Beck-Sickinger, A.G. & Doods, H.N. (1994) The first highly potent and selective non-peptide neuropeptide Y Y1 receptor antagonist: BIBP3226. *Eur. J. Pharmacol.* **271**, R11–R13.

Schwartz, T.W., Fuhlendorff, J., Kjems, L.L., Kirstensen, M.S., Vervelde, M., O'Hare, M., Krstenansky, J.L. & Bjornholm, B. (1990) Signal epitopes in the three-dimensional structure of neuropeptide Y: interaction with Y1, Y2 and pancreatic polypeptide receptors. *Ann. N. York Acad. Sci.* **611**, 35–47.

Schober, D.A. & Gehlert, D.R. (1993) Characterization of [^{125}I]-neuropeptide Y2–36 as a novel radioligand for neuropeptide Y receptors. *Soc. Neurosci. Abst.* **19**, 277.

Schober, D.A., Lundell, I., Schmidt, R., Beavers, L., Gadski, R.A., Statnick, M.A., Gerglund, M., Hoffmann, J.A., Chance, R., Larhammar, D. & Gehlert, D.R. (1995) Pharmacological and biochemical characterization of a novel member of the neuropeptide Y (NPY) receptor family, PP1. *The Physiologist* **38**, A249.

Schwarzer, C., Williamson, J.M., Lothman, E.W., Vezzani, A. & Sperk, G. (1995) Somatostatin, neuropeptide Y, neurokinin B and cholecystokinin immunoreactivity in two chronic models of temporal lobe epilepsy. *Neuroscience* **69**, 831–845.

Seeman, P. (1980) Brain dopamine receptors. *Pharmacol. Rev.* **32**, 229–313.

Serradeil-Le Gal, C., Valette, G., Rouby, P.E., Pellet, A., Oury-Donat, F., Brossard, G., Lespy, L., Marty, E., Neliat, G., deCoitet, P., Maffarand, J.P. & Le Fur, G. (1995) SR 120819A, an orally-active and selective neuropeptide Y Y1 receptor antagonist. *FEBS Lett.* **362**, 192–196.

Sheikh, S.P., Håkanson, R. & Schwartz, T.W. (1989a) Y1 and Y2 receptors for neuropeptide Y. *FEBS Lett.* **245**, 209–214.

Sheikh, S.P., O'Hare, M.M.T., Tortora, O. & Schwartz, T.W. (1989b) Binding of mono-iodinated neuropeptide Y to hippocampal membranes and human neuroblastoma cell lines. *J. Biol. Chem.* **264**, 6648–6654.

Shih, C.D., Chan, J.Y.H. & Chan, S.H.H. (1992) Tonic supression of baroreceptor reflex response by endogenous neuropeptide Y at the nucleus tractus solitarius of the rat. *Neurosci. Lett.* **148**, 169–172.

Sperk, G. (1994) Kainic acid seizures in the rat. *Prog. Neurobiol.* **42**, 1–32.

St-Pierre, J.A., Dumont, Y., Roussi, N., Thakur, M. & Quirion, R. (1994) Characterization of NPY/PYY receptor subtypes in primary hippocampal cell culture. *Soc. Neurosci. Abst.* **20**, 85.

St-Pierre, J.A., Dumont, Y. & Quirion, R. (1995) NPY-positive primary hippocampal cells bear NPY receptors: Anatomical basis for an autoregulation. *The Physiologist* **38**, A253.

Stanley, B.G. (1993) Neuropeptide Y in multiple hypothalamic sites controls eating behavior, endocrine and autonomic systems for body energy balance. In *The Biology of Neuropeptide Y and Related Peptides* (eds Colmers, W.F. & Wahlestedt, C.), pp. 457–510. Totowa, NJ, Humana Press Inc.

Stanley, B.G., Magdalin, W., Seirafi, A., Nguyen, M.M. & Leibowitz, S.F. (1992) Evidence for neuropeptide Y mediation of eating produced by food deprivation and for a variant of the Y1 receptor mediating this peptide's effect. *Peptides* **13**, 581–587.

Tam, S.W. & Mitchell, K.N. (1991) Neuropeptide Y and peptide YY do not bind to brain σ and phencyclidine binding sites. *Eur. J. Pharmacol.* **193**, 121–122.

Terenghi, G., Polak, J.M., Hamid, Q., O'Brien, E., Denny, P., Legon, S., Dixon, J., Minth, C.D., Palay, S.L., Yarsagil, G., Chan-Palay, V. (1987) Localization of neuropeptide Y mRNA in neurons of human cerebral cortex by means of in situ hybridization with a complementary RNA probe. *Proc. Natl Acad. Sci. USA* **84**, 7315–7318.

Terry, R.D. & Davies, P. (1980) Dementia of the Alzheimer type. *Ann. Rev. Neurosci.* **3**, 77–95.

Tong, Y., Chabot, J.C., Dumont, Y., Herzog, H., Selbie, L., Shine, J., Wahlestedt, C., Shen, S.H. & Quirion, R. (1993) Expression of the neuropeptide Y Y1 receptor mRNA in the rat brain: comparison to Y1 receptor autoradiography. *Soc. Neurosci. Abst.* **19**, 727.

Tasgarakis, S., Rees, L.H., Besser, G.M. & Grossman, A. (1989) Neuropeptide Y stimulates CRF-41 release from rat hypothalamus in vitro. *Brain Res.* **502**, 167–170.

Wahlestedt, C. & Reis, D.J. (1993) Neuropeptide Y-related peptides and their receptors: Are the receptor potential therapeutic drug targets? *Annu. Rev. Pharmacol. Toxicol.* **32**, 309–352.

Wahlestedt, C., Yanaihara, N. & Hakanson, R. (1986) Evidence for different pre-and post-junctional receptors for neuropeptide Y and related peptides. *Regul. Pept.* **13**, 307–318.

Wahlestedt, C., Regunathan, S. & Reis, D.J. (1992) Identification of cultured cells selectively expressing Y1-, Y2-, or Y3-type receptors for neuropeptide Y/peptide YY. *Life Sci.* **50**, PL7–PL12.

Wahlestedt, C., Pich, E.M., Koob, G.F., Yee, F. & Heilig, M. (1993) Modulation of anxiety and neuropeptide Y-Y1 receptors by antisense oligodeoxynucleotides. *Science* **259**, 528–531.

Walker, M.W. & Miller, R.J. (1988) ^{125}I-neuropeptide Y and ^{125}I-peptide YY bind to multiple receptor sites in rat brain. *Molec. Pharmacol.* **34**, 779–792.

Walter, J.M., Scherrer, J.F., Flood, J.F. & Morley, J.E. (1994) Effects of localized injections of neuropeptide Y antibody on motor activity and other behaviours. *Peptides* **15**, 607–613.

Weinberg, D.H., Sirinathsinghji, D.J.S., Tan, C.P., *et al.* (1996) Cloning and expression of a novel neuropeptide Y receptor. *J. Biol. Chem.* **271**, 16435–16438.

Whitcomb, D.C., Taylor, I.L. & Vigna, S.R. (1990) Characterization of saturable binding sites for circulating pancreatic polypeptide in rat brain. *Am. J. Physiol.* **259**, G687–G691.

Widdowson, P.S. (1993) Quantitative receptor autoradiography demonstrates a differential distribution of neuropeptide Y Y1 and Y2 receptor subtypes in human and rat brain. *Brain Res.* **631**, 27–38.

Widdowson, P.S. & Halaris, A.E. (1990) A comparison of the binding of [^{3}H]proprionyl-neuropeptide Y to rat and human frontal cortical membranes. *J. Neurochem.* **55**, 956–962.

Widdowson, P.D., Ordway, G.A. & Halaris, A.E. (1992) Reduced neuropeptide Y concentrations in suicide brain. *J. Neurochem.* **59**, 73–80.

Widerlöv, E., Wahlestedt, C., Håkanson, R. & Ekman, R. (1986) Altered brain neuropeptide function in psychiatric illness – with special emphasis on NPY and CRF in major depression. *Clin. Neuropharmacol.* **9**, 572–574.

Widerlöv, E., Heilig, M., Ekman, R. & Wahlestedt, C. (1988) Possible relationship between neuropeptide Y (NPY) and major depression: evidence from human and animal studies. *Nord. J. Psychiatry* **42**, 131–137.

Widerlöv, E., Heilig, M., Ekman, R. & Wahlestedt, C. (1989) Neuropeptide Y: possible involvement in depression and anxiety. In *Neuropeptide Y Nobel Conference Series* (eds Mutt, V., Fuxe, K., Hokfelt, T. & Lundberg, J.M.), pp. 331–342. New York, Raven Press.

CHAPTER 5

EXTRAORDINARY STRUCTURAL DIVERSITY OF NPY-FAMILY RECEPTORS

Dan Larhammar

Table of Contents

5.1 Introduction

Molecular clones are a prerequisite for detailed characterization of all proteins, particularly for receptors, which are often difficult to purify owing to their hydrophobic nature. A DNA clone not only allows production of its encoded receptor in cultured cells for detailed pharmacological characterization but it can also be used as a probe to determine the receptor's mRNA distribution in the body. The specificity of such probes is usually much greater than for antisera, especially if the protein belongs to a multi-member family because an antiserum may cross-react with related proteins. Other possibilities offered by molecular clones are transgenic animals and gene-disrupted animals, which can provide *in vivo* data on receptor functions.

The molecular cloning of receptors that bind to neuropeptide Y (NPY) and its related peptides, peptide YY (PYY) and pancreatic polypeptide (PP), has advanced somewhat more slowly than for many other peptide receptors. Even after the Y1 receptor was cloned (Herzog *et al.*, 1992; Krause *et al.*, 1992; Larhammar *et al.*, 1992) progress has been modest despite expectations from pharmacological studies for up to six more receptor genes, i.e. receptor-types Y2 and Y3 as well as receptors for 'appetite', PYY, PP and PP-fold peptides. At last, reports from several laboratories described clones for additional receptor subtypes, namely the Y2 receptor and a PP receptor, also called Y4 (see Table 1 for all sequence accession codes). The long wait is

Neuropeptide Y and Drug Development
ISBN 0-12-304990-3

Table 1 GenBank accession codes for sequences

Subtype	Species	Accession code for DNA	Accession code for protein	Reference
Y1	Man	M88461 cDNA	P25929	Larhammar et al. (1992)
		M84755 cDNA	P25929	Herzog et al. (1992)
		L07614 prom+exon 1		Herzog et al. (1993)
		L07615 exon 2+3		
		L47167 prom+exon 1a		Ball et al. (1996)
		L47168 prom+exon 1b		
		L47169 prom+exon 1c		
	Rat	Z11504 cDNA	P21555	Eva et al. (1990)
				Corrected by Krause et al. (1992)
		X95507 prom+exon 1		Lundell & Larhammar (unpublished)
	Mouse	Z18280 exons	Q04573	Eva et al. (1992)
		Z18281 exon 1		
		Z18282 exon 2		
		Z18283 exon 3		
		D63818 cDNA		Nakamura et al. (1995)
		D63819 cDNA		
	Xenopus laevis	L25416 cDNA	P34922	Blomqvist et al. (1995)
Y2	Man	U32500 cDNA		Rose et al. (1995)
		U36269 cDNA		Gerald et al. (1995)
		U42766 cDNA		Gehlert et al. (1996)
		gene		Gerald et al. (1995)
	Rat	Z66526 gene		Lundell et al. (1995)
PP1/Y4	Man	U35232 gene		Bard et al. (1995)
	Rat	Z68180 gene		Lundell et al. (1996)
		gene		Bard et al. (1995)
	Mouse	U40189 gene		Gregor et al. (1996)

compensated to some extent by the interesting properties reported for these receptors. The evolutionary relationships and species differences of the receptors are particularly intriguing and can be studied systematically as we already know a great deal about the evolution of their peptide ligands (Larhammar, 1996; Larhammar *et al.*, 1993a,b). Hopefully, clones for the remaining receptor subtypes will not be far down the road.

5.2 Y1 receptors

The first NPY receptor clone was initially published as an orphan receptor (Eva *et al.*, 1990). The clone was isolated by screening a rat forebain cDNA library with a non-degenerate 24-mer oligonucleotide corresponding to a conserved region in TM6 (transmembrane region 6) of heptahelix receptors. The mRNA distribution of the orphan clone in the rat brain (Eva *et al.*, 1990) resembled the Y1-like binding distribution (Aicher *et al.*, 1991), which stimulated other investigators to isolate the corresponding human receptor clone using polymerase chain reaction (PCR)-generated rat probes to screen human brain cDNA libraries. The human clones were demonstrated upon expression in cultured cells to give rise to receptors with Y1 pharmacology (Herzog *et al.*, 1992; Larhammar *et al.*, 1992). Also the rat receptor was found to bind NPY with a binding profile in agreement with Y1 type receptors (Krause *et al.*, 1992).

The human Y1 receptor, when transiently expressed in COS cells (CV-1 origin SV40 (kidney) from African green monkey) displayed virtually equal affinity in the 1–10 nM range for NPY, PYY, and the Y1-selective analogue [Leu^{31},Pro^{34}]NPY in competition with iodinated PYY (Larhammar *et al.*, 1992). The truncated NPY analogue NPY2–36 had about one order of magnitude lower affinity, whereas NPY13–36 and NPY18–36 as well as PP were additional orders of magnitude lower in affinity. This gave the typical rank order of potency for Y1 receptors: PYY≥NPY≥ [Leu^{31},Pro^{34}]NPY>>NPY2–36>>hPP>NPY13–36>NPY18–36. Similar results were reported in stably transfected HEK293 and CHO cells for human Y1 (Herzog *et al.*, 1992), transiently transfected HEK293 cells for rat Y1 (Krause *et al.*, 1992), and stably transfected Chinese hamster ovary (CHO) cells for mouse Y1 receptors (Nakamura *et al.*, 1995).

DNA clones for the mouse Y1 receptor were isolated using rat (Eva *et al.*, 1992) or human (Nakamura *et al.*, 1995) Y1 probes and a *Xenopus laevis* Y1 clone was isolated with a human probe (Blomqvist *et al.*, 1995). The sequence alignment in Figure 1 shows that the Y1 receptor displays the characteristic features of heptahelix receptors for peptide ligands. The two rodent proteins are 98% identical and both are 94% identical to the human sequence. The frog sequence is 80% identical to the three mammals. All four sequences have potential glycosylation sites in the aminoterminal portion (Figure 1) as well as in the second extracellular loop. Four extracellular cysteines presumably form two disulphide loops. All four Y1 sequences have a single intracellular cysteine in the carboxyterminal cytoplasmic portion that is probably used for attachment of palmitate inserted into the cell membrane like in many other heptahelix receptors.

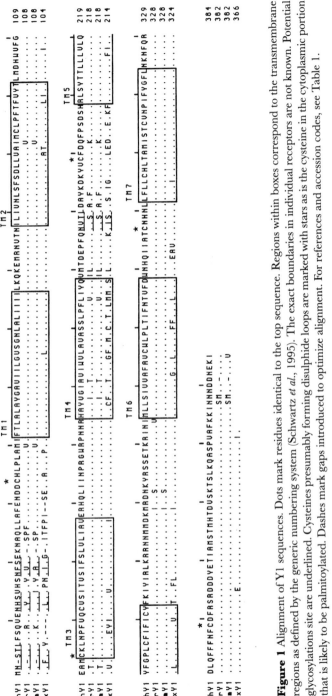

Figure 1 Alignment of Y1 sequences. Dots mark residues identical to the top sequence. Regions within boxes correspond to the transmembrane regions as defined by the generic numbering system (Schwartz *et al.*, 1995). The exact boundaries in individual receptors are not known. Potential glycosylations site are underlined. Cysteines presumably forming disulphide loops are marked with stars as is the cysteine in the cytoplasmic portion that is likely to be palmitoylated. Dashes mark gaps introduced to optimize alignment. For references and accession codes, see Table 1.

Functionally, the human Y1 receptor expressed in COS cells was found to inhibit forskolin-stimulated cAMP accumulation by about 50% in response to 100 nM NPY (Larhammar *et al.*, 1992) and to accelerate $^{45}Ca^{2+}$ influx by about 150% (both NPY and PYY at 100 nM) (Larhammar *et al.*, 1992). Similar results were reported for rat Y1 transiently expressed in HEK293 cells using NPY at 25 nM or 0.25 nM for cAMP response, and at 1 μM for Ca^{2+} response (Krause *et al.*, 1992). The human receptor when stably expressed in HEK293 cells inhibited cAMP accumulation but did not increase intracellular calcium (Herzog *et al.*, 1992). The difference between the rat and human receptors when expressed in the HEK293 cells may be due to different levels of expression. In stably transfected CHO cells, the human receptor increased calcium but failed to inhibit cAMP accumulation, perhaps owing to the lack of the appropriate G-protein isoform in these cells (Herzog *et al.*, 1992). However, the mouse Y1 receptor did inhibit cAMP accumulation in CHO cells (50% inhibition) as well as elevate intracellular Ca^{2+} (Nakamura *et al.*, 1995). Again, the differences between these experiments may be due to the level of expression of the transfected receptor gene. The mouse Y1 receptor was found to activate mitogen-activated protein kinase (MAPK) via a pertussin-toxin (PTX)-sensitive G protein in the transfected CHO cells, probably via phosphoinositide 3-kinase (Nakamura *et al.*, 1995).

The human Y1 mRNA is about 3.5–4 kb and was detected in the neuroblastoma cell line SK-N-MC by Northern hybridization (Larhammar *et al.*, 1992). An *in situ* hybridization study with a riboprobe reported widespread distribution in human fetal and adult organs, e.g. colon, kidney, heart, placenta and adrenal (Wharton *et al.*, 1993). However, a Northern hybridization in the same study detected a single mRNA of only 2.2 kb suggesting that the specificity of the probe for Y1 mRNA may be questioned. Curiously, in the same study the size for NPY mRNA was reported as 3.3 kb, which disagrees with the size seen in a human pheochromocytoma (0.8 kb) as well as the size of the human cDNA clone which ends with a poly(A) tract (Minth *et al.*, 1984).

Rat Y1 mRNA is approximately 4 kb with widespread brain distribution including hippocampus, cerebral cortex and thalamus, as shown by Northern hybridization and *in situ* hybridization (Eva *et al.*, 1990). The mouse Y1 mRNA is of similar size and was detected in brain, heart, kidney, spleen, skeletal muscle and lung, but not in liver and testis (Nakamura *et al.*, 1995). In rat the Y1 mRNA was localized to subregions of hippocampus, thalamus and hypothalamus by *in situ* hybridization (Larsen *et al.*, 1995). In the hypothalamus, substantial Y1 mRNA expression was observed in the arcuate nucleus and in the paraventricular nucleus (PVN) despite low density of Y1 binding sites in both of these regions (Mikkelsen and Larsen, 1992; Larsen *et al.*, 1995). However, it is possible that the Y1 mRNA is not translated into functional receptors or that receptors are transported from the cell body into neurites outside of the PVN. Thus, these findings are still compatible with a separate (non-Y1) PVN receptor for NPY/PYY that mediates the feeding response as indicated by extensive pharmacological evidence (Gehlert, 1994) as well as the failure of Y1 antisense oligonucleotides to block feeding response (Wahlestedt *et al.*, 1993). In the rat spinal cord, *in situ* hybridizations detected Y1 mRNA in 20% of dorsal root ganglion (DRG) cells, predominantly of the small type, at lumbar levels L4 and L5 (Zhang *et al.*, 1994).

Peripheral axotomy caused a decrease of Y1 mRNA in the small neurons and an increase in large neurons. These results suggested that the DRG Y1 receptor is mostly a prejunctional receptor in primary afferent neurons and that it may play a role in the modulation of somatosensory information (Zhang *et al.*, 1994). Low levels of Y1 mRNA have also been reported for rat splenic lymphocytes as documented by a partial cDNA clone, PCR and RNase protection (Petitto *et al.*, 1994). A developmental study by *in situ* hybridization of whole rat embryo sections (Jazin *et al.*, 1993) detected the earliest Y1 mRNA around day 14, both in diencephalon and spinal cord.

The organization of the gene encoding the Y1 receptor has been determined in mouse (Eva *et al.*, 1992) and man (Herzog *et al.*, 1993). It consists of three exons (Figure 2); exon 1 contains the beginning of the 5'-untranslated region (5'UT), exon 2 contains 5'UT and the coding region up to and including TM5, and exon 3 contains the remainder of the coding region and the entire 3'-untranslated region. The first intron is approximately 6 kb in both mouse and man whereas intron 2 is about 100 nucleotides. Recently, two additional promoters with separate initiating 5'UT exons were discovered in the human gene by cDNA cloning and the 5' rapid amplification of cDNA ends (RACE) method (Ball *et al.*, 1996). Exon 1b is located 18.4 kb upstream of exon 2 (12 kb upstream of the previously described promoter) and exon 1c is 23.9 kb upstream of exon 2. The three promoters have different potential binding sites for transcription factors and show differences in tissue distribution, although some tissues use all three promoters, e.g. kidney (Ball *et al.*, 1996).

Additional complexity at the genomic level is indicated by a mouse cDNA clone from bone marrow with a different sequence from amino acid 303 at the beginning of TM7 (Nakamura *et al.*, 1995). This results in a truncated receptor with incomplete TM7. Nevertheless, the binding specificities are identical to the full-length receptor. However, no second messenger responses could be recorded with the truncated receptor why it was proposed to function in NPY internalization. The alternative splicing seems to occur during embryonic development in addition to bone marrow and haematopoietic cells. The novel exon is located more than 15 kb downstream of exon 3. It has not yet been investigated whether the human Y1 gene has the alternative exon. Some human cDNA clones have been found that have retained intron 2 (Lundell *et al.*, 1992). This intron contains termination codons (Herzog, *et al.*, 1993) that will terminate the receptor protein after TM5 and presumably result in a nonfunctional truncated receptor.

5.3 Y2 receptors

With access to clones for one receptor type, it has been possible in several cases to isolate clones rapidly for other receptor types using cross-hybridization as exemplified by opioid receptors and somatostatin receptors. However, clones for the abundant Y2 receptor have resisted detection with Y1 probes. Instead, three different laboratories have recently succeeded by expression screening to isolate Y2 clones using PYY as

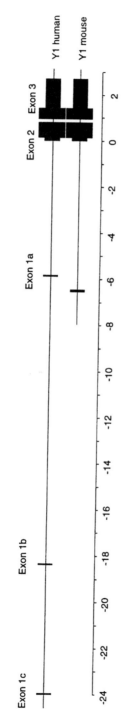

Figure 2 Exon–intron organization of human and mouse Y1 genes. The tall parts of exons 2 and 3 correspond to the translated regions of these exons. Three alternative exon 1 have been found in the human gene (Ball *et al.*, 1996).

radioligand (Gerald *et al.*, 1995b; Gehlert *et al.*, 1996a; Rose *et al.*, 1995). The sequences predicted from these clones (Figure 3) provide the explanation for the lack of cross-hybridization to Y1 probes; the overall sequence identify at the amino-acid level is only 31%, the lowest percentage yet reported for different receptors binding the same peptide.

The human Y2 clones were isolated from expression cDNA libraries of neuro-blastoma cells SMS-KAN (Rose *et al.*, 1995), hippocampus (Gerald *et al.*, 1995b) or total brain (Gehlert *et al.*, 1996a) by screening transfected COS cells for binding to ^{125}I-PYY. The human Y2 receptor was found by all three groups to have affinity for NPY and PYY in the low nanomolar range in competition with ^{125}I-PYY. The truncated analogues NPY2–36, NPY13–36 and NPY18–36 also competed in the low nanomolar range, but with slightly lower affinities than the intact peptides. For instance, NPY18–36 had about six-fold lower affinity as compared to intact NPY (1.8 nM versus 0.30 nM) (Gehlert *et al.*, 1996a). In contrast, the Y1 receptor-selective analogue [Leu^{31},Pro^{34}]NYP had a K_i of about 1 µM. In addition, the Y1 receptor-selective antagonist BIBP3226 (Rudolf *et al.*, 1994) was relatively inactive (Gehlert *et al.*, 1996a). Thus, the pharmacological profile of the cloned receptor conforms well to that of type Y2.

A different approach led to the discovery of a bovine Y2 cDNA clone (Ammar *et al.*, 1995). A retina and pigment epithelium cDNA library was screened for heptahelix receptors and a clone was identified whose human genomic homologue upon expression was found to find NPY with nanomolar affinity and displayed the characteristic Y2 pharmacological profile (Ammar *et al.*, 1995).

Rat Y2 genomic clones have been isolated using the human clone as probe (Gerald *et al.*, 1995a). The pharmacological properties of the rat receptor agree well with the human receptor.

Structurally, the Y2 receptor has the typical heptahelix receptor features including potential glycosylation sites in the amino-terminal portion (Figure 3), two extracellular cysteines that may form a disulphide loop, and a single cysteine in the cytoplasmic tail that probably serves as an attachment site for palmitate. The rat and human receptors are 94% identical (Gerald *et al.*, 1995a) and the bovine and human proteins are 94.5% identical (Ammar *et al.*, 1995). The amino-acid sequence reported by Rose *et al.* differs at one position from that reported by Gehlert *et al.* and Gerald *et al.* (Figure 3). The two reported rat clones (Gerald *et al.*, 1995a) differ at two amino-acid positions (Figure 3). These differences are probably allelic.

When stably expressed in CHO cells, the human Y2 receptor inhibits forskolin-stimulated cAMP accumulation by 50–70% in response to both NPY and PYY at 100 nM (Rose *et al.*, 1995). Stably transfected HEK293 cells were tested with a broad range of peptide concentrations and PYY was found to have EC_{50} at 0.3 nM (Gerald *et al.*, 1995b). Intracellular calcium was increased by PYY (Gerald *et al.*, 1995b) as well as by NPY2–36 and NPY13–36 at 1 µM (Rose *et al.*, 1995).

The human Y2 mRNA is about 4 kb and was observed by Northern hybridization in several brain subregions but surprisingly not in most peripheral organs investigated (Gehlert *et al.*, 1996a; Gerald *et al.*, 1995b; Rose *et al.*, 1995). This suggests that the Y2

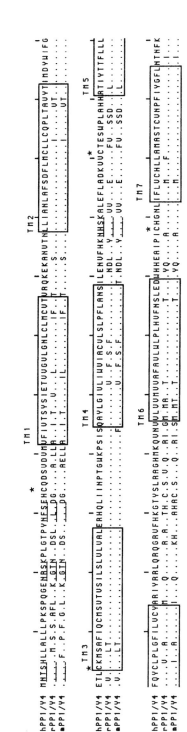

Figure 3 Alignment of Y2 sequences. Dots mark residues identical to the top sequence. The two human sequences hY2A (Gehlert *et al.*, 1996a; Gerald *et al.*, 1995b) and hY2B (Rose *et al.*, 1995) are probably allelic, as are probably the two rat sequences (Gerald *et al.*, 1995a). Regions within boxes correspond to the transmembrane regions as defined by the generic numbering system (Schwartz *et al.*, 1995). The exact boundaries in individual receptors are not known. Potential glycosylation sites are underlined. Cysteines presumably forming disulphide loops are marked with stars as is the cysteine in the cytoplasmic portion, which is likely to be palmitoylated. Dashes mark gaps introduced to optimize alignment. For accession codes, see Table 1.

receptor originally identified in the periphery is distinct from the cloned Y2 receptor. However, this does not exclude the possibility that the peripheral Y2 receptor may also be expressed in the brain. No additional gene was detected with a Y2 probe by Southern hybridization to genomic human DNA after washing at high stringency, indicating that any other Y2-like genes must be fairly divergent from the cloned Y2 receptor at the sequence level (Gehlert et al., 1996a; Gerald et al., 1995b; Rose et al., 1995). The human Y2 mRNA has an unusually long 5'-untranslated region of 1000 nucleotides (Gerald et al., 1995b), the significance of which has not yet been investigated. The human gene has a single intron of approximately 4.5 kb located in the 5'-untranslated region (Ammar et al., 1995).

5.4 Pancreatic polypeptide receptors

Homology-based approaches have led to the discovery of a novel receptor with resemblance to Y1, but with binding preference for PP over PYY and NPY. This receptor was designated PP1 because of its binding profile (Lundell et al., 1995, 1996) or Y4 because it binds NPY-family peptides (Bard et al., 1995b). Lundell et al. (1996) were able to isolate their clone by evaluating the four available Y1 sequences from mammals and Xenopus laevis (Blomqvist et al., 1995) to design DNA primers corresponding to parts of TM2 and TM7. PCR was performed on genomic DNA from several species and a product was obtained in rat that on sequencing revealed a closer identity to Y1 than to all other receptors. The PCR fragment was used to screen a rat total brain cDNA library, but only one truncated clone was obtained. Human and rat genomic libraries provided clones that on sequencing were found to contain an intronless coding region for a receptor, which on expression bound PP with picomolar affinity (Lundell et al., 1995, 1996). Bard et al. (1995a) used a large battery of oligonucleotides corresponding to rat Y1 (TM regions 1, 2, 3, 5 and 7) to screen a human genomic library at low stringency. One clone was identified and its hybridization signal was found to derive exclusively from the TM7 oligonucleotide (Bard et al., 1995a). It encoded a Y1-like receptor with PP binding preference and with a predicted amino-acid sequence identical to receptor PP1 described by Lundell et al. (Figure 4). A rat clone was isolated also by Bard et al. by screening a genomic library with probes from the human receptor's transmembrane regions (Bard et al., 1995a). A genomic clone encoding a mouse PP1/Y4 receptor (called NPYR-D) was isolated with a non-degenerate oligonucleotide corresponding to TM7 of the published Y1 receptors (Gregor et al., 1996).

The human PP1/Y4 receptor binds human PP with a K_i of 0.014 nM (Lundell et al., 1995) and IC_{50} (concentration that gives 50% inhibition) of 0.056 nM (Bard et al., 1995b) in competition with porcine PYY when transiently expressed in COS cells. Both groups also reported affinities in the low nanomolar range for human PYY and NPY. Thus, all three peptides may be physiological ligands to the human PP1/Y4 receptor. The peptide analogue [Leu^{31},Pro^{34}]NPY bound in the 10–20 nM range,

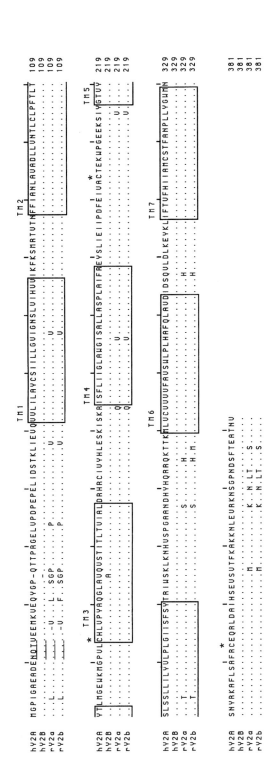

Figure 4 Alignment of PP1/Y4 sequences. Dots mark residues identical to the top sequence. Regions within boxes correspond to the transmembrane regions as defined by the generic numbering system (Schwartz *et al.*, 1995). The exact boundaries in individual receptors are not known. Potential glycosylation sites are underlined. Cysteines presumably forming disulphide loops are marked with stars as is the cysteine in the cytoplasmic portion, which is likely to be palmitoylated. Dashes mark gaps introduced to optimize alignment. For references and accession codes, see Table 1.

which means that it can no longer be considered selective for Y1. Very similar results were obtained for the human receptor in stably transfected CHO cells (Gehlert et al., 1996b).

A large repertoire of truncated PP, PYY and NPY analogues have been tested on the human receptor (Bard et al., 1995b; Gehlert et al., 1996b). For instance, PYY3–36 and NPY3–36 have 10–30-fold higher K_i values than the native peptides. The preferred ligand, PP, is somewhat less affected by amino-terminal truncation. These results show that the PP1/Y4 receptor, like the structurally similar Y1 receptor but in contrast to the Y2 receptor, requires the amino-terminal residues of its ligands for optimal binding. However, it appears to be slightly less dependent on these residues than the Y1 receptor.

The rat and mouse PP1/Y4 clones when expressed in COS cells displayed a binding profile that differed from the human receptor; in fact, radioiodinated PYY showed no specific labelling for the rat receptor in the concentration range tested in one of the studies (Lundell et al., 1996), although it did so in the other report (Bard et al., 1995a). Therefore, Lundell et al. used ^{125}I-PP for the competition experiments; bovine PP gave a K_i of 0.017 nM similar to the human receptor. In contrast, PYY and NPY competed much less efficiently with K_i values of 162 nM and 192 nM, respectively. [Leu^{31},Pro^{34}]NPY had a K_i of 0.74 nM and thus competed better than intact NPY in agreement with the two amino-acid replacements being derived from the PP structure. The rat PP1/Y4 receptor reported by Bard et al. (1995b) did not distinguish as clearly between the three peptides (with ^{125}I-PYY as radioligand); IC$_{50}$ was 0.15 nM for bPP, 0.58 nM for PYY and 1.7 nM for NPY. The affinity of [Leu^{31},Pro^{34}]NPY, with IC$_{50}$ of 0.59 nM, was higher than that of native NPY. The binding properties of the mouse PP1/Y4 receptor agree well with those of the rat receptor reported by Lundell et al. (1996) in that rat PP, in competition with rat ^{125}I-PP, had an IC$_{50}$ of about 0.1 nM, whereas PYY and NPY had values of 500 and 790 nM (Gregor et al., 1996). Again, [Leu^{31},Pro^{34}]NPY competed much better than native NPY with an IC$_{50}$ of 4 nM. Interestingly, the preference for PP over PYY and NPY was much lower when ^{125}I-PYY was used as radioligand with IC$_{50}$ of 0.11, 3 and 3 nM, respectively, for the three peptides. The latter radioligand was reported to have much lower specific binding, only 50%, compared to ^{125}I-PP, which had over 95%. All three studies agree that the modified NPY analogue [Leu^{31},Pro^{34}]NPY binds with high affinity to the PP1/Y4 receptor, thus ruling out this compound as a Y1-specific ligand also in rat and mouse.

Human PP1/Y4 is 42% identical to the human Y1 receptor, displays similar features and seems to undergo the same post-translational modifications (Figures 4 and 5). The TM regions are 53% identical to Y1. Surprisingly, the rat PP1/Y4 receptor is only 75% identical to the human receptor. Southern hybridizations have confirmed that the two receptors are indeed each other's closest homologues, i.e. the genes are orthologous (homologous genes separated as a result of speciation). The rat and mouse receptors are 92% identical (Gregor et al., 1996).

When the human PP1/Y4 receptor was stably expressed in CHO cells, it inhibited forskolin-stimulated cAMP accumulation by 50% in response to human PP at 100 nM with EC$_{50}$ at 7 nM (Lundell et al., 1995). In mouse fibroblasts (thymidine kinase

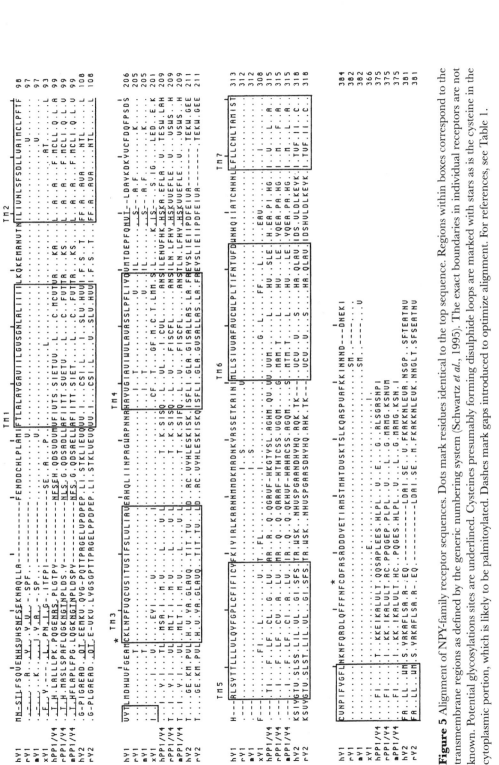

Figure 5 Alignment of NPY-family receptor sequences. Dots mark residues identical to the top sequence. Regions within boxes correspond to the transmembrane regions as defined by the generic numbering system (Schwartz *et al*., 1995). The exact boundaries in individual receptors are not known. Potential glycosylations sites are underlined. Cysteines presumably forming disulphide loops are marked with stars as is the cysteine in the cytoplasmic portion, which is likely to be palmitoylated. Dashes mark gaps introduced to optimize alignment. For references, see Table 1.

negative LMTK-) the inhibition was 80% at a concentration below 1 nM with EC_{50} at 0.07 nM (Bard *et al.*, 1995a). In the latter cells, also the intracellular calcium level in response to 100 nM PP was investigated and was found to increase (Bard *et al.*, 1995a).

The human PP1/Y4 mRNA is about 6 kb and seems to have a narrow tissue distribution as detected by Northern hybridization (Lundell *et al.*, 1995). mRNA was observed in the gastrointestinal tract in the colon, the small intestine and the pancreas as well as in the prostate. Faint bands were observed in some brain subregions after long exposure (Lundell *et al.*, 1995). With reverse transcriptase (RT)-PCR, products were detected in most of the mRNA preparations investigated (Bard *et al.*, 1995a). In rat, mRNA (4.2 kb) was observed by Northern hybridization in the colon at low level and, surprisingly, in the lung and the testis (Lundell *et al.*, 1996). The colon also had a faint shorter mRNA of 1.8 kb. Mouse mRNA (4.2 kb) was observed in the heart and small intestine (Gregor *et al.*, 1996). (Mouse did not have mRNA in the lung whereas rat heart was blank in the report by Lundell *et al.*, thus suggesting clear species differences even between mouse and rat.) The report by Gregor *et al.* also investigated the human mRNA distribution; Northern hybridization detected mRNA in small intestine, colon and prostate in agreement with Lundell *et al.* (1995) and, in addition, in stomach (not investigated by Lundell *et al.*). RT-PCR detected mRNA in various parts of the human brain (Gregor *et al.*, 1996). The presence of PP1/Y4 mRNA in the pancreas and colon is in agreement with the major sites of production of PP (pancreas) and PYY (pancreas and colon).

The 5'-untranslated region of the PP1/Y4 gene has not yet been investigated to see if any introns are present.

5.5 Discussion

The molecular cloning of the Y2 and PP1/Y4 receptors brought two unexpected findings, both of which relate to the functions as well as the evolution of this family of receptors. The first surprise was that Y2 is dramatically different from Y1 (and PP1/Y4) in protein sequence (Figure 5). Only 31% overall identity means that Y1 and Y2 are the most divergent receptors that bind the same peptide ligand. In fact, they both bind two different ligands, i.e. NPY and PYY. Other peptide receptor families generally have higher levels of identity between their members despite binding different ligands. The melanocortin receptors that bind α-MSH (melanocyte-stimulating hormone) (receptor subtype MSH1) and adrenocorticotrophic hormone (ACTH) display 40% identity and these receptors have quite different preferences for the two ligands (MSH is the amino-terminal part of ACTH) (Mountjoy *et al.*, 1992). The five somatostatin receptors have identities of 39% or higher to each other, and differ in their preference for somatostatin-14 and somatostatin-28.

The second surprise from the receptor clones was that the PP receptor PP1/Y4 differs greatly between species in several ways. The human and rat receptors share only 75% overall identity. This percentage is among the lowest for any heptahelix receptor between separate orders of mammals. The low PP1/Y4 identity contrasts with the high percentages for Y1 (94%) and Y2 (94%). However, in one way the PP1/Y4 divergence make sense: the receptor's preferred ligand, PP, is also quite divergent between rat and man with eight replacements out of 36 positions (78% identity). NPY, in contrast, is identical between man and rat, and PYY has only two replacements (see Larhammar, 1996, for review). Among all known mammalian PP sequences, rat and mouse stand out as the most divergent. Therefore, it will be very interesting to see the PP1/Y4 sequence in species representing other orders of mammals. The prediction is that they will be more similar to the human sequence. Preliminary sequence data for the guinea-pig PP1/Y4 receptor indicates that this is indeed the case (H. Eriksson and D. Larhammar, unpublished data).

The PP1/Y4 receptor also differs greatly between species in two other respects: ligand-binding properties and tissue distribution. Although the human and rodent receptors have the same rank order of binding preference, PP>[Leu^{31},Pro^{34}] NPY>PYY>NPY, the K_i values differ greatly between human and rat/mouse. The human receptor binds PP with a K_i of 0.014 nM (Lundell et al., 1995), but also PYY and NPY may be physiological ligands with affinities in the 1–10 nM range (Bard et al., 1995b; Lundell et al., 1995). In contrast, the rat (Lundell et al., 1996) and mouse (Gregor et al., 1996) receptors have a strong preference for PP, and are less likely to respond to PYY and NPY in vivo as these have K_i values of 162 and 192 nM to the rat receptor (Lundell et al., 1996), and IC$_{50}$ values of 500 and 790 nM to the mouse receptor (Gregor et al., 1996). However, the second study of the rat receptor (Bard et al., 1995a) recorded much higher affinities for PYY and NPY (IC$_{50}$ values of 0.58 nM and 1.7 nM) in competition with iodinated PYY, as did the mouse receptor when PYY was used as a radioligand (Gregor et al., 1996). Differences in K_i have been found to depend on the radioligand used for competition (Rosenkilde et al., 1994; Schwartz et al., 1995) and the differential binding to the mouse receptor was hypothesized to be the result of differences in the affinity states recognized by the two radioligands (Gregor et al., 1996). Also, it was noted that iodinated PYY had much lower specific binding than iodinated PP to the mouse receptor. However, this still does not explain the difference in direct binding between the two studies of the rat receptor. It is conceivable that binding properties may differ between batches of radioiodinated PYY.

The PP1/Y4 mRNA is present in several parts of the gastroinestinal tract in man, rat and mouse. Elsewhere some notable differences have been observed: mRNA is present in mouse heart but is absent in rat and human, it is abundant in rat lung and testis but missing in these organs in mouse and human. None of these organs was expected to have PP1/Y4 mRNA. PP receptors have not been characterized in detail in any organ preparation and the extremely low abundance of PP receptor in PC12 cells makes comparisons with the cloned receptor uncertain (Schwartz et al., 1987) and may make detection of mRNA difficult.

The cloned PP receptor shares two prominent features with the Y1 receptor as might be expected from the sequence resemblance (Bard et al., 1995b; Gehlert et al., 1996b). Firstly, PP1/Y4 is dependent on the amino-terminal portion of the peptide ligands for optimal binding (but somewhat less dependent than Y1), and secondly,

PP1/Y4 binds the analogue [Leu^{31},Pro^{34}]NPY, which has been considered to be selective for Y1. Thus, previous binding experiments will have to be re-evaluated in the light of these results. The limited distribution of the PP1/Y4 receptor in both man, rat and mouse suggests that it is unlikely to have interfered significantly with Y1 binding studies. However, certain brain regions have prominent PP binding (Gackenheimer *et al.*, 1995; Whitcomb *et al.*, 1990).

Pharmacologically, the cloned Y1 and Y2 receptors agree very well with previous data *in vivo*, or for isolated organ or tissue preparations. The Y1 receptor requires both ends of NPY and PYY for high-affinity binding whereas Y2 binds and responds to peptide analogues lacking the amino-terminal portion. These differences as well as the divergent sequences will make studies of the molecular interactions between receptors and ligands particularly interesting.

A mutagenesis scan of 14 extracellular Asp residues in the human Y1 receptor identified four that were candidates for interaction with the four basic residues in NPY: D104 in extracellular loop 1; D194 and D200 in loop 2; and D287 in loop 3 (Walker *et al.*, 1994). Surprisingly, we found that the *Xenopus laevis* Y1 receptor has a Gly at the position corresponding to hY1 position D194 (see Figure 5). Assuming that the alignment in Figure 5 in some way reflects the topology of extracellular loop 2, position D194 is a negatively charged residue also in Y2 (Glu) in agreement with the binding model. Position Y1 D200 is also negatively charged in all NPY-family receptors except one, namely rat PP1/Y4, which has valine. Position D287, which may form the third salt bridge, is invariant in all nine sequences. Thus, two of the three candidate positions for salt bridges have occasional losses of negative side chains. [Position D104 in extracellular loop 1 of hY1 has been abandoned as forming a possible salt bridge (Sautel *et al.*, 1995). This position is a Gly in the two Y2 sequences.]

Another series of human Y1 mutant clones has been investigated for interaction with Tyr-36 of NPY by formation of a hydrophobic pocket (Sautel *et al.*, 1995). Out of six mutated positions, three were found to influence NPY binding, namely Y100, F286 and H298. Of these, only Y100 is invariant among the Y1, Y2 and PP1/Y4 sequences. F286 is still hydrophobic in Y2, namely Val, but it is a Glu in both of the PP1/Y4 sequences. H298 seems to vary even more dramatically because it is Gly in both of the PP1/Y4 sequences and Tyr in both of the Y2 sequences.

Taken together, these studies may have found two positions that have roles in binding of NPY-family ligands to all sequenced receptors, namely Y100 and D287, the latter of which may interact with NPY Arg-33 (Walker *et al.*, 1994). The remaining four positions that were found to influence NPY binding to Y1 may account for some of the differences in binding between receptor subtypes, i.e., Y1 positions D194, D200, F286 and H298. Sequences for these receptor types from additional species and sequences for the remaining receptor types, along with pharmacological studies of expressed clones, will shed more light on the interactions of the NPY-family peptides with their receptors.

In conclusion, the clones for the Y2 and PP1/Y4 receptors have raised interesting evolutionary questions owing to their extensive sequence divergence, but in two very different ways: Y2 differs dramatically from Y1 and PP1/Y4, whereas PP1/Y4 differs greatly between species. The novel clones encoding Y2 and Y4/PP1 will be important tools in the continued search for receptor clones. Indeed, clones for candidate NPY-family receptors have already been found. Three zebrafish receptor clones have features suggesting that they correspond to receptor types that are distinct from the three types that have been described in this review. To paraphrase Dobzhansky (1973), these biological surprises will only make sense once we know their evolutionary history.

Acknowledgements

This work was supported by a grant from the Swedish Natural Science Research Council. I thank Ingrid Lundell (Uppsala University), Henrik Eriksson (Uppsala University), Donald R. Gehlert (Lilly Research Laboratories) and Paul Gregor (Bayer) for communication of unpublished results, and Magnus Berglund and Ingrid Lundell for comments on the manuscript.

References

Aicher, S.A., Springston, M., Berger, S.B., Reis, D.J. & Wahlestedt, C. (1991) Receptor-selective analogues demonstrate NPY/PYY receptor heterogeneity in rat brain. *Neurosci. Lett.* **130**, 32–36.

Ammar, D.A., Kolakowski, L.F., Eadie, D.M., Wong, D.J., Ma, Y.-Y., Yang-Feng, T.L. & Thompson, D.A. (1995) A novel neuropeptide Y receptor present in the eye and brain: Cloning, characterization, and expression of the human gene and bovine cDNA. *Receptor Meeting*, Philadelphia, USA.

Ball, H.J., Shine, J. & Herzog, H. (1996) Multiple promoters regulate tissue-specific expression of the human NPY-Y1 receptor gene. *J. Biol. Chem.* **270**, 27 272–27 276.

Bard, J.A., Walker, M.W., Branchek, T. & Weinshank, R.L. (1995a) DNA encoding a human neuropeptide Y/peptide YY/pancreatic polypeptide receptor (Y4) and uses thereof. International patent application WO 95/17906,

Bard, J.A., Walker, M.W., Branchek, T.A. & Weinshank, R.L. (1995b) Cloning and functional expression of a human Y4 subtype receptor for pancreatic polypeptide, neuropeptide Y, and peptide YY. *J. Biol. Chem.* **270**, 26 762–26 765.

Blomqvist, A.G., Roubos, E.W., Larhammar, D. & Martens, G.J. (1995) Cloning and sequence analysis of a neuropeptide Y/peptide YY receptor Y1 cDNA from *Xenopus laevis*. *Biochem. Biophys. Acta* **1261**, 439–441.

Dobzhansky (1973) Nothing in biology make sense except in the light of evolution. *The American Biology Teacher* 125–129.

Eva, C., Keinänen, K., Monyer, H., Seeburg, P. & Sprengel, R. (1990) Molecular cloning of a novel G protein-couple receptor that may belong to the neuropeptide receptor family. *FEBS Lett.* **271**, 81–84.

Eva, C., Oberto, A., Sprengel, R. & Genazzani, E. (1992) The murine NPY-1 receptor gene. Structure and delineation of tissue-specific expression. *FEBS Lett.* **314**, 285–288.

Gackenheimer, S.L., Lundell, I., Schmidt, R., Beavers, L., Gadski, R.A., Berglund, M.,

Schober, D.A., Mayne, N.L., Burnett, J.P., Larhammar, D. & Gehlert, D.R. (1995) Binding of [^{125}I]-[Leu^{31}-Pro^{34}]-peptide YY (LP-PYY) to receptors for neuropeptide Y (Y-1) and pancreatic polypeptide (PP1). *Society for Neuroscience Annual Meeting Abstracts* Vol. 25, 625.4.

Gehlert, D.R. (1994) Subtypes of receptors for neuropeptide Y: implications for the targeting of therapeutics. *Life Sci.* **55**, 551–562.

Gehlert, D.R., Beavers, L., Johnson, D., Gackenheimer, S.L., Schober, D.A. & Gadski, R.A. (1996a) Expression cloning of a human brain neuropeptide Y Y2 receptor. *Mol. Pharmacol.* **49**, 224–228.

Gehlert, D.R., Schober, D.A., Beavers, L., Gadski, R., Hoffman, J.A., Chance, R.E., Lundell, I. & Larhammar, D. (1996b) Characterization of the peptide binding requirements for the cloned human pancreatic polypeptide preferring (PP1) receptor. *Mol. Pharmacol.* **50**, 112–118.

Gerald, C., Walker, M.W., Branchek, T. & Weinshank, R. (1995a) Nucleic acid encoding neuropeptide Y/peptide YY (Y2) receptors and uses thereof. International patent application WO 95/21245.

Gerald, C., Walker, M.W., Vaysse, P.J.-J., He, C., Branchek, T.A. & Weinshank, R.L. (1995b) Expression cloning and pharmacological characterization of a human hippocampal neuropeptide Y/peptide YY Y2 receptor subtype. *J. Biol. Chem.* **270**, 26 758–26 761.

Gregor, P., Millham, M.L., Feng, Y., DeCarr, L.B., McCaleb, M.L. & Cornfield, L.J. (1996) Cloning and characterization of a novel receptor to pancretic polypeptide, a member of the neuropeptide Y receptor family. *FEBS Lett.* **381**, 58–62.

Herzog, H., Baumgartner, M., Vivero, C., Selbie, L.A., Auer, B. & Shine, J. (1993) Genomic organization, localization, and allelic differences in the gene for the human neuropeptide Y Y1 receptor. *J. Biol. Chem.* **268**, 6703–6707.

Herzog, H., Hort, Y.J., Ball, H.J., Hayes, G., Shine, J. & Selbie, L.A. (1992) Cloned human neuropeptide Y receptor couples to two different second messenger systems. *Proc. Natl Acad. Sci. USA* **89**, 5794–5798.

Jazin, E.E., Zhang, X., Söderström, S., Williams, R., Hökfelt, T., Ebendal, T. & Larhammar, D. (1993) Expression of peptide YY and mRNA for the NPY/PYY receptor of the Y1 subtype in dorsal root ganglia during rat embryogenesis. *Dev. Brain Res.* **76**, 105–113.

Krause, J., Eva, C., Seeburg, P.H. & Sprengel, R. (1992) Neuropeptide Y1 subtype pharmacology of a recombinantly expressed neuropeptide receptor. *Mol. Pharmacol.* **41**, 817–821.

Larhammar, D. (1996) Evolution of neuropeptide Y, peptide YY, and pancreatic polypeptide. *Regulatory Peptides* **62**, 1–11.

Larhammar, D., Blomqvist, A.G., Yee, F., Jazin, E., Yoo, H. & Wahlestedt, C. (1992) Cloning and functional expression of a human neuropeptide Y/peptide YY receptor of the Y1 type. *J. Biol. Chem.* **267**, 10 935–10 938.

Larhammar, D., Blomqvist, A.G. & Söderberg, C. (1993a) Evolution of neuropeptide Y and its related peptides. *Comp. Biochem. Physiol.* **106C**, 743–752.

Larhammar, D., Söderberg, C. & Blomqvist, A.G. (1993b) Evolution of the neuropeptide Y family of peptides. In *The Neurobiology of Neuropeptide Y and Related Peptides.* (eds Wahlestedt, C. & Colmers, W.F.), pp. 1–42. Clifton, NJ, Humana Press.

Lundell, I., Blomqvist, A.G., Berglund, M.M., Schober, D.A., Johnson, D., Statnick, M.A., Gadski, R.A., Gehlert, D.R. & Larhammar, D. (1995) Cloning of a human receptor of the NPY receptor family with high affinity for pancreatic polypeptide and peptide. YY. *J. Biol. Chem.* **270**, 29 123–29 128.

Larsen, P.J., Sheikh, S.P. & Mikkelsen, J.D. (1995) Neuropeptide Y Y1 receptors in the rat forebrain: autoradiographic demonstration of [^{125}I][Leu^{31},Pro^{34}]-NPY binding sites and neurons expressing Y1 receptor mRNA. *J. Receptor Signal Transd. Res.* **15**, 457–472.

Lundell, I., Blomqvist, A.G., Yee, F., Yoo, H., Söderberg, C., Wahlestedt, C. & Larhammar, D. (1992) Isolation and characterization of human cDNA clones related to the NPY/PYY Y1 receptor. *Society for Neuroscience Annual Meeting Abstracts* Vol. 22, 193.15.

Lundell, I., Statnick, M.A., Johnson, D., Schober, D.A., Starbäck, P., Gehlert, D.R. & Larhammar, D. (1996) The cloned rat pancreatic polypeptide receptor exhibits profound differences to the orthologous human receptor. *Proc. Natl Acad. Sci. USA* **93**, 5111–5115.

Mikkelsen, J.D. & Larsen, P.J. (1992) A high concentration of NPY (Y1)-receptor mRNA-expressing cells in the hypothalamic arcuate nucleus. *Neurosci. Lett.* **148**, 195–198.

Minth, C.D., Bloom, S.R., Polak, J.M. & Dixon, J.E. (1984) Cloning, characterization, and DNA sequence of a human cDNA encoding neuropeptide tyrosine. *Proc Natl Acad. Sci. USA* **81**, 4577–4581.

Mountjoy, K.G., Robbins, L.S., Mortrud, M.T. & Cone, R.D. (1992) The cloning of a family of genes that encode the melanocortin receptors. *Science* **257**, 1248–1251.

Nakamura, M., Sakanaka, C., Aoki, Y., Ogasawara, H., Tsuji, T., Kodama, H., Matsumoto, T., Shimizu, T. & Noma, M. (1995) Identification of two isoforms of mouse neuropeptide Y-Y1 receptor generated by alternative splicing. *J. Biol. Chem.* **270**, 30 102–30 110.

Petitto, J.M., Huang, Z. & McCarthy, D.B. (1994) Molecular cloning of NPY-Y1 receptor cDNA from rat splenic lymphocytes: Evidence of low levels of mRNA expression and [^{125}I]NPY binding sites. *J. Neuroimmunol.* **54**, 81–86.

Rose, P.M., Fernandes, P., Lynch, J.S., Frazier, S.T., Fisher, S.M., Kodukula, K., Kienzle, B. & Seethala, R. (1995) Cloning and functional expression of a cDNA encoding a human type 2 neuropeptide Y receptor. *J. Biol. Chem.* **270**, 22 661–22 664.

Rosenkilde, M.M., Cahir, M., Gether, U., Hjorth, S.A. & Schwartz, T.W. (1994) Mutations along transmembrane segment II of the NK-1 receptor affect substance P competition with non-peptide antagonists but not substance P binding. *J. Biol. Chem.* **269**, 28 160–28 164.

Rudolf, K., Eberlein, W., Engel, W., Wieland, H.A., Willim, K.D., Entzeroth, M., Wienen, W., Beck-Sickinger, A.G. & Doods, H.N. (1994) The first highly potent and selective non-peptide neuropeptide Y Y1 receptor antagonist: BIBP3226. *Eur. J. Pharmacol.* **271**, R11–R13.

Sautel, M., Martinez, R., Munoz, M., Peitsch, M.C., Beck-Sickinger, A.G. & Walker, P. (1995) Role of a hydrophobic pocket of the human Y1 neuropeptide Y receptor in ligand binding. *Mol. Cell. Endocrinol.* **112**, 215–222.

Schwartz, T.W., Sheikh, S.P. & O'Hare, M.M.T. (1987) Receptors on phaeochromocytoma cells for two members of the PP-fold family – NPY and PP. *FEBS Lett.* **225**, 209–214.

Schwartz, T.W., Gether, U., Schambye, H.T. & Hjort, S.A. (1995) Molecular mechanism of action of non-peptide ligands for peptide receptors. *Curr. Pharmaceut Design* **1**, 355–372.

Wahlestedt, C., Pich, E.M., Koob, G.F., Yee, F. & Heilig, M. (1993) Modulation of anxiety and neuropeptide Y-Y1 receptors by antisense oligonucleotides. *Science* **259**, 528–531.

Walker, P., Munoz, M., Martinez, R. & Peitsch, M.C. (1994) Acidic residues in extracellular loops of the human Y1 neuropeptide Y receptor are essential for ligand binding. *J. Biol. Chem.* **269**, 2863–2869.

Wharton, J., Gordon, L., Byrne, J., Herzog, H., Selbie, L.A., Moore, K., Sullivan, M.H.F., Elder, M.G., Moscoso, G., Taylor, K.M., Shine, J. & Polak, J.M. (1993) Expression of the human neuropeptide tyrosine Y1 receptor. *Proc. Natl Acad. Sci. USA* **90**, 687–691.

Whitcomb, D.C., Taylor, I.L. & Vigna, S.R. (1990) Characterization of saturable binding sites for circulating pancreatic polypeptide in rat brain. *Am. J. Physiol.* **259**, G687–G691.

Zhang, X., Wiesenfeld-Hallin, Z. & Hökfelt, T. (1994) Effect of peripheral axotomy on expression of neuropeptide Y receptor mRNA in rat lumbar dorsal root ganglia. *Eur. J. Neurosci.* **6**, 43–57.

CHAPTER 6

THE IMPORTANCE OF VARIOUS PARTS OF THE NPY MOLECULE FOR RECEPTOR RECOGNITION

Annette G. Beck-Sickinger

Table of Contents

6.1 Neuropeptide Y: sequence and secondary structure

When the sequences of all the members of the vertebrate pancreatic polypeptide (PP) hormone family, also called the neuropeptide Y (NPY) hormone family, are compared, several general characteristics are obvious, such as the chain length of 36 amino acids and the C-terminal amidation. Positions that never change are: Pro at positions 2, 5 and 8, Gly at position 9, Ala at position 12, Tyr at positions 20 and 27, as well as the C-terminal sequence Thr^{32}-Arg-Xaa-Arg-Tyr^{36}-NH_2. The only exceptions are ovine (Ser^2) and alligator (Phe^{36}) PPs. The C-terminal amidation can even be concluded for those hormones whose sequences have been determined by sequencing their structural gene, because in the prohormone sequence a Gly follows the C-terminal residue (Larhammar et al., 1993).

The high number of conserved residues suggests that a similar three-dimensional structure is present in all members of this hormone family. Information about this has been obtained through the work of Blundell and co-workers, who performed X-ray analyses on the avian (turkey) polypeptide (aPP) to identify the three-dimensional structure (Glover et al., 1983). Accordingly, crystalline aPP assumes the so-called hairpin structure. Residues 1–8 form a type II proline helix followed by a loop (residues 9–14), which is bound to an α-helix (amino acids 15–32). The four C-terminal amino acids are arranged flexibly in a loop. The highly conserved residues of the proline helix and the amphiphilic α-helix interact by hydrophobic interactions and lead to the hairpin structure (Figure 1). Comparative circular dichroism measurements of different

Table 1 A selection of peptides frequently used for the pharmacological characterization of NPY receptors

	Y1	Y2	Y3	Y4/PP1	PYY	Feeding
NPY	++	++	++	—	+	++
PYY	++	++	—	+	++	++
NPY2–36	—	++	+	—	++	++
NPY13–36	—	++	+	—	?	—
[Ahx$^{5-24}$]NPY	—	++	?	?	++	?
[Ahx$^{8-20}$]NPY	+	+	?	—	?	?
[Ahx$^{8-20}$, Pro^{34}]NPY	+	—	?	+	?	?
[Pro^{34}]NPY	++	—	+	+	?	+
PP	—	—	—	++	—	—

++ High affinity, + moderate affinity, — no affinity, ? not reported

PPs, NPY and their fragments confirm the high content of α-helical structures, and indicate that the polypeptides from different species investigated so far are built according to the same structural principles (Glover *et al.*, 1985; Krstenansky and Buck, 1987; Tonan *et al.*, 1990).

The conformation of the α-helical segment of NPY could be further confirmed by ^{1}H-nuclear magnetic resonance (NMR) investigations in various solvents, including water, dimethylsulphoxide and trifluoroethanol (Saudek and Pelton, 1990; Mierke *et al.*, 1992). Different numbers of amino acids participating in the helix were, however, found and a helical segment composed of amino acids 11–36, 16–36 and 19–34 is suggested in water, dimethylsulphoxide and trifluoroethanol, respectively. Darbon *et al.* (1992) successfully carried out a ^{1}H-NMR study on NPY monomers in water and the subsequent structural elucidation. In addition to the α-helical segment, long-range NOEs were found that defined the geometry of the residues 11–14 to form the hairpin loop. Owing to the small number of the sequential NOEs, a secondary structure of the segment 1–10 could not be determined. However, the position and orientation of the N-terminal amino acid relative to the C-terminal helix could be established by a series of long-range NOEs. Interestingly, NOEs are always the result of interaction between the side chains, the backbone atoms are not involved. The secondary structure obtained by the NMR investigation is in agreement with the model of Allen *et al.* (1987) obtained by homology modelling.

6.2 Analogues for the characterization of the receptor types

In 1986, Wahlestedt *et al.* predicted the occurrence of two receptor types, the so-called Y1 and Y2 receptors. While the entire NPY molecule is required for the binding to the Y1 receptor, C-terminal segments of NPY (NPY13–36, NPY18–36) show only a slightly diminished affinity and activity (5–10-fold) at the Y2 receptors (Figure 2). Furthermore,

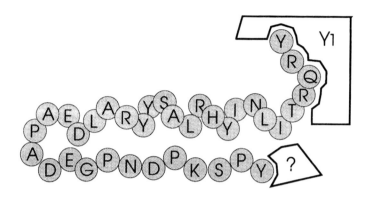

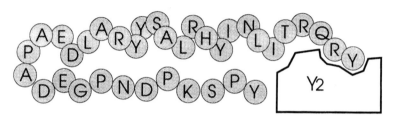

Figure 1 Sequence and schematic structure of the binding of NPY to the Y1 and Y2 receptors.

using discontinuous analogues (Beck *et al.*, 1989; Krstenansky *et al.*, 1989), it was possible to develop highly selective Y2 receptor agonists (Beck-Sickinger *et al.*, 1992). By replacing one or two amino acid residues, Fuhlendorff *et al.* (1990a) succeeded in the preparation of the Y1 receptor selective agonists [Pro³⁴]NPY and [Leu³¹,Pro³⁴]NPY.

Most of the NPY studies using isolated organs or cells have shown the related hormone PYY to be equipotent with NPY. However, in the rat brainstem and heart as well as in the chromaffin cells of bovine adrenal glands, NPY binding sites have been found that bind PYY at least a hundred-fold less strongly (Grundemar *et al.*, 1991; Wahlestedt *et al.*, 1992). These binding sites have been designated as Y3 receptors (Michel, 1991). A great variance in the selectivity is reported by different research groups. While Wahlestedt *et al.* (1992) describe the binding of PP, NPY13–36 (Y2 receptor agonist) and [Leu³¹,Pro³⁴]NPY (Y1 receptor agonist) to Y3 receptors, Dumont *et al.* (1993) found that the NPY loop region is of significance for the affinity to Y3 receptor (Table 1).

A PYY-preferring receptor has been described in the small intestine by the modest preference for PYY over NPY (5–10-fold) (Laburthe *et al.*, 1986). As this receptor binds centrally truncated analogues, such as [Ahx⁵⁻²⁴]NPY (Beck-Sickinger *et al.*, unpublished), this receptor might be a Y2-receptor-like subtype.

Another receptor has been characterized by intracerebroventriclar or hypo-thalamic administration of NPY to rats, which resulted in an increase in feeding behaviour (Stanley and Leibowitz, 1984). As [Pro^{34}]NPY and PYY are equipotent as NPY, and NPY13–36 shows reduced activity, the receptor has been called Y1-like. However, as NPY2–36 fully stimulates the increase of feeding, there are significant differences and a different subtype might be possible as well (Kalra and Crowley, 1992; Stanley *et al.*, 1992).

The sequence of the Y1-receptor from rat (Eva *et al.*, 1990; Krause *et al.*, 1992) and from human (Herzog *et al.*, 1992; Larhammar *et al.*, 1992) tissue has been identified on a molecular level, and the selectivity of the analogues as found in cell lines and tissues could be confirmed. Recently, the human Y2-receptor types (Gerald *et al.*, 1995; Rose *et al.*, 1995) and the human PP1 receptor (Lundell *et al.*, 1995), also called the Y4 receptor (Bard *et al.*, 1995) have been cloned as well. While the pharmacology of the Y2 receptor could be confirmed by the cloned one, some interesting features were found for the PP1/Y4 receptor (Lundell *et al.*, 1996). Human PP is bound with a very high affinity as well as the long C-terminal segments PP2–36 and PP3–36. The affinity for PYY is reduced by 1–2 orders of magnitude while [Pro^{34}]PYY binds almost as effectively as PP. NPY and its segments are less potent than NPY (Gehlert *et al.*, 1996; see also, Larhammar, this volume).

6.3 Structure–activity relationships

Structure–affinity and structure–activity relationships can be used to characterize the interaction between the hormone and its receptor, and to identify the ligand segments that are important. In the case of peptide hormones, the essential segments for recep-tor recognition will be distinguished from the non-essential ones by using shorter peptide sequences. The significance of each sequence position can be assessed by the substitution of amino-acid residues. However, it should not be underestimated that each amino acid has influence on the secondary structure, the dipole moment and the hydrophobicity of the hormone. Consequently, it is very difficult to estimate the importance of different effects and thus to identify the reason for an affinity loss. Principally, however, structure–activity relationship studies furnish valuable informa-tion for the development of small hormone analogues or even non-peptidic lead struc-tures, for the characterization of receptor subtypes and for development of a hormone receptor interaction model. As the Y1 and the Y2 receptors have been characterized a long time ago, most studies were performed using tissues or cell lines that exclusively express those receptors.

6.3.1 Related hormones

The related hormone PYY binds to the Y1 receptor as well as to the Y2 receptor as strongly as NPY, although only 70% of the amino acids are identical (Wieland *et al.*,

1995). By contrast, neither PP nor NPY-OH, an analogue in which the C-terminal tyrosine-amide has been substituted by tyrosine, were recognized by these two receptor types. The feeding receptor recognizes PYY as well, while the Y3 receptor does not bind PYY (Table 1). The PP1/Y4 receptor binds PYY better than NPY, however, both lack affinity compared to PP (Gehlert and Hipskind, 1995).

6.3.2 Segments

The Y1 receptor type can be distinguished from the Y2 receptor by the fact that the former cannot recognize the C-terminal segment and thus only the entire NPY molecule possesses high Y1 receptor affinity. This fact has been verified by many studies, which showed that NPY2–36 possesses only part of the affinity of NPY in the Y1-receptor-mediated systems (Wieland et al., 1995). Shorter segments such as PYY3–36, NPY4–36 or NPY22–36 show a significantly reduced Y1 receptor affinity. All N-terminal segments, such as NPY1–12 or NPY1–24, are completely inactive (Danho et al., 1988). However, C-terminally modified analogues of the 36-mer peptide partially maintain some binding properties on the Y1 receptor system as shown recently (Hoffmann et al., 1996). Various amines, alcohols and modified tyrosine residues have been coupled to NPY1–35 in order to better understand the importance of the C-terminus. It could be confirmed, that the C-terminal tyrosine-amide of NPY is essential for its affinity to the Y1 receptor-type. Obviously, the amino group of the amide part is more important than the oxygen atom of the carbonyl group, as NPY1–35-tyrosinol shows a lower affinity than NPY1–35-tyrosine–thioamide. This is in good agreement with the recently suggested binding mode of Tyr[36] (Sautel et al., 1995). NPY1–35–tyramide could be shown to act as an antagonist in a Ca^{2+} release assay in human neuroblastoma cells. Analogues of NPY1–35–tyramide showed the same structure–affinity relationships as NPY itself, suggesting that there exists a similar binding mode for the agonist and the antagonist (Table 2).

The C-terminal segments 13–36 (Wahlestedt et al., 1986), 16–36 (Colmers et al., 1991), 18–36 (Feinstein et al., 1992; Boublik et al., 1989a,b) and 25–36 (Grundemar and Håkanson, 1990; Beck-Sickinger et al., 1990b) have been identified as agonists in different Y2 receptor assays. In human neuroblastoma cell line SMS-KAN cells NPY2–36 and PYY3–36 bind with about the same affinity as NPY, whereas NPY13–36 and NPY18–36 are about ten times less efficient (Wieland et al., 1995).

By modifying NPY Ac-25–36, it could be shown that the affinity to Y2 receptors still persists even after the exchange of up to six amino acids by alanine, as long as the helix remains stable (Jung et al., 1991). The affinity and activity of NPY Ac-25–36 can be increased by a factor of 20 by substituting the hydrophobic amino acids Leu[30] and Ile[31] by cyclohexylalanine (Chx). As a result, [Chx[30,31]]NPY Ac-25–36 represents a compound with an affinity to the Y2 receptor in the nanomolar range in rabbit kidney membranes and in human LN319 cells (Beck-Sickinger et al., 1993a,b). However, not only its affinity is increased by Chx-containing NPY Ac-25–36 peptides, the activity in the rat vas deferens assay is also increased 6–8 times compared to Ac-25–36. In contrast, peptides, which contain Ala or Gly at positions 28–32 show only little loss of

Table 2 Summary of peptide analogues of NPY with high selectivity or reported antagonistic activity

	Y1 affinity/antagonism	Y2 affinity/antagonism	Feeding receptor affinity/antagonism
PYX-2	—	—	?/+
[D-Trp^{32}]NPY	—	—	?/+
[D-Tyr^{27,36},D-Thr^{32}]NPY27–36	—	—	?/+
[Tyr^{32},Leu^{34}]NPY27–36	+/−	+/?	?
[Pro^{30},Tyr^{32},Leu^{34}]NPY27–36	+/+	+/?	?
([Lys^{29},Pro^{30},Dpr^{31},Tyr^{32},Leu^{34}] NPY28–36)$_2$	+/+	+/?	?
NPY1–35-tyramide	+/+	+/?	?
[ε-Lys^{28}-γ-Glu^{32}]NPY Ac-25–36	—	+/−	?
[desAA$^{10-17}$,Cys^7,Cys^{21}Pro^{34}]NPY	+/−	—	—

— no affinity, +/+ affinity and NPY antagonism, +/− affinity but no NPY antagonism, ? not reported affinity but significant loss of activity. Therefore, we conclude that large hydrophobic residues at positions 28, 30 and/or 31 are involved in transmission of Y2 receptor activity (Figure 2).

While NPY27–36 binds to the Y2 receptor with very low affinity, the modified C-terminal segment [Tyr^{32},Leu^{34}]NPY27–36 increases Y2 receptor affinity by three orders of magnitude. The replacement of Thr^{32} by Tyr^{32} is speculated to imitate Tyr^{1}. However, it also increases the hydrophobicity in this segment, which is important for high Y2 receptor affinity as well. Helicity of the peptide is maintained according to circular dichroism studies (Leban *et al.*, 1995). Further investigations showed that even the modified pentapeptide [Tyr,^{32},Leu^{34}]NPY32–36 showed some affinity (IC$_{50}$ 3500 nM) and optimization led to [His^{32},Leu^{34}]NPY32–36 with an IC$_{50}$ value of 450 nM at rat Y2 receptors (Daniels *et al.*, 1995b; see also, Daniels *et al.*, this volume).

6.3.3 Centrally truncated analogues

Because of the low Y1 receptor affinity of the N- and C-terminal segments, discontinuous analogues, which consist of a short N-terminal segment bound to a longer C-terminal segment via a spacer, have been constructed (Beck *et al.*, 1989). However linear peptides such as [Ahx$^{5-24}$]NPY (Ahx=6-aminohexanoic acid) show only a low affinity at the Y1 receptor. Similar results have been obtained for [Ahx$^{5-17}$]NPY and its analogues (Dumont *et al.*, 1993).

Krstenansky *et al.* (1989) synthesized N- and C-terminally elongated segments and cycled them by disulphide bridges. Thus, [Aoc$^{8-17}$, D-Cys^{7}, Cys^{20}]NPY (Aoc=8-aminooctanoic acid) showed significant Y1 receptor in the mouse brain (Krstenansky *et al.*, 1990) and in human neuroblastoma cell line SK-N-MC cells (Gordon *et al.*, 1990). Kirby *et al.* (1993b) succeeded in optimizing the NPY affinity through the exchange of the configuration, the spacer and the position of cyclization, and synthesized [Gly$^{9-17}$, L-Cys^{7}, Cys^{21}]NPY. However, since a single substitution always leads to a reduction of the affinity, it becomes evident how sensitive the Y1 receptor is against positioning of the N- and C-terminus. Recent investigations showed that linear discontinuous analogues also are able to bind to the Y1 receptor (Rist *et al.*, 1995). However, it is evident that by a given N-terminal length, there exists only one optimal length for the C-terminal segment. For an N-terminus consisting of amino acids 1–5 or 1–6, an optimal C-terminus would consist of the NPY segment 20–36. If the former consists of seven residues, the latter should contain of the fragment NPY21–36. This indicates that the orientation of the N- and C-terminus to each other is of great significance. A long N-terminus requires a short C-terminus and vice versa. If there are eight N-terminal amino acid residues, this can no longer be compensated for and therefore a further helix winding will be required in order to orient the N- and C-terminus towards each other. Analogues with high Y1 receptor affinity are [Ahx$^{8-20}$]NPY and [Ahx$^{8-21}$]NPY. Thus, either Y1 receptor recognizes a discontinuous binding site – perhaps segments of the N-terminal backbone are required – or this segment is capable of stabilizing the receptor conformation of the C-terminus only by having a defined conformation (Figure 3).

Structure–activity relationship studies of Y2 receptor ligands were obtained by the development of novel discontinuous analogues of NPY [Ahx$^{5-24}$]NPY, [Aoc$^{5-24}$]NPY and [Tic$^{5-24}$]NPY (Tic = 1,2,3,4-tetrahydroisoquinoline-3-carboxylic acid), which show high affinity at the rabbit Y2 receptor and at human Y2 receptor expressing cell lines SMS-KAN and LN319 (Beck-Sickinger *et al.*, 1990b, 1993, 1994a). With the availability of these considerably shortened, synthetically easily prepared analogues with a strong affinity to the Y2 receptor, a structure was now available that could systematically be varied, and by which the relevance of each amino-acid residue could be studied. Substitution of each amino acid of [Ahx$^{5-24}$]NPY by L-alanine, glycine and the corresponding D-enantiomer showed that the C-terminal pentapeptide Thr-Arg-Gln-Arg-Tyr-NH$_2$ is very crucial for high Y2 receptor affinity (Beck-Sickinger *et al.*, 1990a). It has also been demonstrated that residues 25–31 can be varied without a significant loss of Y2 receptor affinity as long as the α-helical conformation remains intact. Furthermore, the N-terminal segment can strongly be modified and consequently it serves to stabilize the helix beyond the hydrophobic interactions. This model was refined by the synthesis of analogues containing unusual, non-protein and conformation restricting amino acids, which enabled to study the influence of each residue of [Ahx$^{5-24}$]NPY at the Y2 receptor (recently reviewed by Beck-Sickinger and Jung, 1995).

6.3.4 Systematic scanning in full-length NPY

Substitution of one of the amino acids by L-alanine (Forest *et al.*, 1990), or by a corresponding D-amino acid (Boublik *et al.*, 1989a; Kirby *et al.*, 1993a), leads to a significantly lower affinity or activity at the Y1 receptor, particularly at position 5. In order to characterize the importance of each of the residues in NPY, 36 analogues were synthesized, containing single amino-acid substitutions. For all substitutions, L-alanine was chosen, except for the natural alanyl positions 12, 14, 18 and 23, which were replaced by glycine (Beck-Sickinger *et al.*, 1994b). All the analogues containing substituted amino acids at positions 8–18 show a slightly reduced affinity with up to tenfold higher IC$_{50}$ values, except for Pro^2 and Pro^5. This leads to the speculation that none of these residues is directly involved in interactions in binding pockets of the receptor; however, they influence the affinity conformation by changing the conformation or orientation. At the C-terminal region of the helix containing residues 19–32, both sensitive and less sensitive amino-acid residues are alternately located. It is interesting to note that 1–2 sensitive residues are followed by 2–3 less sensitive ones, so that a wave pattern is formed. Since the sensitive positions Tyr^{20}, Leu^{24}, Tyr^{27} and Ile^{31} correlate with the hydrophobic side of the amphiphilic α-helix, it seems that either the hydrophobicity itself, its influence on the association with the N-terminus or its effect on the relevant amino acids is decisive for the Y1 receptor affinity. The C-terminal pentapeptide seems to be required for the receptor binding at the Y1 receptor. However, Arg^{33} and Arg^{35} are the most sensitive residues and their substitution increases the IC$_{50}$ value by about 10^4-fold. [Ala^{34}]NPY shows only a 10-fold lower affinity, in contrast to the 60-fold lower affinity at the Y2 receptor.

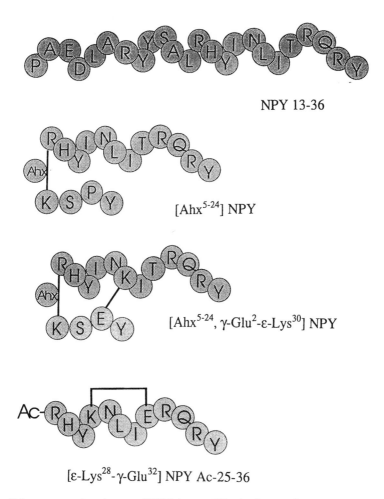

NPY 13-36

[Ahx$^{5-24}$] NPY

[Ahx$^{5-24}$, γ-Glu^2-ε-Lys^{30}] NPY

[ε-Lys^{28}-γ-Glu^{32}] NPY Ac-25-36

Figure 2 Segments and analogues of NPY that are Y2 selective agonists.

Whereas the direct interactions of side chains at the receptors are best investigated using L-alanine substituted analogues, a D-amino-acid scan provides information on the orientation and steric prerequisites. The D-enantiomer-containing analogues in a previously reported D-scan (Kirby *et al.*, 1993a) bound less efficiently to the Y1 receptor compared to NPY and the L-alanine-containing peptides. D-Substitutions at position 2–5 and [D-Tyr^{20}]NPY and [D-Tyr^{21}]NPY showed the strongest reduction of affinity in addition to the substitution within the C-terminal octapeptide. Exchanges of the configuration of any residue of the segment NPY29–36 were not tolerated and caused a more than 100-fold loss of affinity.

The results from the investigations on [Ahx$^{5-24}$]NPY (Beck-Sickinger *et al.*, 1990a) are only partially in agreement with the alanine-scan of full-length NPY (Beck-

Sickinger et al., 1994b) tested in a Y2 receptor assay. All the analogues with alanine substitutions in the segment 1–18 show a five-fold increased IC_{50} value, at the most, except for [Ala^5]NPY and [Ala^8]NPY. In the region of the C-terminal segment the sensitivity of the analogues in which Arg^{19}, Tyr^{20} and Tyr^{27} have been replaced becomes conspicuous. This indicated that the affinity conformation at the Y2 receptor may be stabilized by interactions between Pro^8 and Tyr^{20} as well as between Pro^5 and Tyr^{27}. The importance of the C-terminal pentapeptide for Y2 receptor affinity could be confirmed by this investigation. Whether the differences found signify a species selectivity of Y2 receptor (rabbit versus human) or whether certain substitutions can be compensated in the whole hormone, which is not possible in the case of short peptides, must be investigated.

In both investigations the sensitivity of residues 35 and 36 has been confirmed. An affinity loss of 10^4-fold indicates a direct interaction of Arg^{35}-Tyr^{36}-NH$_2$ with the human Y2 receptor. Since, however, NPY 32–36-NH$_2$ is inactive (Fuhlendorff et al., 1990b), additional amino-acid residues or mimetics are required in order to stabilize the active conformation of the C-terminal part of NPY.

The D-amino-acid scan of NPY1–36 (Kirby et al., 1993a) confirms the results obtained by the D-amino-acid scan of [Ahx$^{5-24}$]NPY (Beck-Sickinger et al., 1990a). None of the residues of the N-terminal or middle segment of NPY is sensitive for D-enantiomer substitution with respect to Y2 affinity. In the C-terminal segment, analogues containing D-amino acids at one position between Leu^{30} and Arg^{35} showed reduced affinity to the Y2 receptors. [D-Arg^{33}]NPY and [D-Gln^{34}]NPY were found to be the compounds with the lowest Y2 receptor affinity, whereas Tyr^{36} can be replaced by D-Tyr with only a moderate loss.

6.3.5 Conformationally constrained analogues

Although small peptides are very flexible in solution, they can adopt a very specific conformation at their receptors. Different receptor subtypes, however, may recognize different conformations of the same peptide. In order to characterize these subtypes, but also to find smaller selective peptides or finally non-peptide drugs, the knowledge of the bioactive conformation of a neuropeptide agonist or antagonist is of main concern in structure–activity studies. In this section, attempts to constrain the conformation of a NPY or segments are described, which include the incorporation of proline, D-amino acids and non-protein amino acids. Replacement of L-amino acids by D-amino acids frequently leads to antagonists. Incorporation of proline or homologues of proline induces a turn structure, which can be an important constraint. Another method to obtain more rigid molecules is the synthesis of cyclopeptides, which stabilizes a reduced number of conformations compared to the linear peptide.

Exchange of a single amino acid by Pro can induce or stabilize a turn conformation. The most famous analogue is [Pro^{34}]NPY, which is a Y1-receptor-selective compound, and still provides the only possibility of losing Y2-receptor affinity, without losing Y1-receptor binding (Fuhlendorff et al., 1990b) of peptide analogues. Recent investigations showed, however, that Pro^{34} is also important for analogues binding to the PP1/Y4 receptor and, for example, [Pro^{34}]PYY shows nanomolar affinity to this type (Gehlert et al., 1996). These results suggest that a turn conformation at the C-terminus is important for receptor recognition of NPY at the Y1 and the PP1/Y4 receptor, whereas the Y2 receptor requires a different orientation of the residues, perhaps an extended helix. The exchange of Tyr^{20} by Pro leads to a significant change in the conformation of NPY – the major helix is destroyed – and to inactive compounds (Fuhlendorff et al., 1990b). Replacement of Ile^{30} by Pro in a modified analogue of NPY27–36 is reported to stabilize a turn formed by Asn^{29} (CO-sidechain) to Ile^{31} (NH-backbone) and to turn an agonist in an Y1-receptor antagonist ([Pro^{30},Tyr^{32},Leu^{34}]NPY27–36) (Leban et al., 1995) (Table 2).

Several analogues of NPY, which contain D-amino acids besides the D-amino-acid scan have been investigated. [D-Trp^{20}]NPY, [D-Trp^{21}]NPY, [D-Tyr^{20}]NPY and [D-Tyr^{21}]NPY are analogues that do not bind to the Y1 receptor (Martel et al., 1990). [D-Trp^{32}]NPY (Balasubramaniam et al., 1994) and [3,5-dichlorobenzyl-Tyr^{27,36}, D-Trp^{32}]NPY Ac-27–36 (PYX2; Tatemoto et al., 1992), which show neither Y1 nor Y2 receptor affinity (Wieland et al., 1995) have been characterized as feeding receptor antagonists (Leibowitz et al., 1992; Dryden et al., 1994). A multiply modified analogue of NPY [D-Tyr^{27,36},D-Thr^{32}]NPY27–36 has been reported to antagonize feeding effects of NPY as well, which suggests that a D-amino acid at position 32 might play an important role in antagonizing the food intake effects of NPY (Myers et al., 1995).

Using cyclic peptides, a number of selective Y2 receptor agonists are reported. By cyclization of the N- and C-terminal segments of the discontinuous analogues, peptides have been obtained which showed strong affinity to the Y2 but no affinity to the Y1 receptor. These highly active Y2 receptor agonists display a selectivity which is 40-fold greater than that of the frequently used NPY13–36. The affinity is neither influenced by the position, site and nature of the rings, nor by the spacer between N- and C-terminal segments. [Aoc$^{5-24}$, Cys^{2}, Cys^{27}]NPY (Krstenansky et al., 1989), [Ahx$^{5-24}$,Glu^{2}-Lys^{30}]NPY (Beck-Sickinger et al., 1992) and [D-Ala$^{6-24}$,Glu^{2} D-Dpr^{27}]NPY (Dpr = 1,3-diaminopropionic acid; Reymond et al., 1992) showed almost the same Y2 receptor selectivity. A change of the configuration of the bridge amino acids, orientation and position of the bridge (Hoffmann et al., 1992, 1993) did not lower the affinity, as long as the helical conformation at the C-terminal segment was not destroyed. Cyclization across the C-terminus as in [Ahx$^{5-24}$,Glu^{31}-Tyr-HMD]NPY (HMD = 1,6-hexamethylenediamine; Beck-Sickinger et al., 1993c) or across the C-terminal amino-acid residues as in [Lys^{33}-Glu^{36}]NPY and [Lys^{30}-Glu^{34}]NPY18–36 (Reymond et al., 1992) drastically reduces the Y2 receptor affinity. Molecular dynamic simulation of [Ahx$^{5-24}$,γ-Glu^{2}-ε-Lys^{30}]NPY showed, that owing to the cyclization a large hydrophobic site, which is formed by the side chains of the residues 28 and 31, becomes accessible to the receptor. Since cyclization via the N-terminus and residue 31 leads to a significantly lower activity (Beck-Sickinger et al., 1993c), we can confirm the results from the Chx-containing analogues of Ac-25–36; the hydrophobic patch is important for signal transduction. Further optimization of the C-terminal dodecapeptide Ac-25–36 finally led to a very rigid, small molecule with very high affinity, selectivity and signal-transduction effects comparable to NPY itself (Rist *et al.*, 1996a): NPY [ε-Lys^{28}-γ-Glu^{32}]NPY Ac-25–36. NMR studies have provided insight in the conformation of NPY at the Y2 receptor by investigating this low-molecular-weight analogue (Rist *et al.*, 1996b). Kirby *et al.* (1995) recently published a series of cyclic 28-mer peptides, which varied in the position and the configuration of the cystine bridge: an analogue with a L-Cys^2/L- or D-Cys^{27} bridge led to Y2-receptor-selective compounds, whereas L-Cys^7/L-Cys^{21} maintained Y1 receptor affinity. Further incorporation of Pro^{34} led to a Y1-receptor-selective cyclopeptide, which was inactive in the feeding assay but was able to lower blood pressure. This suggests again, that the feeding activity is transmitted by a different receptor than the one that increases blood pressure. Dimers, obtained by bridging two molecules of [Pro^{30},Tyr^{32},Leu^{34}]NPY28–36 at position 29 and 31 led to compounds with high Y1 receptor and Y2 receptor affinity. In addition Y1 receptor antagonism has been reported for this type of compound (Daniels *et al.*, 1995a).

While the significance of each side chain for receptor interaction can be investigated by substituting the individual amino acids, information concerning the relevance of the backbone can be obtained by backbone modifications. Introduction of reduced peptide bonds, -CH$_2$NH- instead of -CO-NH-, at distinct positions of NPY has been described by Schwartz (1993). [Gln^{34}-φ[CH$_2$NH]-Arg^{35}NPY and [Arg^{35}-φ[CH$_2$NH]Tyr^{36}]NPY were the peptides that lack Y1-receptor affinity whereas [Gln^{34}-φ[CH$_2$NH]-Arg^{35}NPY and especially [Arg^{33}-φ[CH$_2$NH]-Gln^{34}]NPY are unable to bind to the Y2 receptor. Sensitivity of the backbone residues 34–35 at the Y2 receptor could be confirmed by using retro-inverso analogues (Dürr *et al.*, 1992, 1993). [Ahx$^{5-24}$, Gln^{34}-φ[NHCO]-Arg^{35}]NPY binds to the rabbit kidney membranes with a significantly reduce affinity compared to [Ahx$^{5-24}$]NPY.

6.4 A model of active conformations

The results discussed above indicate that NPY interacts differently with Y1 and Y2 receptors. This is plausible since molecular dynamic simulations reveal several low-energy secondary structures (Beck-Sickinger *et al.*, 1994b). In the following, an attempt is made to develop a model of the receptor active conformations of NPY. With respect to the Y1 receptor binding, the amino acids Arg^{33} and Arg^{35} of NPY are especially sensitive towards a substitution by alanine. Gln^{34} can be replaced by the turn inducing amino acid Pro, whereas neither the helix stabilizing amino acid Ala nor D-Gln or D-Pro are very well tolerated at this position. The conformation and orientation of both N- and C-terminal octapeptide are of importance for the Y1 affinity as could be demonstrated by the D-amino-acid scan, by discontinuous analogues and by cyclic peptides. The most sensitive backbone bonds are those between Arg^{35}-Tyr^{36} and Gln^{34}-Arg^{35}. Replacements of residues, which are possibly involved in the interaction between N- and C-terminal segment, lead to a significant loss of Y1 receptor affinity. Thus, the structure–activity relationships at the Y1 receptor can be aligned with the three-dimensional structures depicted in Plate 3. Accordingly,

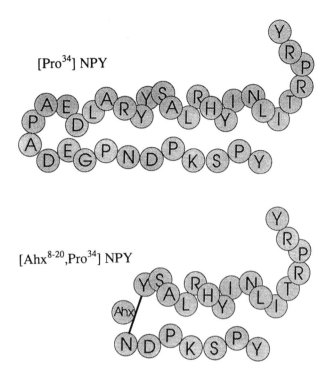

Figure 3 Segments and analogues of NPY that are Y1-selective agonists.

the N-terminus is associated with the C-terminal segment and hydrophobic interactions can be assumed. The C-terminal tetrapeptide adopts a turn-like structure. The correct folding and orientation of which is of utmost importance for the affinity is stabilized by the α-helix, which in turn will be oriented correctly by the N-terminal segment. A different method of stabilization could be performed by π–π interactions of Tyr^{32} and Tyr^{36} as reported for $[Tyr^{32},Leu^{34}]NPY27-36$. While the side chains are responsible for the interactions of the N- and C-terminus, stabilization of the C-terminal turn can be accomplished by hydrogen bonding via peptide bonds of Gln^{34}-Arg^{35} and/or Arg^{35}-Tyr^{36}. This conformation is very close to the original secondary structure of PPs. Since PPs contain histidine or proline at position 34, the C-terminal turn could represent the Y1/PP binding conformation. Various peptide and non-peptide antagonists have been reported recently at the Y1 receptor. They clearly point out that minimal changes can convert an agonist into an antagonist as shown for NPY (agonist) and NPY1–35–tyramide (antagonist) and for $[Tyr^{32},Leu^{34}]NPY27-36$ (agonist) and $[Pro^{30},Tyr^{32},Leu^{34}]NPY27-36$ (antagonist). As all antagonists show modification in the C-terminal segment of the molecule and as the non-peptide antagonist BIBP 3226 that has been derived from the C-terminal dipeptide (Rudolf et al., 1994) was shown to provide a large overlapping binding site with NPY (Sautel et al., 1996), it can be concluded that the C-terminus of NPY is

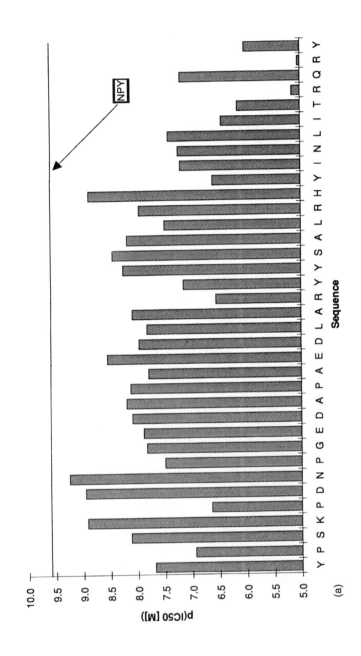

(a)

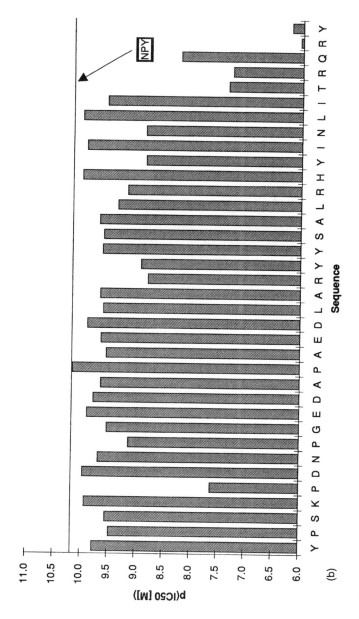

Figure 4 L-Alanine scan of NPY. Affinity of the peptide at (a) SK-N-MC cells (Y1 receptor) and (b) SMS-KAN cells (Y2 receptor) is shown.

important for the binding site to the Y1 receptor. Various approaches to prevent signal transduction are reported.

Summarizing the structure–activity relationships at the Y2 receptor, I conclude that the side chains of Arg^{35} and the aromatic ring of Tyr^{36} are directly involved in the receptor binding. Backbone atoms and/or the correct folding of residues Leu^{30} to Gln^{34} are of major importance. Perhaps the distance between the hydrophobic cluster at positions 28, 30 and 31, which has been suggested for the active site, and the C-terminal dipeptide is of main importance. It has been pointed out that an α-helical conformation is important for the Y2 receptor affinity. A second proposal for the folding of NPY (Plate 1) differs from the first one, so far mainly discussed as a secondary structure (Plate 1), especially regarding the conformation at the C-terminus. In contrast to the NPY conformation with a turn at the C-terminal region containing five amino acid residues, in the second proposed secondary structure the helix is extended to the residue 35. This structure is in accordance with the NMR investigations (Mierke *et al.*, 1992) and with the importance of a pronounced α-helical conformation. The most important side chains, according to the Ala-scan (Arg^{35} and Tyr^{36}), are exposed in this model by the extended α-helix. Therefore, all prerequisites for Y2 receptor affinity, as obtained by structure–affinity studies are fulfilled by this conformation. Consequently, the N-terminus serves only to stabilize the helix. In addition, the Y1 selectivity of $[Pro^{34}]NPY$ as well as the Y2 receptor affinity of $[Gln^{34}]$ PP is in agreement with this structural model. Pro at position 34 breaks the α-helical conformation and stabilizes the Y1 receptor preferred secondary structure, thus it is unable to bind to the Y2 receptor.

References

Allen, J., Novotny, J., Martin, J. & Heinrich, G. (1987) Molecular structure of mammalian neuropeptide Y: analysis by molecular cloning and computer-aided comparison with crystal structure of avian homologue. *Proc. Natl Acad. Sci. USA* **84**, 2532–2536.

Balasubramaniam, A., Sheriff, S., Johnson, M.E., Prabhakaran, M., Huang, Y., Fischer, J.E. & Chance, W.T. (1994) [D-Trp^{32}]neuropeptide Y: a competitive antagonist of NPY in rat hypothalamus. *J. Med. Chem.* **37**, 811–815.

Bard, J.A., Walker, M.W., Branchek, T.A. & Weinshank, R.L. (1995) Cloning and functional expression of a human Y4 subtype receptor for pancreatic polypeptide, neuropeptide Y, and peptide YY. *J. Biol. Chem.* **270**, 26 762–26 765.

Beck, A., Jung, G., Gaida, W., Köppen, H., Lang, R. & Schnorrenberg, G. (1989) Highly potent and small neuropeptide Y agonist obtained by linking NPY 1–4 via spacer to α-helical NPY 25–36. *FEBS Lett.* **244**, 119–122.

Beck-Sickinger, A.G. & Jung, G. (1995) Structure-activity relationship of neuropeptide Y with respect to Y_1 and Y_2-receptors. *Biopolymers* **37**, 123–142.

Beck-Sickinger, A.G., Gaida, W., Schnorrenberg, G., Lang, R. & Jung, G. (1990a) Neuropeptide Y: Identification of the binding site. *Int. J. Pept. Prot. Res.* **36**, 522–530.

Beck-Sickinger, A.G., Jung, G., Gaida, W., Köppen, H., Schnorrenberg, G. & Lang, R. (1990b) Structure-activity relationship of C-terminal neuropeptide Y segments and analogues composed of NPY 1–4 linked to NPY 25–36. *Eur. J. Biochem.* **194**, 449–456.

Beck-Sickinger, A.G., Grouzmann, E., Hoffmann, E., Gaida, W., Van Meier, E.G., Waeber, B. & Jung, G. (1992) A novel cyclic analog of neuropeptide Y specific for the Y_2 receptor. *Eur. J. Biochem.* **206**, 957–964.

Beck-Sickinger, A.G., Dürr, H., Gaida, W. & Jung, G. (1993a) Characterisation of the binding site of neuropeptide Y to the rabbit kidney receptor using multiple peptide synthesis. *Biochem. Soc. Trans.* **20**, 847–850.

Beck-Sickinger, A.G., Hoffmann, E., Gaida, W., Grouzmann, E., Dürr, H. & Jung, G. (1993b) Novel Y2-selective reduced-size agonists of neuropeptide Y. *BioMed. Chem. Lett.* **3**, 937–942.

Beck-Sickinger, A.G., Köppen, H., Hoffmann, E., Gaida, W. & Jung, G. (1993c). Different types of cyclopeptides for the characterisation of the affinity of neuropeptide Y to the Y2-receptor. *J. Receptor Res.* **13**, 215–228.

Beck-Sickinger, A.G., Hoffmann, E., Paulini, K., Reissig, H.-U. Willim, K.-D., Wieland, H.A. & Jung, G. (1994a) High affinity analogues of neuropeptide Y containing conformationally restricted non-proteinogenic amino acids. *Biochem. Soc. Trans.* **22**, 145–149.

Beck-Sickinger, A.G., Wieland, H.A., Wittneben, H., Willim, K.-D., Rudolf, K. & Jung, G. (1994b) Complete L-alanine scan of neuropeptide Y reveals ligands binding to Y_1 and Y_2 receptors with distinguished conformations. *Eur. J. Biochem.* **225**, 947–958.

Boublik, J.H., Scott, N.A., Brown, M.R. & Rivier, J.E. (1989a) Synthesis and hypertensive activity of neuropeptide Y fragments and analogues with modified N- or C-termini of D-substitutions. *J. Med. Chem.* **32**, 597–601.

Boublik, J., Scott, N., Taulane, J. Goodman, M., Brown, M. & Rivier, J. (1989b) Neuropeptide Y and neuropeptide Y18–36 – Structural and biological characterization. *Int. J. Peptide Protein Res.* **33**, 11–15.

Colmers, W.F., Klapstein, G.J., Fournier, A., St-Pierre, S. & Trehere, K.A. (1991) Presynaptic inhibition of neuropeptide Y in rat hippocampal slice *in vitro* is mediated by a Y2 receptor. *J. Pharmacol.* **102**, 41–44.

Danho, W., Triscari, J., Vincent, G., Nakajima, T., Taylor, J. & Kaiser, E.T. (1988) Synthesis and biological evaluation of pNPY fragments. *Int. J. Peptide Protein Res.* **32**, 496–505.

Daniels, A.J., Matthews, J.E., Slepetits, R.T., Jansen, M., Viveros, O.H., Tadepalli, A., Harrington, W., Heyer, D., Landavazo, A., Leban, J.J. & Spaltenstein, A. (1995a) High affinity neuropeptide Y receptor antagonists. *Proc. Natl Acad. Sci. USA* **92**, 9067–9071.

Daniels, A.J., Matthews, J.E., Viveros, O.H., Leban, J.J., Cory, M. & Heyer, D. (1995b) Structure-activity relationship of novel pentapeptide neuropeptide Y receptor antagonist is consistent with a noncontinuous epitope for ligand-receptor binding. *Mol. Pharmacology* **48**, 425–432.

Darbon, H., Bernassau, J.-M., Deleuze, C., Chenu, J., Roussel, A. & Cambillau, C. (1992) Solution conformation of human neuropeptide Y by ^1H nuclear magnetic resonance and restrained molecular dynamics. *Eur. J. Biochem.* **209**, 765–771.

Dryden, S., Frankish, H. Wang, Q. & Williams, G. (1994) Neuropeptide Y and energy balance: one way ahead for the treatment of obesity? *Eur. J. Clin. Invest.* **24**, 293–308.

Dumont, Y., Satoh, H., Cadieux, A., Taoudi-Benchekroun, M., Pheng, L.-H., St. Pierre, S., Fornier, A. & Quirion, R. (1993) Evaluation of truncated neuropeptide Y analogues with modifications of the tyrosine residue in position 1 on Y1, Y2 and Y3 receptor sub-types. *Eur. J. Pharmacol.* **238**, 37–45.

Dürr, H., Gaida, W., Schnorrenberg, G., Beck-Sickinger, A.G. and Jung, G. (1992) Continuous versus discontinuous analogues of neuropeptide V. In *Innovation and Perspectives in Solid Phase Synthesis, Peptides, Polypeptides and Oligonucleotides, Macro-organic Reagents and Catalysts* (ed. Epton, R.), 2nd International Symposium, pp. 367–370.

Dürr, H., Wieland, H., Beck-Sickinger, A.G., Jung, G. (1993) Retro-inverso analogs of neuropeptide Y. In *Peptides 1992*, Proc. 22nd Eur. Pept. Symp. (eds. Schneider C. & Eberle, A.), pp. 609–610. Leiden, Escom.

Eva, C., Keinänen, K., Monyer, H., Seeburg, P. & Sprengel, R. (1990) Molecular cloning of a novel G protein coupled receptor that may belong to the neuropeptide receptor family. *FEBS Lett.* **271**, 80–84.

Feinstein, R.D., Boublik, J.H., Kirby, D.A., Spicer, M.A., Craig, A.G., Malwicz, N.A., Scott, N.A., Brown, M.R. & Rivier, J.E. (1992) Structural requirements for neuropeptide Y18–36-evoked hypotension: A systematic study. *J. Med. Chem.* **35**, 2836–2843.

Forest, M., Martel, J.-C., St. Pierre, S., Quirion, R. & Fournier, A. (1990) Structural study of the N-terminal segment of neuropeptide tyrosine. *J. Med. Chem.* **33**, 1615–1619.

Fuhlendorff, J., Gether, U., Aakerlund, L., Langeland-Johansen, N., Thøgersen, H., Melberg, S.G., Olsen, U.B., Tharstrup, O. & Schwartz, T.W. (1990a) [Leu^{31},Pro^{34}] Neuropeptide Y: A specific Y1 receptor agonist. *Proc. Natl Acad. Sci. USA* **87**, 182–186.

Fuhlendorff, J., Langeland-Johansen, N., Melberg, S.G., Thøgersen, H. & Schwartz, T.W. (1990b) The antiparallel pancreatic polypeptide fold in the binding of neuropeptide Y to Y1 and Y2 receptors. *J. Biol. Chem.* **265**, 11 706–11 712.

Gehlert, D.R. (1994) Subtypes of receptors for neuropeptide Y: implications for the targeting of therapeutics. *Life Sci.*, **55**, 551–562.

Gehlert, D.R. & Hipskind, P.A. (1995) *Curr. Pharm. Design* **1**, 327–336.

Gehlert *et al.* (1996) Characterization of the peptide binding requirements for the cloned human pancreatic polypeptide-preferring receptor. *Mol. Pharmacol.* **50**, 112–118.

Gerald, C., Walker, M.W., Vaysse, P.J.J., He, C.G., Branchek, T.A. & Weinshank, R.L. (1995) Expression cloning and pharmacological characterization of a human hippocampal neuropeptide Y/peptide YY Y2 receptor subtype. *J. Biol. Chem.* **270**, 26 758–26 761.

Glover, I., Haneef, I., Pitts, J., Wood, S., Moss, D., Tickle, I. & Blundell, T. (1983) *Biopolymers* **22**, 293–304.

Glover, I.D., Barlow, D.J., Pitts, J.E., Wood, S.P., Tickle, I.J., Blundell, T.L., Tatemoto, K., Kimmel, J.R., Wollmer, A., Strassburger, W. & Zhang, Y.-S. (1985) Conformational studies on the pancreatic polypeptide hormone family. *Eur. J. Biochem.* **142**, 379–385.

Gordon, E.A., Kohout, T.A. & Fishman, P.H. (1990) Characterization of functional neuropeptide Y receptors in a human neuroblastoma cell line. *J. Neurochem.* **55**, 506–513.

Grundemar, L. & Håkanson, R. (1990) Effects of various neuropeptide Y/peptide YY fragments on electrically-evoked contractions of the rat vas deferens. *Br. J. Pharmacol.* **100**, 190–192.

Grundemar, L., Wahlestedt, C. & Reis, D.J. (1991) Long-lasting inhibition of the cardiovascular response to glutamate and the baroreceptor reflex elicited by neuropeptide Y injected into the nucleus tractus solitarius. *J. Pharmacol. Exp. Ther.* **258**, 633–638.

Herzog, H., Hort, Y., Ball, H.J., Hayes, G., Shrine, J. & Selbie, L.A. (1992) Cloned human neuropeptide Y receptors couples to two different messenger systems. *Proc. Natl Acad. Sci. USA* **89**, 5794–5798.

Hoffmann, E., Beck-Sickinger, A.G., Gaida, W. & Jung, G. (1992) Variations on a highly selective cyclic analog of neuropeptide. In *Innovation and Perspectives in Solid Phase Synthesis, Peptides, Polypeptides and Oligonucleotides, Macro-organic Reagents and Catalysts* (ed. Epton, R.), 2nd International Symposium, pp. 89–93. Andover, Intercept.

Hoffmann, E., Grouzmann, E., Beck-Sickinger, A.G. & Jung, G. (1993) Large hydrophobic residues influence the secondary structure and receptor affinity of C-terminal neuropeptide Y analogues. In C. Schneider, A. Eberle (eds.), *Peptides 1992*, Proc. 22nd Eur. Pept. Symp. (eds Schneider, C. & Eberle, A.), pp. 589–590. Leiden, Escom.

Hoffmann, S., Rist, B., Willim, K.D., Videnov, G., Jung, G. & Beck-Sickinger, A.G. (1996) Structure-affinity studies of C-terminally modified analogs of neuropeptide Y led to a novel class of peptidic Y$_1$ receptor antagonists. *Reg. Peptides* (in press).

Jung, G., Beck-Sickinger, A.G., Dürr, H., Gaida, W. & Schnorrenberg, G. (1991) α-Helical, small molecular size analogues of neuropeptide Y: structure-activity-relationships. *Biopolymers* **31**, 613–619.

Kalra, S.P. & Crowley, W.R. (1992) Neuropeptide Y: a novel neuroendocrine peptide in the control of pituitary hormone secretion and its relation to luteinizing hormone. *Front. Neuroendocrinol.* **13**, 1–46.

Kirby, D.A., Boublik, J.H. & Rivier, J.E. (1993a) Neuropeptide Y: Y1 and Y2 affinities of the complete series of analogues with single D-residue substitutions. *J. Med. Chem.* **36**, 3802–3808.

Kirby, D.A., Koerber, S.C., Craig, A.G., Feinstein, R.D., Delmas, L., Brown, M.R. & Rivier, J.E. (1993b) Defining structural requirements for neuropeptide Y receptors using truncated and conformationally restricted analogues. *J. Med. Chem.* **36**, 385–393.

Kirby, D.A., Koerber, S.C., May, J.M., Hagaman, C., Cullen, M.J., Pelleymounter, M.A. & Rivier, J.E. (1995) Y1 and Y2 receptor selective neuropeptide Y analogues: evidence for a Y1 receptor subclass. *J. Med. Chem.* **38**, 4579–4586.

Krause, J., Eva, C., Seeburg, P.H. & Sprengel, R. (1992) Neuropeptide Y1 subtype pharmacology of a recombinantly expressed neuropeptide receptor. *Mol. Pharmacol.* **41**, 817–821.

Krstenansky, J.L. & Buck, S.H. (1987) The synthesis, physical characterization and receptor binding affinity of neuropeptide Y (NPY). *Neuropeptides* **10**, 77–85.

Krstenansky, J.L., Owen, T.J., Buck, S.H., Hagaman, K.A. & McLean, L.R. (1989) Centrally truncated and stabilized porcine neuropeptide Y analogues: design, synthesis and mouse brain receptor binding. *Proc. Natl Acad. Sci. USA* **86**, 4377–4381.

Krstenansky, J.L., Owen, T.J., Payne, M.H., Shatzer, S.A. & Buck, S.H. (1990) C-Terminal modifications of neuropeptide Y and its analogs leading to selectivity for the mosue brain receptor over the porcine spleen receptor. *Neuropeptides* **17**, 117–120.

Laburthe, M., Chenut, B., Rouyer-Fessard, C., Tatemoto, K., Couvineau, A., Servin, A. & Amiranoff, B. (1986) Interaction of peptide YY with rat intestinal epithelial plasma-membranes: binding of the radioiodinated peptide. *Endocrinology* **118**, 1910–1917.

Larhammår, D., Blomqvist, A.G., Yee, F., Jazin, E., Yoo, H. & Wahlestedt, C. (1992) Cloning and functional expression of a human neuropeptide Y/peptide YY receptor of the Y1 type. *J. Biol. Chem.* **267**, 10935–10938.

Larhammår, D., Söderberg, C. & Blomqvist, A.G. (1993) Evolution of the neuropeptide Y family of peptides. In *Biology of Neuropeptide Y* (eds Colmers, W.F. & Wahlestedt, C.). Totowa, NJ, Humana Press.

Leban, J.J., Heyer, D., Landavazo, A., Matthews, J., Aulabaugh, A. & Daniels, A.J. (1995) Novel modified carboxy terminal fragments of neuropeptide Y with high affinity for Y_2 type receptors and potent functional antagonism at a Y_1 type receptor. *J. Med. Chem.* **38**, 1150–1157.

Leibowitz, S.F., Xuereb, M. & Kim, T. (1992) Blockade of natural and neuropeptide Y-induced carbohydrate feeding by a receptor antagonist PYX-2. *Neuroreport 1992*, 3.

Lundell, I., Blomqvist, A.G., Berglund, M., Schober, D.A., Johnson, D., Statnick, M., Gadski, R.A., Gehlert, D.R. & Larhammår, D. (1995) Clotting of a human receptor of the NPY receptor family with high affinity for pancreatic polypeptide and peptide YY. *J. Biol. Chem.* **270**, 29123–29128.

Lundell, I., Statnick, M.A., Johnson, D., *et al.* (1996) The cloned rat pancreatic polypeptide receptor exhibits profound differences to the orthologous human. *Proc. Natl. Acad. Sci. USA* **93**, 5111–5115.

Martel, J.C., Fournier, S.S., Dumont, F., Forest, M. & Quirion, R. (1990) Comparative structural requirements of brain neuropeptide Y binding sites and vas deferens neuropeptide Y receptors. *Mol. Pharmacol.* **38**, 494–502.

Michel, M.C. (1991) Receptors for neuropeptide Y: multiple subtypes and multiple second messengers. *Trends Pharmacol. Sci.* **12**, 389–394.

Mierke, D.F., Dürr, H., Kessler, H. & Jung, G. (1992) Neuropeptide Y: Optimized solid-phase synthesis and conformational analysis in trifluroethanol. *Eur. J. Biochem.* **206**, 39–48.

Myers, R.D., Wooten, M.H., Ames, C.D. & Nyce, J.W. (1995) Anorexic action of a new potential neuropeptide Y antagonist [D-Tyr^{27,36}, D-Thr^{32}]-NPY (27–36) infused into the hypothalamus of the rat. *Brain Res. Bull.* **37**, 237–245.

Reymond, M.T., Delmas, L., Koerber, S.C., Brown, M.R. & Rivier, J.E. (1992) Truncated, branched, and/or cyclic analogues of NPY: Importance of the PP-fold in the design of specific Y2 receptor ligands. *J. Med. Chem.* **35**, 3653–3659.

Rist, B., Wieland, H.A., Willim, K.D. & Beck-Sickinger, A.G. (1995) A rational approach for the development of reduced-size analogues of neuropeptide Y with high affinity to the Y_1 receptor. *J. Pept. Sci.* **1**, 341–348.

Rist, B., Wieland, H.A., Willim, K.D. and Beck-Sickinger, A.G. (1996) Structure-affinity studies of cyclic analogues of neuropeptide Y. In *Innovation and Perspectives in Solid Phase Synthesis, Peptides, Polypeptides and Oligonucleotides, Macro-organic Reagents and Catalysts* (ed. Epton, R.), 4th International Symposium (in press).

Rist, B., Zerbe, O., Ingenhoven, N. *et al.* (1996b) Modified, cyclic analog of neuropeptide Y is the smallest full agonist at the human Y_2-receptor. *FEBS Lett.* (in press).

Rose, P.M., Fernandez, J.S., Lynch, J.S., Frazier, S.T., Fisher, S.M., Kodukula, K., Kienzle, B. & Seetha, R. (1995) Cloning and functional expression of a cDNA encoding a human type 2 neuropeptide Y receptor. *J. Biol. Chem.* **270**, 22 661–22 664.

Rudolf, K., Eberlein, W., Engel, W., Wieland, H.A., Willim, K.D., Entzeroth, M., Wienen, W., Beck-Sickinger, A.G. & Doods, H.N. (1994) The first highly potent and selective non-peptide neuropeptide Y Y_1 receptor antagonist: BIBP 3226. *Eur. J. Pharmacol.* **271**, R11–R13.

Saudek, V. & Pelton, J.T. (1990) Sequence-specific ^{1}H-NMR assignment and secondary structure of neuropeptide Y in aqueous solution. *Biochemistry* **29**, 4509–4515.

Sautel, M., Martinez, R., Munoz, M., Peitsch, M.C., Beck-Sickinger, A.G. & Walker, P. (1995) Role of hydrophobic residues of the human Y_1 neuropeptide Y receptor in ligand binding. *Mol. Cell. Endocrinol.* **112**, 215–222.

Sautel, M., Rudolf, K., Wittneben, H., Herzog, H., Martinez, R., Munoz, M., Eberlein, W., Engel, W., Walker, P. & Beck-Sickinger, A.G. (1996) *Mol. Pharmacol.* **50**, 285–292.

Schwartz, T.W. (1993) Molecular characteristics of NPY receptor subtypes. *Neuropeptide Y Meeting*, Cambridge, Lecture.

Stanley, B.G. & Leibowitz, S.F. (1984) Neuropeptide Y: Stimulation of feeding and drinking by injections into paraventricular nucleus. *Life Sci.* **35**, 2635–2642.

Stanley, B.G., Magdalin, W., Seirafi, A., Nguyen, M.M. & Leibowitz, S.F. (1992) Evidence for neuropeptide Y mediation of eating produced by food deprivation and for a variant of the Y1 receptor mediating this peptide's effect. *Peptides* **13**, 581–587.

Tatemoto, K., Mann, M. & Shimizu, M. (1992) Synthesis of receptor antagonists of neuropeptide Y. *Proc. Natl Acad. Sci. USA* **89**, 1174–1178.

Tonan, K., Kawata, Y. & Hamaguchi, K. (1990) Conformation of isolated fragments of pancreatic polypeptide. *Biochemistry* **29**, 4424–4429.

Wahlestedt, C., Yanaihara, N. & Håkanson, R. (1986) Evidence for different pre- and post-junctional receptors for neuropeptide Y and related peptides. *Reg. Peptides* **13**, 307–318.

Wahlestedt, C., Regunathan, S. & Reis, D.J. (1992) Identification of cultured cells selectively expressing Y1-, Y2- or Y3-type receptors for neuropeptide Y/peptide YY. *Life Sci.* **50**, PL 7–12.

Wieland, H.A., Willim, K.D. & Doods, H.N. (1995) Receptor binding profiles of NPY analogues and fragments in different tissues and cell lines. *Peptides* **16**, 1389–1394.

CHAPTER 7

PEPTIDE ANTAGONISTS OF NEUROPEPTIDE Y: DESIGN, STRUCTURE AND PHARMACOLOGICAL CHARACTERIZATION

Alejandro J. Daniels, Dennis Heyer and Andrew Spaltenstein

Table of Contents

7.1 Background

Neuropeptide Y (NPY) is a linear 36-amino-acid peptide amide first isolated from porcine brain (Tatemoto *et al.*, 1982). NPY is an abundant neuropeptide, widely distributed throughout the peripheral and central nervous systems (Adrian *et al.*, 1983; Lundberg *et al.*, 1984; Gray and Morley, 1986). On the basis of pharmacological effects observed in experimental animals after central or peripheral administration of NPY, the peptide has tentatively been implicated in the regulation of a wide variety of biological functions, such as vascular tone, feeding behaviour, mood and hormone secretion amongst others (Wahlestedt and Reis, 1993).

NPY is a member of the pancreatic polypeptide (PP) family of peptide hormones (Glover *et al.*, 1985; Schwartz *et al.*, 1990). A high-resolution X-ray analysis of one member of this family, avian pancreatic polypeptide (aPP), has been reported (Blundell *et al.*, 1981; Glover *et al.*, 1983), and a tertiary structure, referred to as the PP-fold (or the hair-pin loop), for the PP family was proposed. The PP-fold consists of

Neuropeptide Y and Drug Development
ISBN 0-12-304990-3

a polyproline-like helix (residues 1–8) that is closely packed against an amphiphilic α-helix (residues 13–32). The two antiparallel helices are linked by a β-turn (residues 9–12), while the C-terminal region (residues 33–36) adopts no regular structure and extends away from the molecule. Residues considered to be essential for maintaining the integrity of the PP-fold are also found in analogous positions in NPY, suggesting that the neuropeptide adopts a similar secondary structure motif (Fuhlendorff *et al.*, 1989; Schwartz *et al.*, 1990). Using the X-ray coordinates for aPP, a computer-generated three-dimensional model of NPY in which the PP-fold is maintained was reported (Allen *et al.*, 1987). More recently, nuclear magnetic resonance (NMR) solution structures of NPY (Darbon *et al.*, 1992) and bovine pancreatic polypeptide (bPP) (Li *et al.*, 1992) were determined, and both were shown to contain the PP-fold motif present in the crystal structure of aPP.

The biological actions of NPY are mediated through 7-transmembrane G-protein-coupled receptors and at least three types have been described based on the relative affinity of different NPY receptor agonists. Y1 receptors require essentially the full NPY sequence of amino acids for activation and have a high affinity for the analogue [Leu^{31},Pro^{34}]NPY, whereas Y2 receptors can be activated by both NPY and the shorter carboxy-terminal fragment, NPY13–36, but have a low affinity for [Leu^{31},Pro^{34}]NPY (Wahlestedt *et al.*, 1986; Fuhlendorff *et al.*, 1990). The third type (Y3) recognizes all three of the above peptides but is insensitive to the NPY homologue, peptide YY (Michel, 1991; Wahlestedt *et al.*, 1992). In addition, a hypothalamic 'feeding' receptor, distinct from all of the above, has been proposed (Gehlert, 1994). The Y1 and Y2 receptors have been cloned and expressed in stable cell lines (Larhammar *et al.*, 1992; Gerald *et al.*, 1995; Rose *et al.*, 1995). Recently, the cloning of an additional Y-type receptor (PP1), which is preferentially activated by PP, has been reported (Bard *et al.*, 1995; Lundell *et al.*, 1995).

A direct demonstration of a physiological and pathophysiological role for NPY had, until recently, been hampered by the lack of specific, high-affinity NPY receptor antagonists. In this chapter we describe, through a structure-based and rational design effort, the discovery of potent, peptide NPY receptor agonists and antagonists.

7.2 Design of small peptide antagonists of neuropeptide Y

Our interest in discovering peptide agonist/antagonists of NPY focused initially on developing pharmacological tools to elucidate the physiological and pathophysiological roles of NPY. In addition, such peptides could provide the basis for designing small molecules as therapeutic agents for treating a potentially wide range of NPY-related disease states.

At the outset of this work the precise molecular determinants governing NPY binding to its receptors were unclear, although some general principles had emerged from extensive structure–activity/affinity studies on NPY and large NPY fragments (Boublik *et al.*, 1990; Wahlestedt and Reis, 1993). For example, both the N- and C-terminal amino acids of NPY were found to be essential for strong receptor binding and activity, consistent with the published NPY model in which these regions are held in close proximity. In native NPY this proximity is enforced by the PP-fold, which aligns amino acids located in the C- and N-termini into the correct spatial orientation for presentation to the receptor (Fuhlendorff et al., 1989; Schwartz et al., 1990).

To explore the relative importance of the N- and C-termini further, we independently generated a molecular model of NPY (Plate 13) and focused specifically on the region spanning these amino-acid residues. To further support this model, we prepared a series of NPY fragments and analyzed their ability to displace radiolabeled NPY from rat brain receptors. Figure 1 illustrates the characterization of this binding assay showing a typical saturation isotherm for the binding of [^{3}H]NPY to rat brain membranes. The non-linear regression analysis (Lundon ReceptorFit Saturation Two-Site Software) best fits a single binding site, suggesting a homogeneous population of receptors in this membrane preparation (Daniels et al., 1995a). Displacement of [^{3}H]NPY by NPY, NPY analogs and fragments of NPY are shown in Table 1, and the data is consistent with both the N- and C-terminal regions playing a role in receptor affinity, in agreement with previously published data (Wahlestedt and Reis, 1993).

To determine the minimum requirements for binding to NPY receptors, we prepared a series of small peptides containing elements of the N- and C-terminal regions of NPY. Analysis of the NPY model suggested that peptides containing 4–5 residues, in an extended backbone conformation, bridged the distance between Tyr-1 and Tyr-36 (approximately 14 Å).

The initial indication that small peptides could bind to rat brain NPY receptors came from the observation, shown in Table 2, that the commercially available cardioactive tetrapeptide FMRF-NH$_2$ (**13**) interacted with NPY receptors, albeit weakly (IC$_{50}$=40 μM). Further inspection of the NPY model supported a relationship between FMRH-NH$_2$ and a composite of N- and C-terminal residues of NPY. This led to the preparation of YRQRY-NH$_2$ (**14**), corresponding to the NPY N-terminal Tyr and the C-terminal sequence NPY33–36, which displayed comparable binding (IC$_{50}$=62 μM). However, a 20-fold increase in affinity was obtained by replacing Gln with Met (**15**). Substitution of Met-3 with the common Met replacements Leu and norleucine (Nle), compounds **16** and **17**, afforded peptides with similar affinity.

YRLRY-NH$_2$ (**16**) was used as the reference peptide to examine the effect of substitutions at positions 1 and 5. Replacement of the N-terminal Tyr by D-Tyr or His resulted in a 3–5-fold increase in affinity (**21** and **32**). These observations parallel results found for the full-length NPY analogs **5** and **6** (Table 1), where replacement of Tyr-1 with His or D-Tyr had minimal effect on affinity. Other aromatic (**31**), but not aliphatic (**34**), residues were tolerated at the N-terminus as was the corresponding des-NH$_2$ analogue (**54**). N-Acetylation of **21** (compound **53**) reduced affinity ten-fold. The structure–affinity pattern found for the pentapeptide series agrees well with previously reported structural requirements at the N-terminus of NPY (Boublik et al., 1989, 1990; Forest et al., 1990) and centrally truncated NPY analogs (Beck-Sickinger et al., 1990a). In contrast, substitution of the C-terminal Tyr by either aromatic or aliphatic amino acids uniformly afforded analogues (**35–39**) with significantly reduced affinity.

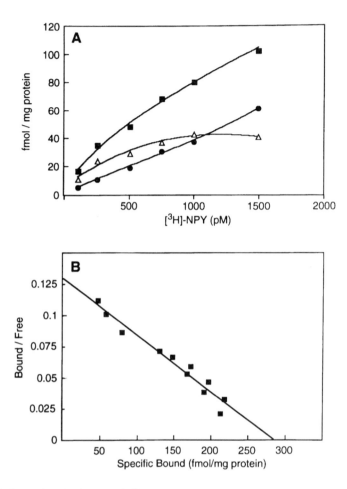

Figure 1 Saturation isotherms of [³H]propionyl NPY binding to rat brain membranes. (Reproduced from *Mol. Pharmacol.* 1995: **48**, 425–432.) (A) Binding of [³H]NPY to brain membranes incubated with increasing concentrations of the radiolabeled peptide. ■, Total binding; ●, non-specific binding; △, specific binding (the difference between total and non-specific binding). For further details, see Daniels *et al.* (1995a). (B) Scatchard analysis of the saturation experiments. The results represent a typical saturation experiment repeated ($n > 10$) with different membrane preparations; $K_d = 0.36 \pm 0.1$ nM, $B_{max} = 306 \pm 53$ fmol mg^{-1} protein (mean $\pm$ SE; $n = 15$). The Hill slope for the NPY displacement curve is consistent with a single binding site ($n_H = 0.99 \pm 0.01$).

Overall, the data strongly suggest that the N- and C-terminal Tyr in compounds such as YRLRY-NH₂ function as surrogates for Tyr-1 and Tyr-36 of NPY.

The more potent analog D-YRLRY-NH₂ (compound **21**) was used as a reference to examine further the effect of substitution at position 3. This series (**22–30**) revealed that, with the exception of Phe and Met analogs (**27** and **28**), all other replacements

Table 1 Displacement of specifically bound [^{3}H]NPY from rat brain membranes by NPY, NPY analogues and NPY fragments

Compound	Peptide-NH$_2$	IC$_{50}$ (nM) rat brain (Y2)
1	NPY	0.5
2	[Leu^{31},Pro^{34}]NPY	2.6
3	NPY13–36	15
4	NPY2–36	3
5	[D-Tyr^1]NPY	1.5
6	[His^1]NPY	1.5
7	NPY1–20	>>50 000
8	NPY20–36	26
9	NPY25–36	1000
10	NPY26–36	2500
11	NPY27–36	30 000
12	NPY32–36	>>50 000

Membranes were incubated with 0.2 nM [^{3}H]NPY ($\leqslant K_d$) for 60 min at 37°C as previously described (Daniels *et al.*, 1995a). Results are presented as the IC$_{50}$ calculated from non-linear regression analysis of the concentration-dependent displacement data. The abbreviations for the amino acids are in accord with the recommendations of the International Union of Pure and Applied Chemistry/International Union of Biochemistry Joint Commission on Biochemical Nomenclature [(1984) *Eur. J. Biochem.* **138**, 9–37]. The symbols represent the L-isomer except where indicated otherwise.

significantly reduced affinity. The poor affinity of the Gln-3 analog (compound **14**) would be consistent with a recent study (Beck-Sickinger *et al.*, 1994) in which Gln-34 of NPY appears not to be essential for receptor binding. Gln-34 may play a role in stabilizing specific amino-acid side-chain/backbone conformations or secondary structure in NPY, neither of which have relevance to the pentapeptide analogs.

The relative importance of the two Arg residues in this series was determined by varying the position, nature and number of positively charged amino acids. Replacement of Arg-4 in **16** by Lys (compound **40**) reduced binding 21-fold, however; only a minor change in affinity was found for the corresponding Lys-2 analog (compound **41**). Substitution of both Arg residues by Lys (compound **42**) weakened binding still further. Replacement of Arg-2 by His in either the His-1 or D-Tyr-1 series (compounds **45** and **46**) lowered affinity by about six-fold. Analogs where Arg-2 was replaced with a neutral residue such as Tyr (compound **47**) maintained binding, but the Gly analog (compound **43**) showed poor affinity. Apparently, there is no strict requirement for Arg, or, in fact, any positively charged residue at position 2. These results differ significantly from full-length or large C-terminal fragments of NPY, where both Arg-33 and Arg-35 are needed for high affinity and activity (Baeza and Unden, 1990; Beck-Sickinger *et al.*, 1990a,b,c, 1994). The effect of substitution by the

Table 2 Displacement of specifically bound [³H]NPY from rat brain membranes by small peptide amides

Compound	Peptide-NH$_2$	IC$_{50}$ (µM) rat brain (Y2)	Compound	Peptide-NH$_2$	IC$_{50}$ (µM) rat brain (Y2)
13	FMRF	40	**34**	TRLRY	17
14	YRQRY	62	**35**	YRMRF	9
15	YRMRY	3	**36**	YRLRH	98
16	YRLRY	1.5	**37**	D-YRLRW	29
17	YRNleRY	4	**38**	D-YRLRH	94
18	YRVRY	35	**39**	D-YRLRP	>100
19	YRPRY	31	**40**	YRLKY	32
20	YRHRY	30	**41**	YKLRY	3
21	D-YRLRY	0.6	**42**	YKLKY	93
22	D-YRGRY	33	**43**	YGMRY	50
23	D-YRSRY	21	**44**	YFMRY	10
24	D-YRTRY	32	**45**	HHLRY	3
25	D-YRIRY	13	**46**	D-YHLRY	3.5
26	D-YRARY	35	**47**	D-YYLRY	0.5
27	D-YRFRY	6	**48**	D-YRL-D-RY	2.5
28	D-YRMRY	2	**49**	D-Y-D-RLRY	6
29	D-YRDRY	>100	**50**	H-D-RLRY	0.6
30	D-YRERY	>100	**51**	YRLR-D-Y	9
31	WRLRY	2.5	**52**	Ac-YRLRY	5
32	HRLRY	0.5	**53**	Ac-D-YRLRY	11
33	D-HRLRY	3	**54**	des-NH$_2$-YRLRY	2

Comparative potencies of novel pentapeptides in displacing [³H]NPY from rat brain membranes (procedure as described in Table 1). Ac, acetyl; Nle, norleucine.

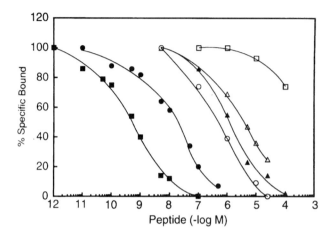

Figure 2 Inhibition isotherms for the specific binding of [³H]NPY to rat brain membranes as a function of competitor concentration. The amount of [³H]NPY bound at each concentration of competitor is expressed as a percentage of [³H]NPY specifically bound in the absence of competitor. ■, NPY (**1**); ●, NPY13–36 (**3**); ○, HRLRY-NH₂ (**32**); ▲, D-YRLRY-NH₂ (**21**); △, YRLRY-NH₂ (**16**); ❑, NPY32–36: TRQRY-NH₂ (**12**). (Reproduced from *Mol. Pharmacol.* 1995: **48**, 425–432.)

corresponding D-amino acids was also examined (compounds **48–51**). No clear trends emerged from this series, although the tolerance for D-amino acids diminished some-what from the N- to the C-terminus. Several laboratories have shown that D-amino-acid substitution in large (Boublik *et al.*, 1990) and centrally truncated fragments of NPY weakens but often does not eliminate bioactivity, particularly at the C-terminal tyrosine (Kirby *et al.*, 1993).

The displacement of [³H]NPY bound to rat brain membranes by our most potent pentapeptides is shown in Figure 2 and compared to the inactive C-terminal fragment NPY32–36.

Having established that these small peptides interact with NPY rat brain recep-tors, we next evaluated their activity in a Y1-type-receptor-mediated functional assay (Daniels *et al.*, 1992). Figure 3A shows a typical increase in cytosolic Ca^{2+} in human erythroleukemic (HEL) cells in response to NPY. The preferential mobilization of intracellular Ca^{2+} in these cells by the selective Y1 receptor agonist [Leu³¹,Pro³⁴]NPY relative to the Y2 agonist NPY13–36 is illustrated in Figure 3B. Compound **32**, at 1 μM, did not induce cytosolic calcium increase on its own; however, it inhibited by 50% the response to a subsequent addition of NPY (Figure 3C, C2). Moreover, the dose–response curves for the NPY-induced Ca^{2+} mobilization in the presence or absence of compound **32** indicated that this pentapeptide was a competitive antag-onist of NPY in HEL cells (Figure 3D). Pentapeptides that displayed the highest affinity at the rat brain receptor were tested in this system and the results, presented in Table 3, show that HRLRY-NH₂ (**32**) was the compound with the highest

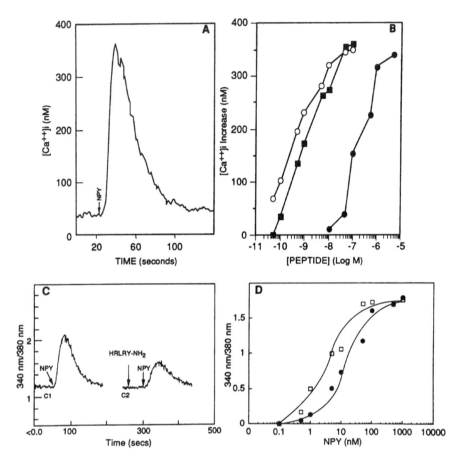

Figure 3 Characterization of the inhibitory effect of HRLRY-NH$_2$ (compound **32**) on the NPY-induced increase in cytosolic Ca^{2+} in fura-2 loaded HEL cells. (A) Effect of NPY (100 nM) on the increase in cytosolic Ca^{2+} in HEL cells. (Reproduced from *Mol. Pharmacol.* 1992: **41**, 767–771.) (B) Comparative potencies of NPY (■), the Y1-receptor-specific agonist [Leu^{31},Pro^{34}]NPY (○) and the Y2-receptor agonist NPY13–36 (●) on the increase in cytosolic Ca^{2+} in HEL cells. (Reproduced from *Mol. Pharmacol.* 1992: **41**, 767–771.) (C) C1: cytosolic Ca^{2+} increase in response to a half-maximal concentration (5 nM) of NPY. C2: cytosolic Ca^{2+} response of 5 nM NPY 30 s after addition of 1 μM HRLRY-NH$_2$ to the medium. C1 and C2 represent separate cuvettes. (Reproduced from Mol. Pharmacol. 1995: **48**, 425–432.) (D) Dose–response curves for the NPY-induced increase in cytosolic Ca^{2+} in the presence (●) and absence (□) of 1.0 μM HRLRY-NH$_2$. The inhibitor was added to the medium 30 s prior to stimulation with NPY (5 nM). (Reproduced from *Mol. Pharmacol.* 1995: **48**, 425–432.) Results in panels C and D are presented as the 340/380 nm fluorescence ratio, and represent a typical experiment repeated with different cell preparations and with similar results (for detailed experimental procedure, see Daniels *et al.*, 1992).

Table 3 Inhibition of NPY-induced increase in cytosolic Ca^{2+} in HEL cells by pentapeptide amides

Compound	Structure	IC_{50} (μM) HEL cell (Y1)
32	HRLRY	0.5
21	D-YRLRY	1
16	YRLRY	10
15	YRMRY	3

Results are expressed as the concentration of peptide that inhibits 50% (IC_{50}) of the increase in the 340/380 nm fluorescence ratio in fura-2 loaded cells induced by a half-maximal concentration of (5 nM) of NPY (for procedure, see Daniels *et al.*, 1992).

antagonistic activity, while compounds that displayed poor affinity at the 'Y2' receptor were inactive (e.g. compound 19).

In conclusion, the pentapeptides of the YRLRY-NH$_2$ type appear to represent the discontinuous epitope Tyr-1. Arg-35 and Tyr-36 -NH$_2$ (Plate 14). Incorporation of these residues into appropriately substituted pentapeptides is sufficient to allow interaction, with modest affinity, to NPY rat brain 'Y2' receptors. Furthermore, they competitively antagonize the NPY-induced increase in cytosolic Ca^{2+} in the Y1-receptor-mediated HEL cell assay. Importantly, these linear peptides suggested a simple model for a minimum, essential pharmacophore and provided a useful starting point for the design of more potent and selective peptide antagonists.

7.3 High-affinity peptide ligands

7.3.1 Discovery and structural characterization of potent agonists

To improve the relatively modest affinity for NPY receptors of our small peptide ligands, we attempted to optimize the orientation of the Tyr and Arg residues. NMR analysis of the pentapeptide ligands was consistent with a mixture of rapidly interconverting conformers. Thus, as an approach to restricting the flexibility of these molecules, we incorporated a larger segment of the C-terminal region of NPY on to the N-terminus of the lead compound, YRLRY-NH$_2$ (**16**) (Leban *et al.*, 1995). The added residues could increase affinity by providing additional positive interactions directly with the receptor and/or promote the formation of secondary structural features, such as a turn or helix, thus orienting the critical side chains of **16** into a more favourable binding conformation.

This approach is illustrated in Table 4 by compounds **54–60**, in which residues 31–25 of NPY are sequentially added to the N-terminus of pentapeptide **16** (YRLRY-NH$_2$). In this series, affinity for rat brain NPY receptors peaks at the decapeptide **58**

Table 4 Displacement of specifically bound [^{3}H]NPY from rat brain membranes and mobilization of intracellular Ca^{2+} in HEL cells by NPY, NPY fragments and N-terminally extended pentapeptides

Compound	Peptide-NH$_2$	IC$_{50}$ (nM) rat brain (Y2)	ED$_{50}$(nM) HEL cell (Y1)
1	NPY	0.5	4
3	NPY13–36	15	
11	YINLITRQRY	30 000	
16	YRLRY	1500	
54	IYRLRY	3000	
55	LIYRLRY	400	
56	NLIYRLRY	300	
57	INLIYRLRY	40	150
58	YINLIYRLRY	8	9
59	HYINLIYRLRY	12	
60	RHYINLIYRLRY	12	
61	YINLITRLRY	2000	
62	YINLLYRQRY	400	
63	YSPK-Aha-YINLIYRLRY	15	41
64	[Tyr^{32},Leu^{34}]NPY	83	50*

Rat brain binding data are presented as the IC$_{50}$ calculated from non-linear regression analysis of the concentration-dependent displacement data (procedure as described in Table 1). Mobilization of calcium in HEL cells is expressed as the concentration of peptide that produces a half-maximal increase in the 340/380 nm fluorescence ratio in fura-2 loaded cells. For compound **62**, we have observed, in a parallel series, that substitution of Ile-5 by Leu had little effect on rat brain receptor binding.
* The maximal response of compound **64** was only 60% of the maximal response to NPY (for procedure, see Daniels *et al.*, 1995a).

(YINLIYRLRY-NH$_2$), which represents a 3700-fold enhancement relative to the native sequence NPY 27–36 (compound **11**). Neither individual replacement of Thr-6 by Tyr nor Gln-8 by Leu afforded high-affinity analogs: apparently both modifications are required (compare **58** to **61** and **62**).

In addition to strong affinity for rat brain NPY receptors, **58** also proved to be a potent agonist in the Y1-receptor-mediated HEL cell assay (Figure 4). Furthermore, following intravenous (iv) administration, compound **58** was found to be half as potent as NPY in inducing an increase in blood pressure in normotensive rats (not shown). These results are noteworthy and suggest that, contrary to literature reports (Wahlestedt *et al.*, 1986; Sheikh *et al.*, 1989), full-length NPY, particular the N-terminus, is not required for high activity at Y1 receptors.

It has previously been demonstrated that appending an N-terminal segment of NPY (residues 1–4) linked by a flexible spacer on to NPY25–36 produces potent Y2-

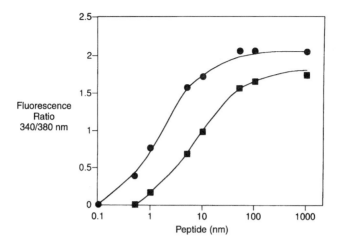

Figure 4 Dose–response curves for the NPY (●; ED_{50} = 3.3 nM) and YINLIYRLRY-NH$_2$ (compound **58**) (■; ED_{50} = 8.7 nM) induced increase in cytosolic Ca^{2+} in fura-2 loaded HEL cells. Results are presented as the 340/380 nm fluorescence ratio.

receptor-selective agonists (Beck *et al.*, 1989). Our efforts to further improve the potency of **58** by employing this strategy (compound **63**) resulted in a marked reduction in Y1-receptor activity, although Y2-receptor affinity was unaffected (Table 4). Moreover, replacement of the C-terminal pentapeptide sequence in full-length NPY by **16** ([Tyr^{32}, Leu^{34}]NPY; compound **64**) did not result in improved activity at the Y1 receptor or affinity for Y2 receptors. It is interesting to note that, while **58** is much more active than NPY27–36 (**11**), a corresponding enhancement in activity or affinity was not observed in **64**, the full-length analog of NPY.

The dramatic improvement in the affinity/activity of the native C-terminal decapeptide of NPY (**11**) following introduction of the critical Tyr-6 and Leu-8 residues (compound **58**) is not clearly understood. However, circular dichroism (CD) spectroscopy of **58** in methanol indicates that these two residues induce a significant increase in helicity (Figure 5a). It has been proposed that the C-terminal α-helical domain of NPY provides an additional receptor recognition site and may play a role in receptor-subtype selectivity (Krstenansky, 1993). Additionally, Tyr-6 may serve as a surrogate for Tyr-1 of NPY, either by directly interacting with the receptor (Allen *et al.*, 1987) or by assisting in stabilizing a bioactive conformation at the C-terminus (Forest *et al.*, 1990). The hypothesis that there is a functional relationship between Tyr-6 of **58** and Tyr-1 of NPY is appealing; however, additional structure–activity data needs to be generated to evaluate this proposal further. It appears that whatever the precise function of the N-terminus of NPY in inducing strong interactions with Y1 and Y2 receptors, these features already appear to be incorporated into the short, C-terminally modified NPY sequence of **58**.

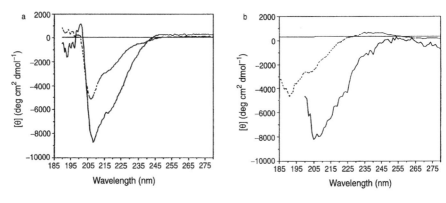

Figure 5 Far ultraviolet region of the CD spectra of (a) YINLIYRLRY-NH$_2$ (compound **58**, solid line) and YINLITRQRY-NH$_2$ (compound **11**, dashed line) in methanol and (b) INPIYRLRY-NH$_2$ (compound **66**) as a function of solvent. Solid lines correspond to 10 mM peptide in 10 mM sodium phosphate buffer, pH 7.5, and dashed lines correspond to 10 mM peptide in methanol. The CD spectrum in aqueous buffer correspond to a mixture of predominantly unfolded conformers. Type C spectra are observed in methanol, corresponding to the presence of predominantly helical conformers. (Reproduced from *J. Med. Chem.* 1995: **38**, 1150–1157.)

7.3.2 Discovery of potent antagonists

Having achieved our initial goal of developing high-affinity small peptides for NPY receptors, we explored strategies for converting compounds, such as **58**, into antagonists. Since there exists no general principle for developing antagonists from agonists, we decided to employ a strategy that focused on the rational modification of the three-dimensional structure of **58**. Toward this end the solution structure of compound **58** was examined by ^{1}H-NMR and CD spectroscopy. In methanol, the NMR data supported the presence of only one major conformer (Plate 15a). The most prominent features of this structure were the presence of an α-helix from residues 3–10 and an Asx-turn (Abbadi *et al.*, 1991), highlighted by a hydrogen bond between the Asn-3 side-chain carbonyl oxygen and the backbone amide N-H of Ile-6. In addition, the tyrosine residues at positions 1, 6 and 10 are closely associated on one face of the helix.

To complement ^{1}H-NMR studies, an extended molecular dynamics simulation of **58** was carried out. The starting geometry for **58** was generated using coordinates taken from the partially helical, C-terminal decapeptide portion (residues 27–36) of the NPY model shown in Plate 13. The residues corresponding to Thr-32 and Gln-34 were replaced with Tyr and Leu, respectively, and subjected to an unconstrained molecular dynamics simulation. The structures obtained from this simulation (a representative structure is shown in Plate 15b) share several important features with those observed by ^{1}H-NMR, specifically the formation of an Asx turn and close association of the aromatic tyrosine rings.

The ^{1}H-NMR and molecular dynamics experiments suggested modifications of **58**

138

Table 5 Effect of NPY peptide antagonists in the displacement of specifically bound [^{3}H]NPY from rat brain membranes and on the inhibition of the NPY-induced increase in cytosolic Ca^{2+} in HEL cells.

Compound	Peptide	IC_{50}(nM) rat brain (Y2)	IC_{50}(nM) HELcell (Y1)
65	YINPIYRLRY-NH$_2$	44	100
66	INPIYRLRY-NH$_2$	170	9
67	YINLLYRPRY-NH$_2$	2700	>100
68	INPIFRLRY-NH$_2$	480	10
69	INPI(4-Phe)FRLRY-NH$_2$	520	5
70	INPI(2,6-Cl$_2$-Bnz)YRLRY-NH$_2$	50	2
71	INPIYRLR(2,6-Cl$_2$-Bnz)Y-NH$_2$	1300	10
72	INPIYRLR(3,4-Cl$_2$)F-NH$_2$	560	100
73	INPI-D(Y)RLRY-NH$_2$	4700	>>100
74	INPIY-D(R)LRY-NH$_2$	>50 000	>>100
75	INP(Aib)YRLRY-NH$_2$	260	9
76	IQPIYRLRY-NH$_2$	1400	90
77	INPIYRLRY-OCH$_3$	710	10
78	INPIYRLRY-NHEt	>1000	50
79	INPIYRLRY-OH	6500	>>100
80	IN(3,4-Dehydro)PIYRLRY-NH$_2$	40	2.3

Procedures for brain binding and HEL cell Ca^{2+} experiments were carried out as described in Tables 1 and 3, respectively.

that might increase potency through stabilization of particular structure features. For example, the sequence Asn-Pro-Xxx is especially prone to formation of an Asn-turn (Pichon-Pesme *et al.*, 1989). As shown in Table 5, substitution of Leu-4 by Pro afforded YINPIYRLRY (**65**), which maintained good binding affinity to the Y2 receptor (IC_{50} = 44 nM). More importantly, however, **65** inhibited the NPY-induced mobilization of intracellular Ca^{2+} in HEL cells (IC_{50} ≈ 100 nM) and, in contrast to **58**, induced no observable increase in intracellular Ca^{2+} by itself at concentrations up to 1 μM. Thus, this modification effectively converted a potent agonist into a pure antagonist at the Y1-type NPY receptor. Deletion of the N-terminal Tyr from **65** increased antagonistic activity an additional ten-fold (compound **66**, IC_{50} = 9 nM) with a corresponding six-fold reduction in affinity at the Y2 receptor. In good correlation, **66** effectively displaced radio-labeled NPY from Y1-type receptors in SK-N-MC (human neuroblastoma) cells (IC_{50} = 3 nM). Figure 6A shows the inhibition of the NPY-induced cytosolic calcium increase by compound **66**. This inhibition is competitive in nature as illustrated in Figure 6B. The inhibition isotherms for the displacement of ^{3}H-NPY from rat brain membranes, presented in Figure 7, compares the affinities of our most potent nona- and deca-peptide agonists, and antagonists with NPY and its C-terminal decapeptide, NPY27–36.

A comparison of the ^{1}H-NMR solution structure of **65** (not shown) and **58** revealed few differences apart from a proline-induced kink (Yun *et al.*, 1991) in the first turn of

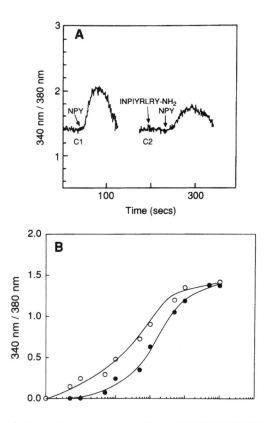

Figure 6 Characterization of the antagonistic effect of INPIYRLRY-NH$_2$ (**66**) on the NPY-induced increase in cytosolic calcium in fura-2 loaded HEL cells. (A) C1: cytosolic calcium increase in response to a half-maximal concentration of NPY (5 nM). C2: cytosolic calcium response to 5 nM NPY, 30 s after the addition of 5 nM of compound **66** to the medium. (B) Dose–response curves for the NPY-induced increase in cytosolic calcium in the presence (●) and absence (○) of 5 nM inhibitor. Results are presented as the 340/380 nm fluorescence ratio and represent typical experiments repeated with different cell preparations with similar results. C1 and C2 represent separate cuvettes. (Reproduced from *J. Med. Chem.* 1995: **38**, 1150–1157.)

the helix defined by residues 3–10. While it is conceivable that subtle distortions of an α-helical recognition element may, in part, be responsible for the observed antagonism of **65**, there is no direct evidence for this.

The judicious introduction of a proline into the backbone of **58** to afford the antagonist **65** led us to examine alternative positions for Pro substitution. Of special interest was the decapeptide analog of [Leu^{31},Pro^{34}]NPY, a well-known potent and selective Y1-receptor agonist (Fuhlendorff *et al.*, 1990). To this end, the Leu-5, Pro-8 analog of **58** (compound **67**), was prepared but no agonistic, and only modest antagonistic activity (30% inhibition at 100 nM), was observed in the Y1-receptor-mediated HEL cell Ca^{2+} assay along with poor affinity for rat brain Y2 receptors.

140

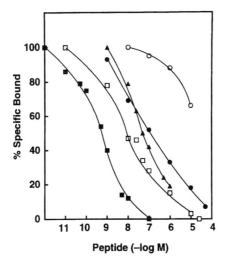

Figure 7 Inhibition isotherms for the specific binding of [³H]NPY to rat brain membranes as a function of competitor concentration. The amount of [³H]NPY specifically bound at each concentration of competitor is expressed as a percentage of [³H]NPY specifically bound in the absence of competitor. ■, NPY (**1**); ❑, YINLIYRLRY-NH₂ (**58**); ▲, YINPIYRLRY-NH₂ (**65**); ●, INPIYRLRY-NH₂ (**66**); ○, YINLITRQRY-NH₂ (**11**). For details refer to Leban *et al.*, 1995. (Reproduced from *J. Med. Chem.* USA 1995: **38**, 1150–1157.)

To further probe the structure activity/affinity of the potent Y1 antagonist **66**, several analogs were prepared and representative examples shown in Table 5. Our hypothesis that these C-terminal analogs of NPY serve to orient the critical Tyr and Arg residues (positions 5, 9 and 8, respectively) via formation of an α-helix (initiated by a Asx-turn), is supported by this set of compounds (the CD spectrum of **66**, shown in Figure 5b, is consistent with the presence of a helical structure). A wide range of aromatic residues are tolerated at positions 5 and 9 (compounds **68–72**). However, in contrast to the pentapeptides described in Table 2, D-stereochemistry at position 5 yields an inactive compound (**73**). D-Substitution at other positions (**74**) also yields inactive compounds, which are, presumably, unable to adopt the desired helical conformation. In contrast, helix-stabilizing residues, such as Aib (compound **75**) maintain good potency. The contribution to enhanced activity provided by an Asx-turn is supported by the glutamine analog **76**, which is an order of magnitude less active than **66**. Interestingly, a primary C-terminal carboxamide is not required for good Y1-receptor antagonism (compounds **77** and **78**), although the carboxylic acid derivative, **79**, is inactive. Finally, replacement of proline at position three by other cyclic amino acids led, with the exception of the dehydroproline derivative **80**, to weak or inactive compounds in the rat brain and HEL cell assays. Compound **80** proved to be one of the most potent antagonists uncovered in this series.

7.4 Peptide dimers as potent NPY antagonists

7.4.1 Nonapeptide dimers

The incorporation of amino acids present in the C-terminal α-helical segment of NPY on to the N-terminus of the weak pentapeptide antagonist, YRLRY (**16**) afforded a high-affinity ligand for NPY Y1 and Y2 receptors (compound **58**). Stabilization of the Asn-turn observed in compound **58** led to the antagonists **65** and **66**. This turn represented an attractive structural motif for introducing conformational constraints, therefore, in an effort to improve antagonist potency, we attempted to stabilize it further by covalently linking the side chains flanking the essential proline through disulfide and lactam bridges (Figure 8a).

Synthesis of a series of disulfide- (Leban *et al.*, 1996) and lactam-bridged analogs of **66** afforded both the desired monomeric compounds along with the corresponding dimers (Figure 8b). Table 6 shows the ability of these compounds, compared to that of NPY and NPY analogs, to displace specifically bound [^{3}H]NPY from rat brain membranes and [^{125}I]NPY from SK-N-MC neuroblastoma cells.

Relative to the reference antagonist **66**, the affinity of the monomeric disulfide **81** for the Y2 receptor (rat brain) dropped by a factor of two, while the monomeric lactam **82** displayed a 40-fold higher affinity. More interestingly, the dimeric structures **83–86** (Figure 9) showed significantly higher affinities than compound **66**, for both Y2 (rat brain) and Y1 (SK-N-MC cells) receptors. Thus, these dimers appear to be potent, albeit non-selective, NPY receptor ligands.

We examined next the ability of these dimers and their monomeric counterparts to inhibit the NPY-induced increase in cytosolic calcium in HEL cells (Table 7). While the potency of the monomeric lactam **82** was three-fold greater than that of **66**, the dimers displayed significantly higher inhibitory activity. These results are in good correlation with the SK-N-MC binding data presented in Table 6. Figure 10 (left panel) illustrates the potent inhibitory effect of 0.5 nM GW1229 when added to HEL cells in suspension, 30 s prior to the stimulation with a half-maximal concentration of NPY (5 nM). Furthermore, inhibition by GW1229 appears to be competitive as suggested from the NPY dose–response curve in the presence and absence of the inhibitor (Figure 10, right panel). None of the dimers displayed agonistic activity as no increase in cytosolic calcium was observed in response to their addition to the cell suspension prior to NPY (even up to 1 μM), indicating that these compounds would behave as pure antagonists at the Y1-type receptor expressed in HEL cells.

7.4.2 Antagonism of the pressor effects of NPY by GW1229

7.4.2.1 *Ex vivo*: isolated rat kidney perfusion

The vasculature of the perfused isolated rat kidney contracts intensively in response to a bolus injection of NPY or [Leu^{31},Pro^{34}]NPY but not to NPY13–36, producing an

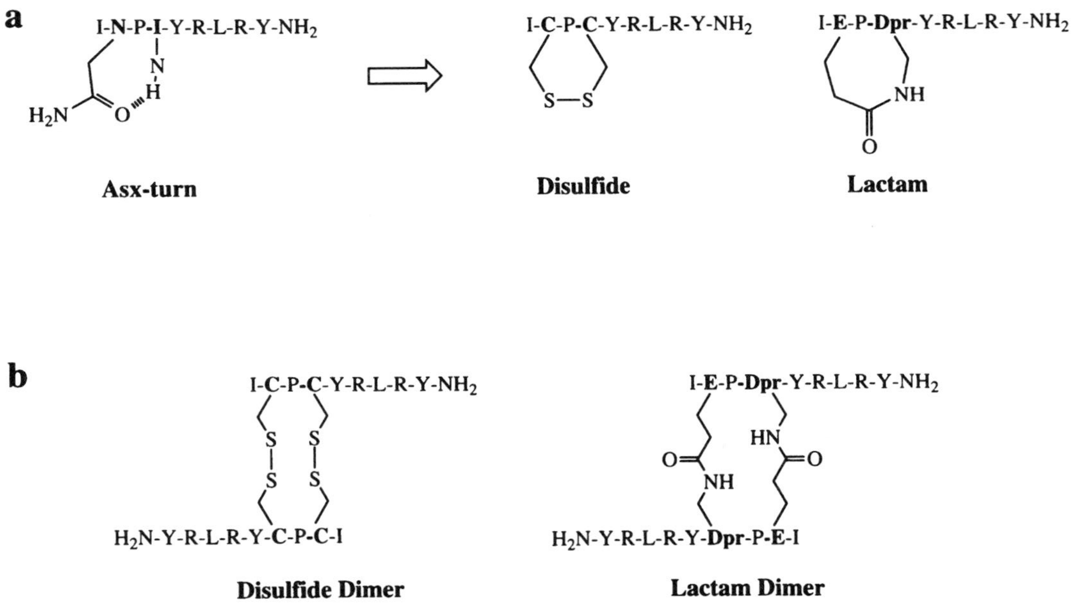

Figure 8 (a) Covalently modified analogs of the Asx-turn motif. (b) Disulfide and lactam dimers; disulfide dimers are equal mixtures of parallel and antiparallel isomers. Dpr, (L)-2,3-diaminopropionic acid.

Table 6 Effect of NPY peptide monomer and dimer antagonists in the displacement of specifically bound [³H]NPY from rat brain membranes and [¹²⁵I]NPY from SK-N-MC neuroblastoma cells

Compound	Peptide-NH₂	IC_{50}(nM) rat brain (Y2)	IC_{50}(nM) SK-N-MC (Y1)
66	INPIYRLRY	170	3
81	GW176	390	
82	GW1027	4.3	
83	GW383	8.8	2.9
84	GW1229	0.02	0.2
85	GW1120	1.3	0.73
86	GW530	5	0.45

Brain membranes were incubated with 0.2 nM [³H]NPY and SK-N-MC cells with 0.7 nM [¹²⁵I]NPY (see Daniels *et al.*, 1995b). Results are expressed as the IC_{50} calculated from non-linear regression analysis of the concentration-dependent displacement data. Analysis of the SK-N-MC cell data, shows a single binding site with a K_d=0.7±0.07 nM and a B_{max}=39.1±7.9 fmol/10^6 cells (mean±SE; n=5) and a Hill slope close to unity (n_H=0.89±0.17) consistent with a single binding site. Parameters for the rat brain assay are shown in the legend to Figure 1. GW383, GW1229 and GW1120 were previously referred to as 383U91, 1229U91 and 1120W91, respectively (Daniels *et al.*, 1995b).

immediate increase in perfusion pressure (Daniels *et al.*, 1995b). Figure 11 (left panel) shows the time course of the pressor effect of a single bolus injection of a half-maximal dose (50 pmol) of NPY. Stimulation with a 50 pmol bolus of NPY while the preparation is being infused with GW1229 at a concentration of 5 nM (right panel) results in a marked inhibition of the pressor effect of NPY. All of the dimers inhibited the NPY-induced vasoconstriction in this system with comparable potencies (not shown). Supporting the specificity of these compounds for NPY receptors, increases in kidney-perfusion pressure induced by methoxamine (α1-adrenoceptor agonist), isoproterenol (β-adrenoceptor agonist) or by depolarization with KCl, are not affected by the presence of these antagonists.

7.4.2.2 *In vivo*: mean arterial blood pressure in normotensive rats

NPY is a potent vasoconstrictor *in vivo*, elevating arterial blood pressure in rats (Zukowska-Grojec and Wahlestedt, 1993). Figure 12 shows the *in vivo* NPY receptor-blocking effect of compound GW1229. iv infusion of GW1229 into anesthetized Sprague–Dawley rats, dose-dependently inhibited the pressor response produced by a bolus iv injection of an ED_{50} dose of NPY (1 nmol kg⁻¹). The antagonistic effect of GW1229 was selective for NPY receptors, since the pressor response induced by a bolus iv injection of norepinephrine (3 nmol kg⁻¹) is not altered. It is noteworthy that resting mean arterial blood pressure (MAP) was not significantly affected by GW1229

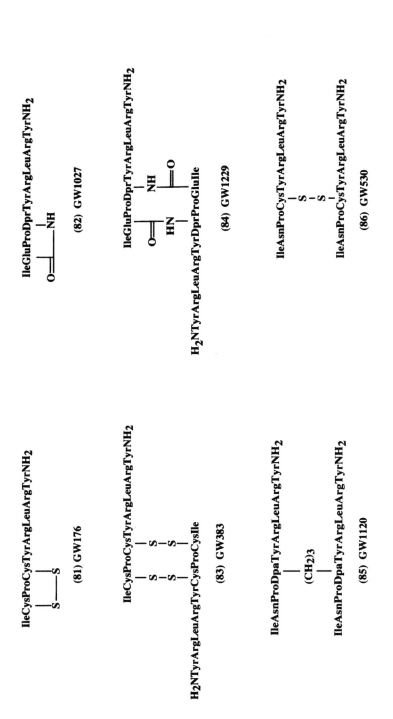

Figure 9 Peptide dimer and monomer antagonists. Dpa, (+)-2,6-diaminopimelic acid; Dpr, (L)-2,3-diaminopropionic acid. Compound **83** was obtained as an equal mixture of parallel and antiparallel isomers. GW383, GW1229 and GW1120 were previously referred to as 383U91, 1229U91 and 1120W91, respectively (Daniels *et al.*, 1995b).

Table 7 Inhibition of NPY-induced increase in cytosolic Ca^{2+} in HEL cells by peptide monomers and dimers

Compound	Peptide-NH_2	IC_{50}(nM) HEL cell (Y1)
66	INPIYRLRY	10
81	GW176	25
82	GW1027	3
83	GW383	0.5
84	GW1229	0.3
85	GW1120	0.4
86	GW530	0.5

HEL cell Ca^{2+} experiments were carried out as described in Table 3.

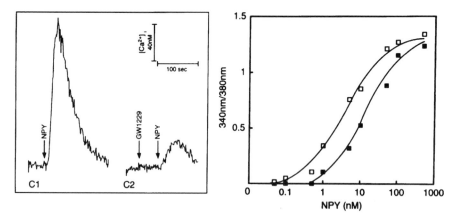

Figure 10 Inhibition of the NPY-induced increase in cytosolic calcium in fura-2 loaded HEL cells by GW1229 (compound **84**). (Left) C1: cytosolic calcium response to a half-maximal dose of NPY (5 nM). C2: cytosolic calcium response to NPY 30 s after the addition of 0.5 nM compound **84**. C1 and C2 represent separate cuvettes. (Right) NPY dose–response curves in the presence (■) and absence (□) of **84** at 0.25 nM. (Reproduced from *Proc. Natl Acad. Sci. USA* 1995: **92**, 9067–9071.)

(−9 ± 7% at the highest dose), strongly suggesting that endogenous NPY is not a major contributor to the cardiovascular tone in anesthetized normotensive rats. Further characterization of the hemodynamic effects of GW1229 in the rat have been reported recently (Tadepalli *et al.*, 1996).

The inhibitory potency of the dimers in HEL cells correlates well with their potency in antagonizing the pressor effect of NPY in anesthetized rats, thus HEL cells may constitute a good model to screen for NPY receptor antagonists as potential antihypertensive agents.

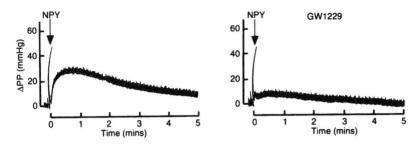

Figure 11 Inhibition of the NPY-induced increase in perfusion pressure in the isolated rat kidney. The kidneys were perfused at constant flow rate for 30 min before the first challenge with a bolus injection of 50 pmol of NPY in 0.1 ml of perfusion media (left panel). Following a 30 min recovery period, GW1229 was infused for 5 min at a concentration of 5 nM. After 4 min of infusion with GW1229, the kidney was challenged again with 50 pmol of NPY (right panel). The infusion was discontinued 1 min after the stimulation with NPY. Results represent a typical experiment repeated at least twice with identical results. An $IC_{50}=2.2\pm0.6$ nM was calculated from the dose–response curve ($n=3$) for the inhibition of the increase in perfusion pressure in response to 50 pmol NPY. (Reproduced from *Proc. Natl Acad. Sci. USA* 1995: **92**, 9067–9071.)

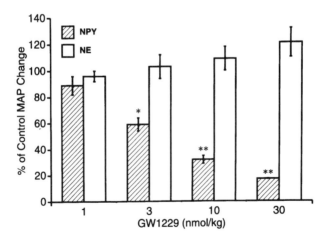

Figure 12 Effect of GW1229 on the pressor responses induced by NPY and norepinephrine (NE) in inactin-anesthetized rats. GW1229 was administered as an intravenous infusion at half log incremental doses (0.1–10 nmol kg^{-1} min^{-1}) over a 10 min period. Porcine NPY (1 nmol kg^{-1}) and NE (3 nmol kg^{-1}) were administered as an intravenous bolus, 1 min after the end of the compound infusion and peak changes in mean arterial blood pressure (MAP) were recorded. Note the absence of any effect on the pressor response to iv NE. Control MAP changes to NPY and NE were 28 ± 1 and 56 ± 8 mmHg, respectively. Results are shown as percent change of control (mean $\pm$ SE; $n = 5$). *$P < 0.05$; **$P < 0.01$. (Reproduced from *Proc. Natl Acad. Sci. USA* 1995: **92**, 9067–9071.)

7.4.3 Selectivity of GW1229 for NPY receptors

The selectivity of GW1229 for NPY receptor types warrants further discussion. The results presented in Table 6 show that GW1229 displays high affinity for both rat brain membranes (predominantly Y2 receptors) and SK-N-MC human neuro-blastoma cells (Y1 receptors) indicating little or no NPY receptor selectivity. However, we have recently observed (Matthews, *et al.*, 1995) that GW1229, up to concentrations of 1 μM, failed to antagonize the inhibitory effect of NPY in the electrically evoked contraction of the rat vas deferens, a standard Y2-receptor-mediated functional assay (Grundemar and Håkanson, 1990; Jörgensen, *et al.*, 1990). Moreover, we have also observed that GW1229 is several orders of magnitude less effective ($IC_{50}=2$ μM) in displacing specifically bound [^{125}I]PYY from Y2-type receptors expressed in KAN-TS (a subclone of SMS-KAN neuroblastoma cells) human neuroblastoma cells when compared with rat brain membranes (Matthews *et al.*, 1995). While this chapter was in preparation, in agreement with our results, the ineffectiveness of GW1229 in the rat vas deferens and the low affinity in SK-N-BE2 neuroblastoma cells (Y2 receptors) was reported (Hegde *et al.*, 1995). These recent results would rather indicate that GW1229 is a selective Y1-receptor antagonist. The high affinity of GW1229 for the homogenous population of NPY receptors present in our rat brain membrane preparation, suggests that the brain receptor may correspond to a subtype of central Y2 receptors, different from those present in the rat vas deferens and in the human neuroblastoma cell lines.

7.4.4 Solution structure of GW1229: insight into the mechanism of binding

In order to examine the factors contributing to the enhancement in activity and affin-ity for the extended peptide dimers **83–86**, a structural study on the most potent peptide in this series, GW1229, was carried out. The ^{1}H-NMR of GW1229 in methanol revealed a helical structure that extended the full length of the lactam-bridged polypeptide (Plate 16). By comparison, a recent NMR study of NPY (Darbon *et al.*, 1992) describes a well-defined α-helix extending from Arg-19 to Gln-34, with the last two or three residues not involved in the helix. This is consistent with the X-ray structure of aPP, which also contains a disordered C-terminal region (Blundell *et al.*, 1981). Thus, we suggest that a helix stabilization effect, which serves to orient the peptide chains (including the critical -Arg-Tyr-NH$_2$ C-terminal moiety), contributes to the enhanced affinity of these ligands. This conclusion is supported by claims that increased helicity at the C-terminus may be responsible for improved affinity at NPY receptors (Jung *et al.*, 1991). Such an effect has been proposed for the high-affinity ligand **58** (Leban *et al.*, 1995) in which an Asx-turn-induced α-helix dramatically improves affinity relative to the unstructured native C-terminal NPY sequence (residues 27–36; see Figure 5 and Plate 15). With respect to the tether/linkers exam-ined, the cyclic lactam in GW1229 appears to be optimal. Several other lactam-bridged dimers of the GW1229 type have been prepared and their Y2 affinity is at

List of abbreviations (for plate section)

I–VI   1–6 cortical layers
amy   amygdaloid complex
AO   anterior olfactory nuclei
AP   area postrema
AV   anteroventral thalamic nucleus
AVVL   anteroventral thalamic nucleus, ventrolateral part
CA1   Field CA1 of Ammon's horn of the hippocampus
CA3   Field CA3 of Ammon's horn of the hippocampus
Ce   cerebellum
Cl   claustrum
CM   central medial thalamic nucleus
CPU   caudate putamen (striatum)
Cx   cerebral cortex
DG   dentate gyrus
E   ependymal and subependymal layer of the olfactory bulb
EP1   external plexiform layer of the olfactory bulb
Fr   frontal cortex
Ge   geniculate nuclei
GrA   granule cell layer accessory olfactory bulb
Hi   hippocampus
Hy   hypothalamic nuclei
IO   inferior olive
LD   laterodorsal thalamic nucleus
LS   lateral septal nucleus
MD   mediodorsal thalamic nucleus
Mol   molecular layer of the dentate gyrus
MM   mammillary nucleus
NS   non-specific binding
or   oriens layer of the hippocampus
OV   olfactory ventricle
par   parietal cortex
pir   piriform cortex
py   pyramidal cell layer of the hippocampus
rad   stratum radiatum of the hippocampus
Re   reuniens thalamic nucleus
Rh   rhomboid thalamic nucleus
SC   superior colliculus
SN   substantia nigra
Sol   nucleus of the solitary tract
st   stria terminalis
TE   temporal cortex
Th   thalamic nuclei
TS   triangular septal nucleus
TT   tenia tecta
Tu   olfactory tubercle
VP   ventral pallidum

RAT

$[^{125}I][Leu^{31},Pro^{34}]PYY$

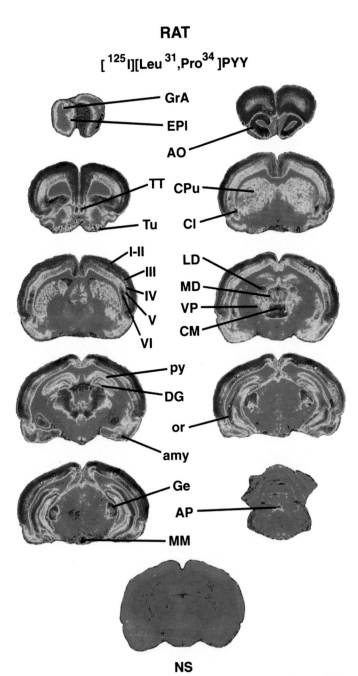

Plate 1 Photomicrographs of the autoradiographic distribution of $[^{125}I][Leu^{31},Pro^{34}]PYY/Y1-$ like binding sites at various levels of the rat brain. Adjacent coronal sections were incubated with 30–45 pM $[^{125}I][Leu^{31},Pro^{34}]PYY$ in the presence or absence of 1 μM pNPY in order to determine non-specific binding. See list of abbreviations for details of anatomical identification.

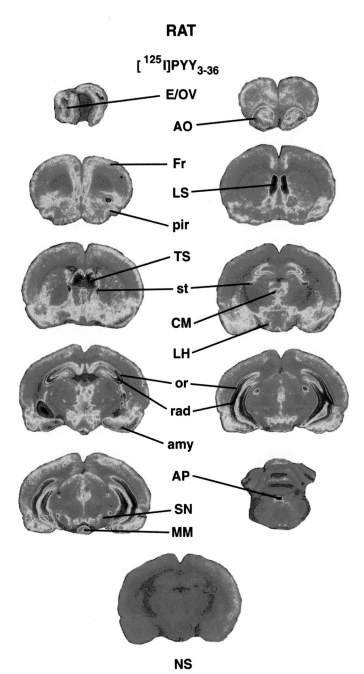

RAT

$[^{125}I]PYY_{3-36}$

E/OV

AO

Fr

LS

pir

TS

st

CM

LH

or

rad

amy

AP

SN

MM

NS

Plate 2 Photomicrographs of the autoradiographic distribution of $[^{125}I]PYY3-36/Y2$-like binding sites at various levels of the rat brain. Adjacent coronal sections used in Plate 1 were incubated with 30–45 pM $[^{125}I]PYY3-36$ in the presence or absence of 1 μM pNPY in order to determine non-specific binding. See list of abbreviations for details of anatomical identification.

RAT

$[^{125}I]Leu^{31},Pro^{34}]PYY$ $[^{3}H]BIBP3226$

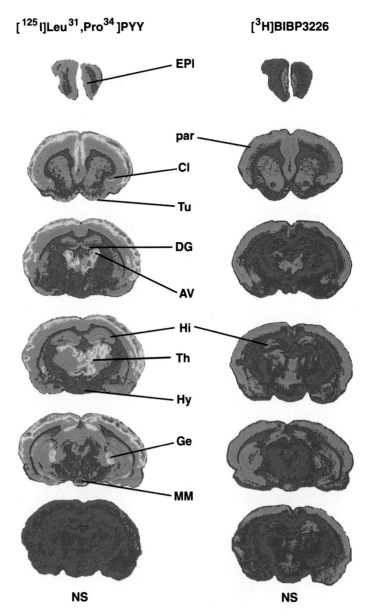

EPI

par

CI

Tu

DG

AV

Hi

Th

Hy

Ge

MM

NS   NS

Plate 3 Photomicrographs of the comparative autoradiographic distribution of $[^{125}I][Leu^{31},Pro^{34}]PYY$ (Y1 agonist) and $[^{3}H]BIBP$ 3226 (Y1 receptor antagonist) binding sites at various levels of the rat brain. Adjacent coronal sections were incubated with either 30 pM $[^{125}I][Leu^{31},Pro^{34}]PYY$ or 5 nM $[^{3}H]BIBP$ 3226 in the presence or absence of 1 μM pNPY in order to determine non-specific binding. See list of abbreviations for details of anatomical identification.

RAT

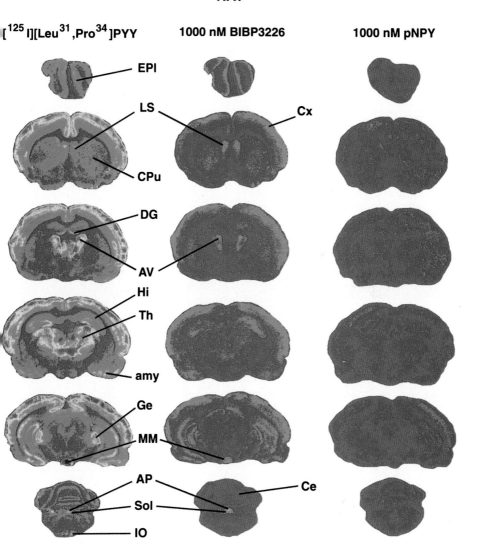

| [^{125}I][Leu^{31},Pro^{34}]PYY | 1000 nM BIBP3226 | 1000 nM pNPY |

EPI
LS
Cx
CPu
DG
AV
Hi
Th
amy
Ge
MM
AP
Ce
Sol
IO

Plate 4 Photomicrographs of the autoradiographic distribution of [^{125}I][Leu^{31},Pro^{34}] PYY/BIBP 3226-insensitive binding sites at various levels of the rat brain. Adjacent coronal sections were incubated with 35 pM [^{125}I][Leu^{31},Pro^{34}]PYY (Y1 agonist) in the presence or absence of 1 µM BIBP 3226 (Y1 antagonist). Non-specific binding was determined in the presence of 1 µM pNPY. See list of abbreviations for details of anatomical identification.

RAT

$[^{125}I]$BH-NPY   1000 nM [Leu^{31},Pro^{34}]PYY   1000 nM pNPY
                     1000 nM PYY$_{3\text{-}36}$

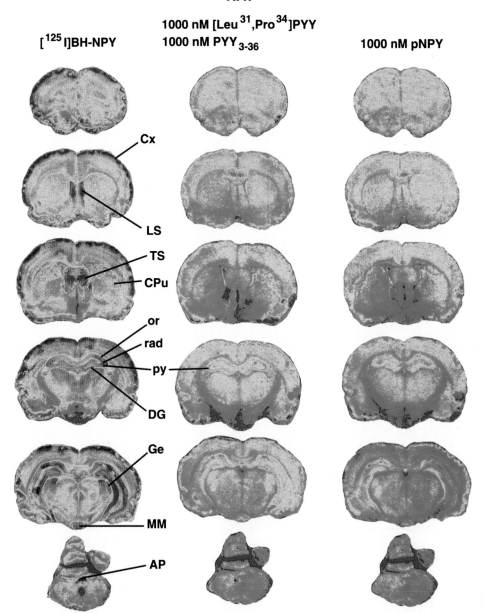

Cx
LS
TS
CPu
or
rad
py
DG
Ge
MM
AP

Plate 5 Photomicrographs of the comparative autoradiographic distribution of $[^{3}H]$BH-NPY alone and in the presence of Y1 and Y2 receptor blockers, thus revealing the possible distribution of the Y3 receptor type in the rat brain. Adjacent coronal sections were incubated with 40 pM $[^{3}H]$BH-NPY in the presence or absence of 1 μM of both [Leu^{31},Pro^{34}]PYY and PYY3–36. Non-specific binding was determined in the presence of 1 μM pNPY. See list of abbreviations for details of anatomical identification.

MOUSE

$[^{125}I][Leu^{31},Pro^{34}]PYY$

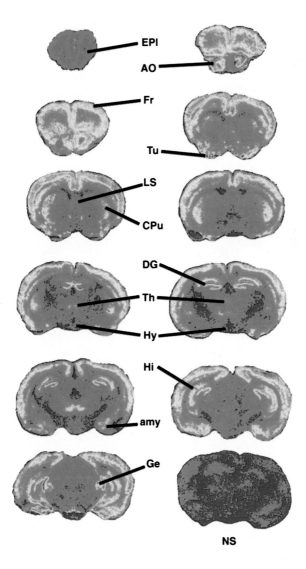

Plate 6 Photomicrographs of the autoradiographic distribution of $[^{125}I][Leu^{31},Pro^{34}]PYY/Y1$-like binding sites at various levels of the mouse brain. Adjacent coronal sections were incubated with either 35 pM $[^{125}I][Leu^{31},Pro^{34}]PYY$ in the presence or absence of 1 μM pNPY in order to determine non-specific binding. See list of abbreviations for details of anatomical identification.

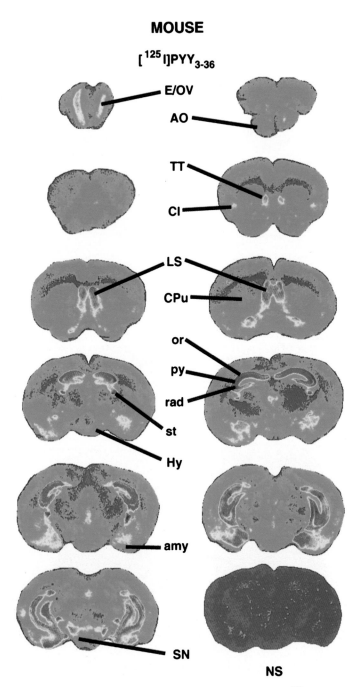

Plate 7 Photomicrographs of the autoradiographic distribution of [^{125}I]PYY3–36/Y2-like binding sites at various levels of the mouse brain. Adjacent coronal sections were incubated with 35 pM [^{125}I]PYY3–36 in the presence or absence of 1 μM pNPY in order to determine non-specific binding. See list of abbreviations for details of anatomical identification.

GUINEA PIG

[^{125}I][Leu^{31},Pro^{34}]PYY

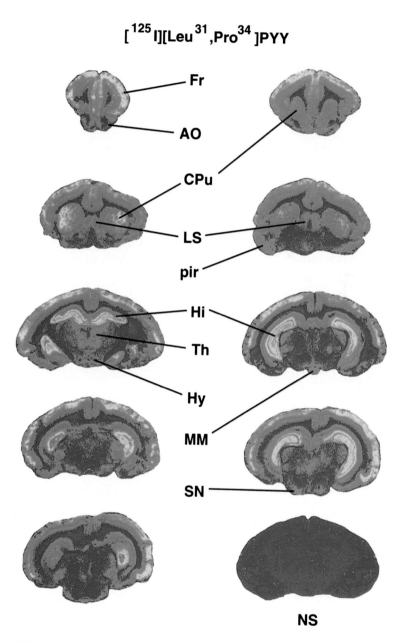

NS

Plate 8 Photomicrographs of the autoradiographic distribution of [^{125}I][Leu^{31},Pro^{34}]PYY/Y1-like binding sites at various levels of the guinea-pig brain. Adjacent coronal sections were incubated with 35 pM [^{125}I][Leu^{31},Pro^{34}]PYY in the presence or absence of 1 μM pNPY in order to determine non-specific binding. See list of abbreviations for details of anatomical identification.

GUINEA PIG

$[^{125}I]PYY_{3-36}$

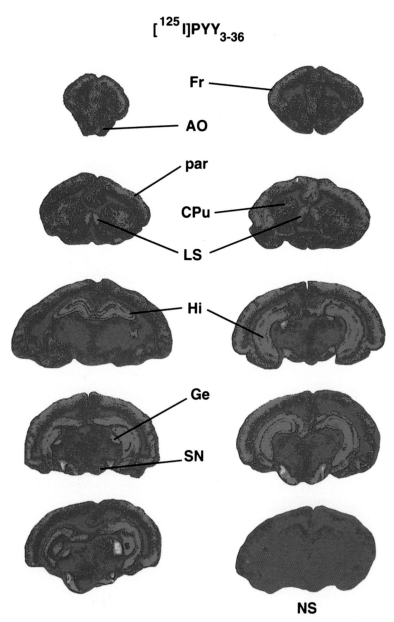

Plate 9 Photomicrographs of the autoradiographic distribution of $[^{125}I]PYY3-36/Y2$-like binding sites at various levels of the guinea-pig brain. Adjacent coronal sections were incubated with 35 pM $[^{125}I]PYY3-36$ in the presence or absence of 1 μM pNPY in order to determine non-specific binding. See list of abbreviations for details of anatomical identification.

GUINEA PIG

$[^{125}\text{I}][\text{Leu}^{31},\text{Pro}^{34}]\text{PYY}$ 1000 nM BIBP3226   1000 nM pNPY

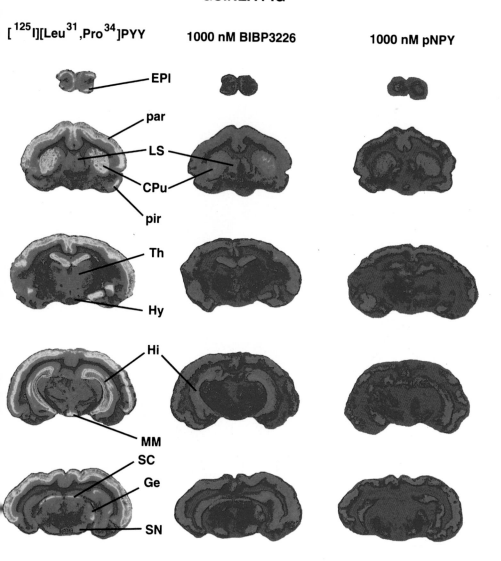

EPI
par
LS
CPu
pir
Th
Hy
Hi
MM
SC
Ge
SN

Plate 10 Photomicrographs of the autoradiographic distribution of $[^{125}\text{I}][\text{Leu}^{31},\text{Pro}^{34}]$ PYY/BIBP 3226-insensitive binding sites at various levels of the guinea-pig brain. Adjacent coronal sections were incubated with 35 pM $[^{125}\text{I}][\text{Leu}^{31},\text{Pro}^{34}]$PYY (Y1 receptor agonist) in the presence or absence of 1 μM BIBP 3226 (Y1 receptor antagonist). Non-specific binding was determined by the presence of 1 μM pNPY. See list of abbreviations for details of anatomical identification.

MONKEY

$[^{125}I][Leu^{31},Pro^{34}]PYY$

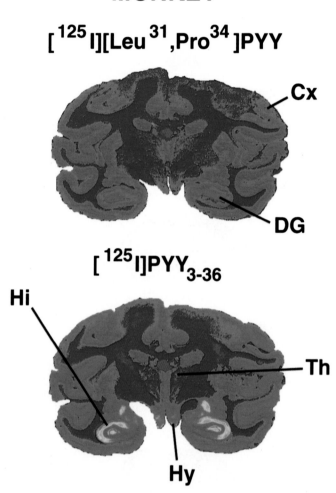

$[^{125}I]PYY_{3\text{-}36}$

Plate 11 Photomicrographs of the comparative autoradiograhic distribution of $[^{125}I][Leu^{31},Pro^{34}]PYY/Y1$-like and $[^{125}I]PYY3–36/Y2$-like binding sites at the level of the hippocampal formation of the monkey brain. Adjacent coronal sections were incubated with 35 pM of either $[^{125}I][Leu^{31},Pro^{34}]PYY$ or $[^{125}I]PYY3–36$ in the presence or absence of 1 µM pNPY in order to determine non-specific binding. See list of abbreviations for details of anatomical identification.

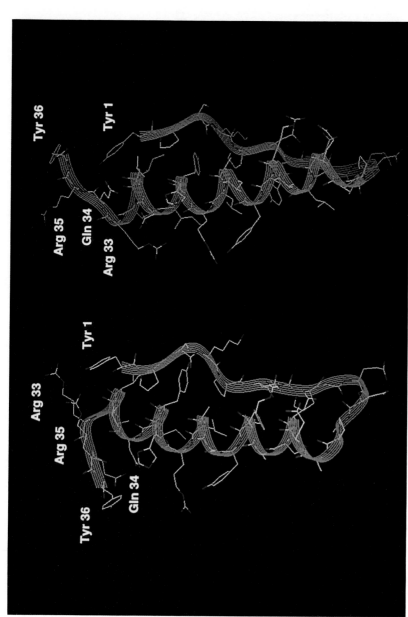

Plate 12 Different conformations of NPY binding to the Y1 receptor (left) or the Y2 receptor (right) according to molecular modelling (Beck-Sickinger et al., 1994b).

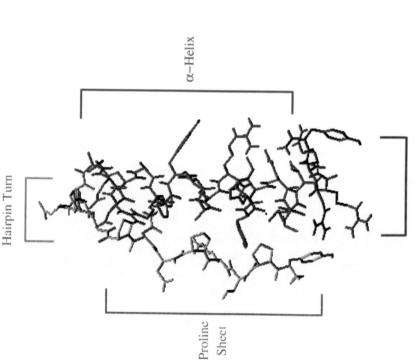

aPP $\longrightarrow$ NPY

NPY Sequence

Tyr–Pro–Ser–Lys–Pro–Asp–Asn–Pro–Gly–
Glu–Asp–Ala–Pro–Ala–Glu–Asp–Met–Ala–
Arg–Tyr–Tyr–Ser–Ala–Leu–Arg–His–Tyr–
Ile–Asn–Leu–Ile–Thr–Arg–Gln–Arg–Tyr–NH2

α–Helix

Hairpin Turn

Unstructured

Proline
Sheet

Plate 13 Computer-derived model of neuropeptide Y (NPY) based on the crystal structure of avian pancreatic polypeptide (aPP). For the detailed procedure used in generating this model, see Leban *et al.* (1995).

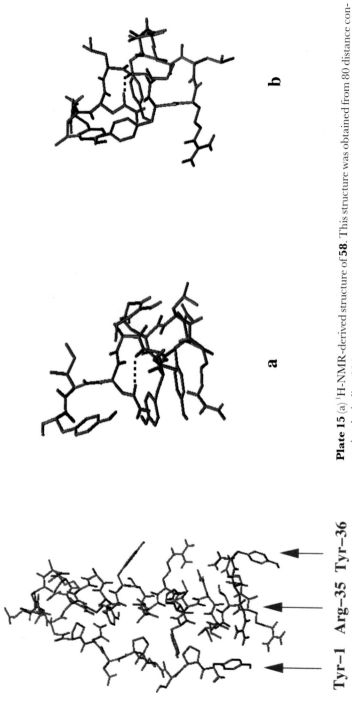

Tyr–1 Arg–35 Tyr–36

Plate 14 A model for minimum structural requirements for binding to NPY receptors. The essential amino-acid residues, Tyr-1, Arg-35 and Tyr-36, are highlighted in green.

a

b

Plate 15 (a) ¹H-NMR-derived structure of **58**. This structure was obtained from 80 distance constraints including 32 inter-residue NOEs, 33 intraresidue NOEs, 6 H-bonds, and 9 torsional constraints using the program DGEOM (Blaney *et al.*, 1990) (b) Structure of **58** generated from an unconstrained molecular dynamics simulation. A representative, minimized structure (*t*=600 ps) is shown and is typical of those observed from 160 ps until the end of the simulation. The Asn-turn is highlighted by residues in blue (Asn-3, Leu-4 and Ile-5). The Tyr residues are shown in green. Dashed lines represent the hydrogen bond of the Asn-turn from Asn-3 (CO) to Ile-5 (NH).

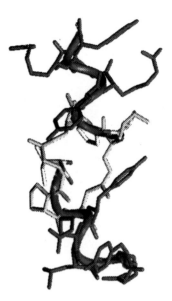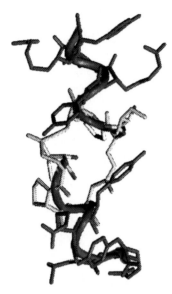

Plate 16 Stereo view of a representative ^{1}H-NMR-derived structure of the dimeric lactam GW1229. The lactam bridge is shown in yellow and the YRLRY pentapeptide amide moieties are shown in blue. The structure was obtained using the program DGEOM (Blaney *et al.*, 1990) from 103 distance constraints, including 45 inter-residue NOEs, 46 intra-residue NOEs and 12-H bonds. A total of ten structures satisfying the distance constraints were calculated and then further energy minimized.

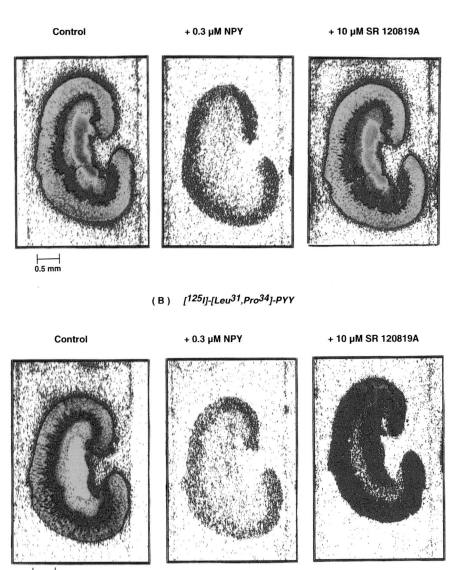

Plate 17 Autoradiograms in rabbit kidney sections using SR 120819A, [125I]PYY3–36 and [125I][Leu31,Pro34]PYY as ligands. Each ligand, [125I]PYY3–36 (A) or [125I][Leu31,Pro34]PYY (B), was incubated alone (control) or in the presence of 0.3 μM NPY (non-specific binding) or 10 μM SR 120819A. Magnification: 2. Graduation colour bar: lower ▁▃▅▇ higher intensity of labeling.

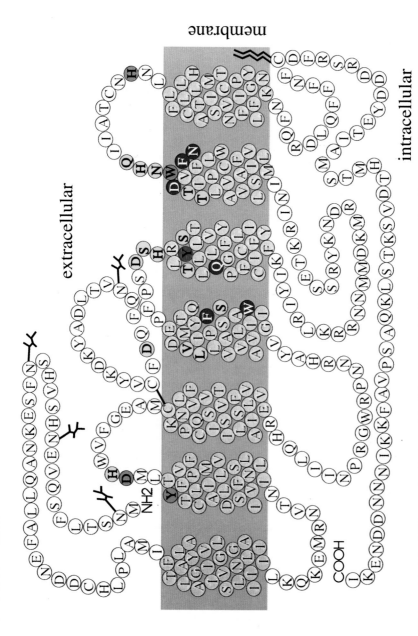

Plate 18 A model of the hY1-receptor. Amino acids of the receptor that have been mutated to Ala are marked. Those mutations that showed reduced affinity for only NPY are marked in blue, whereas Y211, which affected the binding of only BIBP 3226, is marked in pink. Mutations reducing the binding of both NPY and BIBP 3226 are marked in purple, mutants affecting the binding of neither NPY or BIBP 3226 are marked in yellow.

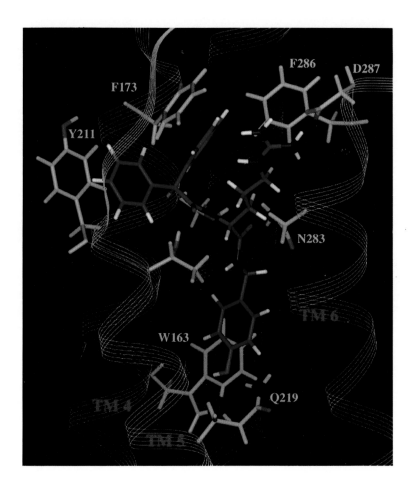

Plate 19 A model of BIBP 3226 binding to the hY1-receptor. Transmembrane helices of the hY1-receptor are indicated by a solid ribbon in yellow and labeled in red. Amino-acid side chains of the human Y1 receptor suggested to interact with the antagonist BIBP 3226 (in green) are shown in yellow.

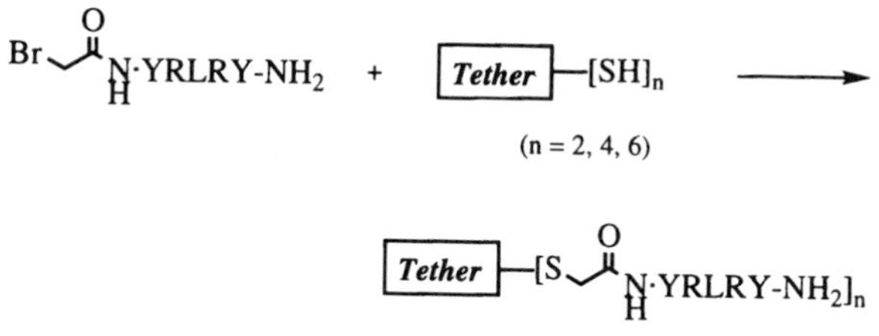

Figure 13 General synthetic route for preparation of dimeric and multimeric analogs of the pentapeptide amide antagonist YRLRY (16).

least 100-fold weaker than that of GW1229 (A. Spaltenstein, unpublished results). Finally, the solution structure of GW1229 and its unprecedented affinity at rat brain receptors, agrees well with a recently proposed model, which correlates a helical conformation of NPY, extending to the C-terminal tyrosine, with structure–activity relationships for binding at a Y2-type receptor (Beck-Sickinger and Jung, 1995).

7.5 Pentapeptide dimers and multimers

Having observed the dramatic effect of dimerization on affinity and activity at NPY receptors with analogs of the nonapeptide 66, an investigation into other di- and multimeric systems was initiated. We chose the pentapeptide amide YRLRY (compound 16) as the starting point and prepared a variety of structurally diverse dimers as well as some tetra- and hexameric derivatives. These compounds were prepared following the procedure illustrated in Figure 13, and were then evaluated in the rat brain and HEL cell assays. The results for a representative set of compounds are presented in Table 8.

Compounds containing bridges that may place the two peptide chains in fairly close proximity, such as cis-alkene 88, lead to a drop in activity of up to ten-fold, while those having moderately rigid tethers spanning a larger number of atoms (such as compound 89) afford analogues of comparable potency (relative to the monomeric reference peptides 16 and 87). On the other hand, compounds with either highly flexible spacers (90) or those that geometrically enforce longer distances (91) lead to significantly more potent analogs. The range of affinity observed for this set of pentapeptide dimers (about 100-fold) indicates that binding to Y2 rat brain receptors is highly dependent on the spatial arrangement of the peptide chains, determined by the tether. A further 50-fold improvement in affinity was found for the tetra- and hexameric compounds 92 and 93.

Interestingly, a different trend is observed with Y1 receptors (HEL cells) where an even more substantial enhancement in activity occurs upon dimerization. The activity at this receptor was largely independent of the nature of the tether, with each dimer displaying a 50–100-fold enhancement relative to the reference monomers. Similar to what was observed in the rat brain assay, the tetra- and hexamer display an additional 20-fold higher activity.

149

Table 8 Effect of dimeric and multimeric pentapeptide antagonists in the displacement of specifically bound [3H]NPY from rat brain membranes and on the inhibition of the NPY-induced increase in cytosolic Ca2+ in HEL cells

Compound	Monomers	$IC_{50}(\mu M)$ rat brain (Y2)	$IC_{50}(\mu M)$ HEL cell (Y1)
16	YRLRY	3	10
87	Br–C(=O)–N(H)-YRLRY	5	30
	Dimers and Multimers		
	Tether		
88	(tether structure)	30	0.5
89	(tether structure)	4	0.25
90	(tether structure)	0.5	0.1
91	(tether structure)	0.25	0.1
92	(tether structure)	0.005	0.0025
93	(tether structure)	0.006	0.006

Results are presented on a per-molecule and not a per-peptide chain basis. Brain and HEL cell asays were carried out as described on Tables 1 and 3, respectively.

7.5.1 Pentapeptide dimers: proposed mechanism of binding

Throughout our efforts to design potent antagonists of NPY, we have observed that ligand dimerization generally results in a modest to large improvement in affinity and activity. Among the possible reasons commonly proposed for enhanced receptor affinity upon ligand dimerization are: (1) increased local concentration of the ligand at the receptor; (2) co-operative binding to multiple sites on the same receptor; or (3) co-operative cross-linking of two receptors (Cheronis *et al.*, 1992; Lees *et al.*, 1994; Mammen *et al.*, 1995). However, the specific contribution by each of these mechanisms is difficult to assess. For example, considering the pentapeptide dimers shown in Table 8, the modest improvement in affinity in the rat brain assay observed for **90** and **91** would be consistent with an increased local concentration effect (Lees *et al.*, 1994), however, the 50-fold enhancement in Y1-receptor activity for the dimers **88–91** precludes such a simple explanation. Interestingly, the lack of sensitivity with respect to tether/linkage geometry, coupled with the relatively large enhancement in activity at the Y1 receptor, is inconsistent with any previously proposed mechanism. Rather, we suggest an 'induced conformation' mechanism, wherein the peptide residues may synergistically stabilize a preferred binding conformation. Such a mechanism would be related to the commonly observed α-helix bundle formation found in proteins (Weber and Salemme, 1980). On the other hand, the much wider variation in affinity ($\geqslant$100-fold) at the Y2 receptor is not easily interpreted, and may be consistent with a combination of cross-linking and local concentration effects.

Conclusion

We have described the first structure-based peptide design of potent peptide antagonists. The compounds described here, particularly GW1229, represent a first generation of high-affinity NPY receptor antagonists, which will help unveil the participation of NPY in important physiological functions. In addition, these compounds may assist in the development of novel therapeutic agents to treat central as well as peripheral pathologies associated with an NPYergic transmission hyperactivity.

The peptides described in this report suggest a simple model for a minimum, essential pharmacophore that could provide a useful starting point for the design of potent and selective small peptide and non-peptide antagonists. To this end, the structure of the recently reported NPY antagonist BIBP3226 (Rudolf *et al.*, 1994) is consistent with this model.

Acknowledgements

We wish to thank the following scientists for their contributions to this research effort: J.J. Leban, A. Landavazo, G. Painter, M. Cory, C.W. Andrews, J. Bentley, L. Kuyper, L. Taylor, W. Chestnut and A. Aulabaugh (Chemistry). J.E. Matthews, R.J. Slepetis, M. Jansen, W. Harrington, A. Tadepalli, M. Hashim and O.H. Viveros (Pharmacology).

References

Abbadi, A., Mcharfi, M., Aubry, A., Prelimat, S., Boussard, G. & Marraud, M. (1991) Involvement of side functions in peptide structures: The Asx turn. Occurrence and conformational aspects. *J. Am. Chem. Soc.* **113**, 2729–2735.

Adrian, T.E., Allen, J.M., Bloom, S.R., Ghatei, M.A., Rossor, M.N., Roberts, G.W., Crow, T.J., Tatemoto, K. & Polak, J.M. (1983) Neuropeptide Y distribution in human brain. *Nature (Lond.)* **306**, 584–586.

Allen, J.M., Novotny, J., Martin, J. & Heinrich, G. (1987) Molecular structure of mammalian neuropeptide Y: Analysis by molecular cloning and computer-aided comparison with crystal structure of avian homologue. *Proc. Natl Acad. Sci. USA* **84**, 2532–2536.

Baeza, C.R. & Unden, A. (1990) Binding of analogues of the neuropeptide Y model peptide NPY 1–4–ahx-25–36 to rat cerebral cortex. In *Peptides: Chemistry, Structure and Biology* (eds Giralt, E. & Andreu, D.), pp. 649–651. The Netherlands, ESCOM Science Publishers B.V.

Bard, J.A., Walker, M.W., Branchek, T.A. & Weinshank, R.L. (1995) Cloning and functional expression of a human Y4 subtype receptor for pancreatic polypeptide, neuropeptide Y and peptide YY. *J. Biol. Chem.* **270**, 26 762–26 765.

Beck, A., Jung, G., Gaida, W., Koppen, H., Lang, R. & Schnorrenberg, G. (1989) Highly potent and small neuropeptide Y agonist obtained by linking NPY1–4 via spacer to α-helical NPY25–36. *FEBS Lett.* **244**, 119–122.

Beck-Sickinger, A.G. & Jung, G. (1995) Structure activity relationships of neuropeptide Y analogues with respect to Y1 & Y2 receptors. *Biopolymers* **37**, 123–142.

Beck-Sickinger, A.G., Jung, G., Gaida, W., Koppen, H. & Schnorrenberg, G. (1990a) Structure–activity relationships of c-terminal neuropeptide Y peptide segments and analogues composed of sequence 1–4 linked to 25–36. *Eur. J. Biochem.* **194**, 449–456.

Beck-Sickinger, A.G., Gaida, W., Schnorrenberg, G., Lang, R. & Jung, G. (1990b) Neuropeptide Y: identification of the binding site. *Int. J. Pept. Protein Res.* **36**, 522–530.

Beck-Sickinger, A.G., Gaida, W., Schnorrenberg, G. & Jung, G. (1990c) Systematic point mutation of high affinity analogue neuropeptide Y 1–4–ahx-25–36. In *Peptides: Chemistry, Structure and Biology* (eds Giralt, E. & Andreu, D.), pp. 646–648. The Netherlands, ESCOM Science Publishers B.V.

Beck-Sickinger, A.G., Wieland, W.K., Wittneben, H., Willim, K.D., Rudolf, K. & Jung, G. (1994) Complete L-alanine scan of neuropeptide Y reveals ligands binding to Y1 and Y2 receptors with distinguished conformations. *Eur. J. Biochem.* **225**, 947–958.

Blaney, Crippen, Dearing & Dixon. (1990) Quantum chemistry exchange programme 590, E.I. Wilmington DE, Dupont & Co.

Blundell, T.L., Pitts, J.E., Tickle, I.J., Wood, S.P. & Wu, C.-W. (1981) X-ray analysis (1.4 Å resolution) of avian pancreatic polypeptide: small globular protein hormone. *Proc. Natl Acad. Sci. USA* **78**, 4175–4179.

Boublik, J.H., Scott, N.A., Brown, M.R. & Rivier, J.E. (1989) Synthesis and hypertensive activity of neuropeptide Y fragments and analogues with modified n- or c-termini or d-substitutions. *J. Med. Chem.* **32**, 597–601.

Boublik, J.H., Spicer, M.A., Scott, N.A., Brown, M.R. & Rivier, J.E. (1990) Biologically active neuropeptide Y analogues. *Ann. N. York Acad. Sci.* **511**, 27–34.

Cheronis, J.C., Whalley, E.T., Nguyen, K.T., Eubanks, S.R., Allen, L.G., Duggan, M.J., Loy, S.D., Bonham, K.A. & Blodgett, J.K. (1992) A new class of bradykinin antagonists. Synthesis and in vitro activity of bissuccinimidoalkane peptide dimers. *J. Med. Chem.* **35**, 1563–1572.

Daniels, A.J., Matthews, J.E., Viveros, O.H. & Lazarowski, E.R. (1992) Characterization of the neuropeptide Y-induced intracellular calcium release in human erythroleukemic cells. *Mol. Pharmacol.* **41**, 767–771.

Daniels, A.J., Matthews, J.A., Viveros, O.H., Leban, J.J., Cory, M. & Heyer, D. (1995a) Structure–activity relationship of novel pentapeptide neuropeptide Y receptor antagonists is consistent with a noncontinuous epitope for ligand-receptor binding. *Mol. Pharmacol.* **48**, 425–432.

Daniels, A.J., Matthews, J.E., Slepetis, R.J., Jansen, M., Viveros, O.H., Tadepalli, A.,

Harrington, W., Heyer, D., Landavazo, A., Leban, J.J. & Spaltenstein, A. (1995b) High-affinity neuropeptide Y antagonists. *Proc. Natl Acad. Sci. USA* **92**, 9067–9071.

Darbon, H., Bernassau, J.-M., Deleuze, C., Chenu, J., Roussel, A. & Cambillau, C. (1992) Solution structure of human neuropeptide Y by ^{1}H nuclear magnetic resonance and restrained molecular dynamics. *Eur. J. Biochem.* **209**, 765–771.

Forest, M., Martel, J.-C., St-Pierre, S., Quirion, R. & Fournier, A. (1990) Structural study of the n-terminal segment of neuropeptide tyrosine. *J. Med. Chem.* **33**, 1615–1619.

Fuhlendorff, J., Johansen, N.L., Melberg, S.G., Thoegersen, H. & Schwartz, T.W. (1989) The antiparallel pancreatic polypeptide fold in the binding of neuropeptide Y to Y1 and Y2 receptors. *J. Biol. Chem.* **265**, 11 706–11 712.

Fuhlendorff, J., Gether, U., Aakerlund, L., Langeland-Johansen, N., Thoegersen, H., Melberg, S.G., Olsen, U.B., Thastrup, O. & Schwartz, T.W. (1990) [Leu^{31},Pro^{34}] Neuropeptide Y: a specific Y1 receptor agonist. *Proc. Natl Acad. Sci. USA* **87**, 182–186.

Gehlert, D.R. (1994) Subtypes of receptors for NPY: implications for the targeting of therapeutics. *Life Sci.* **55**, 551–562.

Gerald, C., Walker, M.W., Vaysee, P.J.J., He, C.G., Branchek, T.A. & Weinshank, R.L. (1995) Pharmacological characterization of a human hippocampal neuropeptide Y peptide YY Y2 receptor subtype. *J. Biol. Chem.* **270**, 26 758–26 761.

Glover, I., Haneef, I., Pitts, J.E., Wood, S.P., Moss, D., Tickle, I.J. & Blundell, T.L. (1983) Conformational flexibility in a small globular hormone: x-ray analysis of avian pancreatic polypeptide at 0.98 Å resolution. *Biopolymers* **22**, 293–304.

Glover, I., Barlow, D.J., Pitts, J.E., Wood, S.P., Tickle, I.J., Blundell, T.L. Tatemoto, K., Kimmel, J.R., Wollmer, A., Strassburger, W. & Zhang, Y.-S. (1985) Conformational studies on the pancreatic polypeptide family. *Eur. J. Biochem.* **142**, 379–385.

Gray, T.S. & Morley, J.E. (1986) Neuropeptide Y: anatomical distribution and possible function in mammalian nervous system. *Life Sci.* **38**, 389–401.

Grundemar, L. & Håkanson, R. (1990) Effects of various neuropeptide Y/peptide YY fragments on electrically evoked contractions of the rat vas deferens. *Br. J. Pharmacol.* **100**, 190–192.

Hegde, S.S., Bonhaus, D.W., Stanleyt, W., Eglen, R.M., Moy, T.M., Loeb, M., Shetty, S.G., Desouza, A. & Krstenansky, J. (1995) Pharmacological evaluation of 1229U91, a novel high affinity and selective neuropeptide Y-Y1 receptor antagonist. *J. Pharm. Exp. Ther.* **275**, 1261–1266.

Jörgensen, JCh., Fuhlendorff, J. & Schwarz, T.W. (1990) Structure–function studies on neuropeptide Y and pancreatic polypeptide – evidence for two PP-fold receptors in vas deferens. *Eur. J. Pharmacol.* **186**, 105–114.

Jung, G., Beck-Sickinger, A.G., Durr, H., Gaida, W. & Schnorrenberg, G. (1991) α-Helical, small molecular size analogues of neuropeptide Y: structure–activity-relationships. *Biopolymers* **31**, 613–619.

Kirby, D.A., Boublik, J.H. & Rivier, J.E. (1993) Neuropeptide Y: Y1 and Y2 affinities of the complete series of analogues with single d-residue substitutions. *J. Med. Chem.* **36**, 3802–3808.

Krstenansky, J.L. (1993) Designing selective analogs for peptide receptors: neuropeptide Y as an example. In *Methods in Neuroscience* (ed. Conn, P.M.), Vol. 12, pp. 388–403. San Diego, CA, Academic Press, Inc.

Larhammår, D., Blomqvist, A.G., Yee, F., Jazin, E., Yoo, H.Y. & Wahlestedt, C. (1992) Cloning and functional expression of a human neuropeptide Y peptide YY receptor of the Y1-type. *J. Biol. Chem.* **267**, 10 935–10 938.

Leban, J.J., Heyer, D., Landavazo, A., Matthews, J.E., Aulabaugh, A. & Daniels, A.J. (1995) Novel modified carboxy terminal fragments of neuropeptide Y with high affinity for Y2-type receptors and potent functional antagonism at a Y1-type receptor. *J. Med Chem.* **38**, 1150–1157.

Leban, J.J., Spaltenstein, A., Landavazo, A., Chestnut, W., Aulabaugh, A., Taylor, L. & Daniels,

A.J. (1996) Synthesis, structure and stability of novel peptide dimeric disulfides. *Int. J. Peptide Protein Res.* **47**, 161–166.

Lees, W.J., Spaltenstein, A., Kingery-Wood, J.E. & Whitesides, G. (1994) Polyacrylamides bearing pendant α-sialoside groups strongly inhibit agglutination of particulate biological systems. *J. Med. Chem.* **37**, 3419–3433.

Li, X., Sutcliffe, M.J., Schwartz, T.W. & Dodson, C.M. (1992) Sequence specific ^{1}H NMR assignments and solution structure of bovine pancreatic polypeptide. *Biochemistry* **31**, 1245–1253.

Lundberg, J.M., Terenius, I., Hökfelt, T. & Tatemoto, K. (1984) Comparative immunohistochemical and biochemical analysis of pancreatic polypeptide-like peptides with special reference to presence of neuropeptide Y in central and peripheral neurons. *J. Neurosci.* **4**, 2376–2386.

Lundell, I., Blomqvist, A.G., Berglund, M.M., Schober, D.A., Johnson, D., Statnick, M.A., Gadski, R.A., Gehlert, D.A. & Larhammår, D. (1995) Cloning of a human receptor of the NPY family with high affinity for pancreatic polypeptide and peptide YY. *J. Biol. Chem.* **270**, 29 123–29 128.

Mammen, M., Dahmann, G. & Whitesides, G.M. (1995) Effective inhibitors of hemagglutination by influenza virus synthesized from polymers having active ester groups. Insight into mechanism of inhibition. *J. Med. Chem.* **38**, 4179–4190.

Matthews, J.E., Jansen, M., Slepetis, R.S., Rash, V.A. & Daniels, A.J. (1995) Novel high affinity NPY antagonist identifies different subclasses of Y2-type NPY receptors. *Soc. Neurosci. Abstr.* **21**(2), 1593.

Michel, M.C. (1991) Receptors of neuropeptide Y: multiple subtypes and multiple second messengers. *Trends Pharmacol. Sci.* **12**, 389–394.

Pichon-Pesme, V., Aubry, A., Abbadi, A., Mcharfi, M., Boussard, G. & Marraud, M. (1989) The Asx-turn structure in Asn and Asp-containing peptides. In *Peptides: Proceedings of the Twentieth European Peptide Symposium* (eds Jung, G. & Bayer, E.), pp. 507–509. Berlin, Walter de Gruyter.

Rose, P.M., Fernandes, P., Lynch, J.S., Frazier, S.T., Fisher, S.M., Kodukula, K. Kienzle, B. & Seethala, R. (1995) Cloning and functional expression of a cDNA encoding a human type 2 neuropeptide Y receptor. *J. Biol. Chem.* **270**, 22 661–22 664.

Rudolf, K.W., Eberlein, W., Engel, W., Wieland, H.A., Willim, K.D., Entzeroth, M., Wienen, W., Beck-Sickinger, A.G. & Doods, H.N. (1994) The first highly potent and selective non-peptide neuropeptide Y Y1 receptor antagonist: BIBP3226. *Eur. J. Pharmacol.* **27**, R11–R13.

Schwartz, T.W., Fuhlendorff, J., Kjems, L.L., Kristensen, M.S., Vervelde, M., O'Hare, M., Krstenansky, J.L. & Bjoernholm, B. (1990) Signal epitopes in the three-dimensional structure of neuropeptide Y. Interaction with Y1, Y2 and pancreatic polypeptide receptors. *Ann. N. York Acad. Sci.* **611**, 35–47.

Sheikh, S.P., Håkanson, R. & Schwartz, T.W. (1989) Y1 and Y2 receptors for neuropeptide Y. *FEBS Lett.* **245**, 209–214.

Tadepalli, A.S., Harrington, W.W., Hashim, M., Matthews, J., Leban, J.J., Spaltenstein, A. & Daniels, A.J. (1996) Hemodynamic characterization of a novel neuropeptide Y receptor antagonist. *J. Cardiovasc. Pharm.* **27**, 712–718.

Tatemoto, K., Carlquist, M. & Mutt, V. (1982) Neuropeptide Y – a novel brain peptide with structural similarities to peptide YY and pancreatic polypeptide. *Nature (Lond.)* **296**, 659–660.

Wahlestedt, C. & Reis, D.J. (1993) Neuropeptide Y-related peptides and their receptors: are the receptors potential therapeutic drug targets? *Annu. Rev. Pharmacol. Toxicol.* **32**, 309–352.

Wahlestedt, C., Yanaihara, N. & Håkanson, R. (1986) Evidence for different pre- and postjunctional receptors for neuropeptide Y and related peptides. *Regul. Pept.* **13**, 307–318.

Wahlestedt, C., Regunathan, S. & Reis, D.J. (1992) Identification of cultured cells selectively expressing Y1-, Y2- or Y3-type receptors of neuropeptide Y/peptide YY. *Life Sci.* **50**, 7–12.

Weber, P.C. & Salemme, F.R. (1980) Structural and functional diversity in 4-α-helical proteins. *Nature (Lond.)* **287**, 82–84.

Yun, R.H., Anderson, A. & Hermans, J. (1991) Proline in α-helix: stability and conformation studied by dynamics simulation. *Proteins Struct. Funct. Genet.* **10**, 219–228.

Zukowska-Grojec, Z. & Wahlestedt, C. (1993) Origin and actions of neuropeptide Y in the cardiovascular system. In *The Biology of Neuropeptide Y and Related Peptides* (eds Colmers, W.F. & Wahlestedt, C.) pp. 315–388. Totowa, NJ, Humana Press.

-------------------- CHAPTER 8 --------------------

SR 120819A OR THE FIRST GENERATION OF ORALLY ACTIVE Y1-RECEPTOR ANTAGONISTS

Claudine Serradeil-Le Gal

Table of Contents

8.1 Introduction

Neuropeptide Y (NPY) is one of the most abundant neuropeptides, and it is widely distributed throughout the central and peripheral nervous system in mammals (Lundberg and Tatemoto, 1982; Tatemoto, 1982; Gray and Morley, 1986). A huge amount of data accumulated during the past decade has highlighted the key role of NPY in a variety of physiological responses, especially concerning cardiovascular regulation, food intake, metabolism, behavioral, sexual and endocrine functions (see Chapters 1–3 of this book; for reviews, see Stanley, 1993; Grundemar and Hakanson, 1994; Frankish *et al.*, 1995). Moreover, the direct or indirect implications of NPY in various diseases or pathological states, such as hypertension, unstable angina, myocardial infarction, obesity, bulimia, anxiety, epilepsy, depression, memory, pain, etc. suggest that NPY may be a promising therapeutic target (Heilig, 1993; Wahlestedt and Reis, 1993; Gehlert, 1994; Grundemar, 1995; Wettstein *et al.*, 1995).

Pharmacological studies using synthetic NPY analogues or fragments, the recent progress made in molecular biology with the cloning of Y1 (Herzog *et al.*, 1992; Larhammar *et al.*, 1992), Y2 (Gerald *et al.*, 1995; Rose *et al.*, 1995) and Y4 (or PP1) (Bard *et al.*, 1995; Lundell *et al.*, 1995) receptors, and the use of receptor antisense oligonucleotides (Erlinge *et al.*, 1993; Akabayashi *et al.*, 1994; Heilig, 1995) have shown

Neuropeptide Y and Drug Development
ISBN 0-12-304990-3

that multiple receptor types (the so-called Y1, Y2, Y3, PP1 or Y4, PYY-preferring and 'appetite' receptors) support the diverse actions of NPY and those of the two closely related hormones, peptide YY (PYY) and pancreatic polypeptides (PP) (Tatemoto *et al.*, 1982).

In particular, an important role could be attributed to Y1 receptors in regulating the cardiovascular functions (Walker *et al.*, 1991; Dermott *et al.*, 1993). Through post-synaptic peripheral Y1 receptors, NPY, PYY and the selective Y1 receptor agonist, [Leu^{31},Pro^{34}]NPY induced vasoconstriction in crucial areas, such as coronary and cerebral blood vessels, and even amplified the action of other vasoconstrictor agents like noradrenaline (Clarke *et al.*, 1987; Edvinsson *et al.*, 1987; Potter, 1988).

Among various central effects, the Y1 receptors probably mediate anxiolysis whereas, a Y1-like subtype may support the powerful stimulation of NPY in food intake (Heilig, 1993; Stanley, 1993; Bouali *et al.*, 1994; Currie and Coscina, 1995; Kirby *et al.*, 1995). These facts illustrate both the complexity and the heterogeneity of NPY receptors.

Accordingly, the discovery of selective agonist or antagonist molecules is the first step in understanding the role of NPY, its receptor functions and in establishing an accurate receptor classification. Obviously, the design of potent, specific, orally-active compounds is the following stage for further addressing the physiopathological role of NPY and for designing potential therapeutical agents. In this field, the recent years have marked a turning point with the design of the first potent and selective NPY Y1-receptor antagonists, BIBP 3226 (Rudolf *et al.*, 1994) and SR 120819A (Serradeil-Le Gal *et al.*, 1994a, 1995). To our knowledge, SR 120819A represents the first genera-tion of orally active NPY Y1-receptor antagonists yet described and constitutes, in that respect, a promising tool for exploring NPY functions and developing therapeu-tic agents.

This chapter gives an overview of the original biochemical and pharmacological profile of SR 120819A in several animal and human models *in vitro* and *in vivo*. In addi-tion, this report clearly illustrates the usefulness of this selective Y1-receptor ligand in acutely discriminating the NPY receptors and in selectively mapping Y1 binding sites in complex tissues expressing mixed populations of NPY/PYY receptors.

All the methods given in this manuscript are described in the Materials and Methods section of the following papers (Serradeil-Le Gal *et al.*, 1993, 1995, 1996).

8.2 The discovery of SR 120819A

SR 120819A (1-[2-[2-(2-naphthylsulfamoyl)-3-phenylpropionamido]-3-[4-[N-[4-(dimethylaminomethyl)-*cis*-cyclohexylmethyl]amidino]phenyl]propioyl]-pyrrolidine (R, R) stereoisomer) (Figure 1) was obtained by the optimization of a lead compound. The initial lead compound, with a modest 10 μM potency, has been optimized by rational design and three-dimensional modeling based on the known interactions of NPY and [Leu^{31},Pro^{34}]NPY with NPY receptors in different species (Allen *et al.*, 1987;

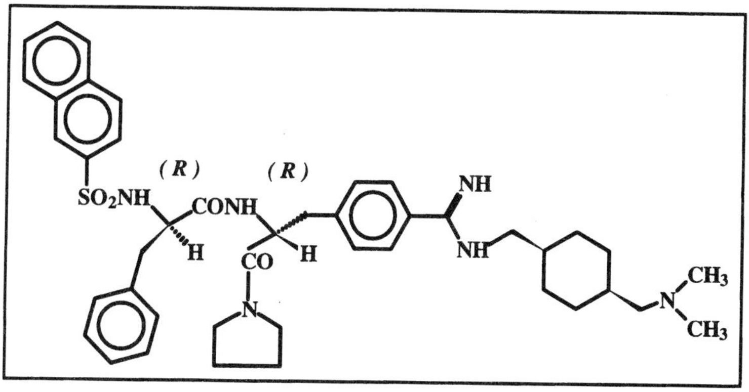

Figure 1 Chemical structure of SR 120819A.

Darbon *et al.*, 1992; Kirby *et al.*, 1993; Walker *et al.*, 1994). This fruitful strategy has led to the design of SR 120819A (and analogs) able to bind selectively Y1 receptors with high affinity. This (R,R) *cis* molecule corresponds to the most active enantiomer. As previously described, the *trans* isomer of SR 120819A, called SR 120107A (Figure 2), is a NPY Y1-receptor antagonist with lower affinity and potency than SR 120819A *in vitro* and *in vivo* (Serradeil-Le Gal *et al.*, 1994a). These structures mimic the C-terminal part of NPY in which Tyr-36, and both Arg-33 and Arg-35 play a major role in receptor binding (Walker *et al.*, 1994; Sautel *et al.*, 1995). As a general remark, a pharmacophore involving an hydrophobic region together with a strong basic center (constituted by the benzamidin group for SR compounds), seem to be a common feature required for the binding to NPY receptors, i.e. BIBP 3226 (Rudolf *et al.*, 1994), Benextramine or its analogs (Chaurasia *et al.*, 1994), and derived histamine H2-receptor agonists related to arpromidine, such as He 90482 and its analogs (Michel and Motulsky, 1990; Knieps *et al.*, 1995) (Figure 2).

8.3 Biochemical profile of SR 120819A

8.3.1 Affinity and selectivity of SR 120819A for Y1 receptors *in vitro*

The cloning of NPY receptors Y1 (Herzog *et al.*, 1992; Larhammar *et al.*, 1992), Y2 (Gerald *et al.*, 1995; Rose *et al.*, 1995) and Y4 (or PP1) (Bard *et al.*, 1995; Lundell *et al.*, 1995) in different species demonstrated that they all belong to the seven transmembrane domain G-protein-coupled receptors. As already reported for several peptide ligand receptors, marked differences exist in the amino-acid sequence of Y1 receptors according to species: mouse, rat and human (Eva *et al.*, 1992; Herzog *et al.*,

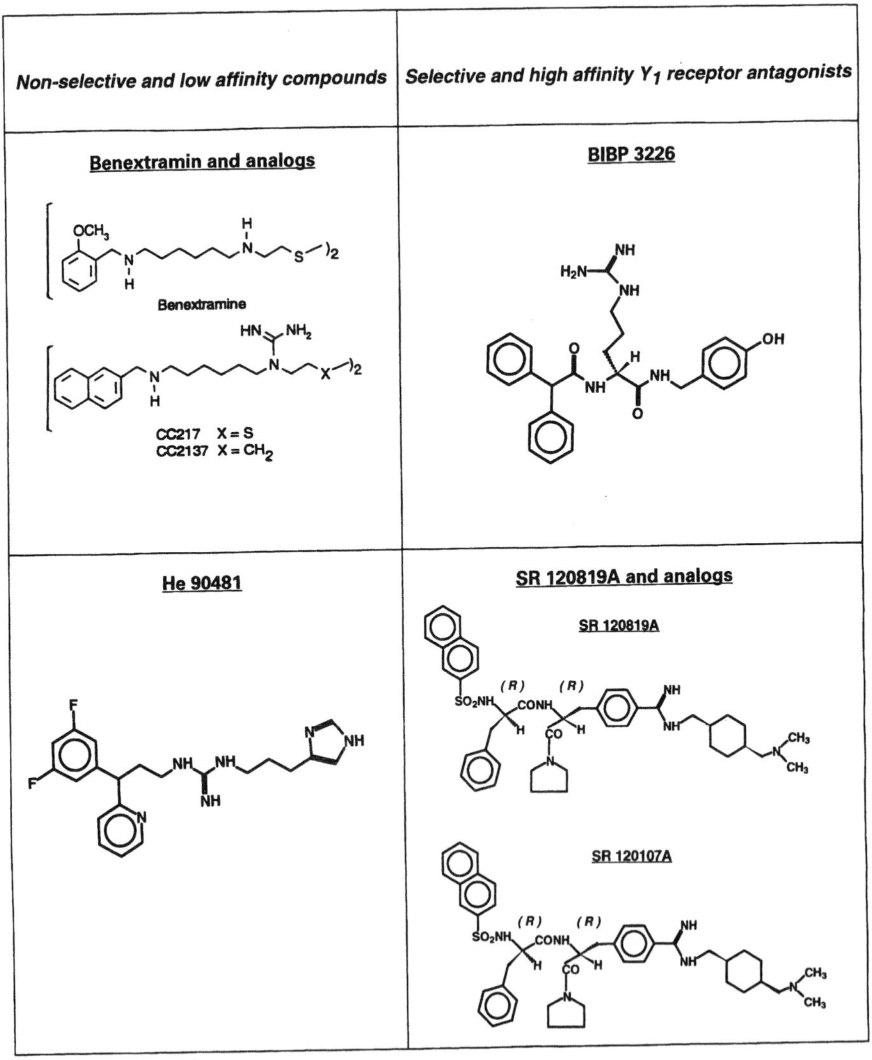

Figure 2 Chemical structures of non-peptide NPY receptor ligands.

1992; Larhammar *et al.*, 1992). Therefore, special attention was paid to the investigation of SR 120819A at human NPY receptors using the human neuroblastoma cell line, SK-N-MC, which only expresses Y1 receptors (Fuhlendorff *et al.*, 1990; Feth *et al.*, 1991).

As shown in Table 1, SR 120819A exhibited similar affinity for Y1 receptors from rat, guinea-pig and human origin. SR 120819A inhibited [125I]PYY (or [125I]NPY) binding to SK-N-MC cells in a concentration-dependent manner and displayed rather similar affinity to that of the recently described non-peptide compound, BIBP

160

Table 1 Affinity and selectivity profile of SR 120819A for NPY Y1, Y2 and Y3 receptors *in vitro*

	Binding studies					Functional test
Type	Y1			Y2		Y3
Results	K_i (nM)			Inhibition (%) at 10 μM		Inhibition (%) at 1 μM
Tissues	Rat Brain cortex	Guinea-pig Brain cortex	Human SK-N-MC cells	Rabbit Cortex kidney	Human Brain cortex	Rat Colon
Ligands						Agonist
[^{125}I]NPY	15±6	22±6	21±8	5±3	2±2	NPY
[^{125}I]PYY	11±3	20±5	17±6	0±3	3±1	5±2

K_i values are calculated according to the equation of Cheng and Prusoff (1973). Studies are performed as described in Materials and Methods in Serradeil-Le Gal et al. (1995).

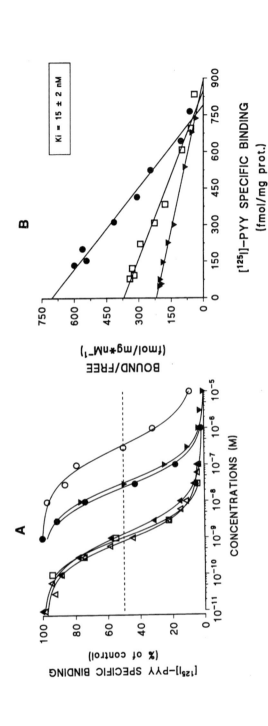

Figure 3 Binding studies with SR 120819A in human neuroblastoma SK-N-MC cells. (A) Inhibition of [^{125}I]PYY binding by NPY (□), PYY (△), [Leu^{31},Pro^{34}]NPY (▲), NPY13–36 (○), SR 120819A (●) and BIBP 3226 (▼) in SK-N-MC membranes. (B) Scatchard plots of [^{125}I]PYY binding to human SK-N-MC membranes without (●) of with 15 (□) and 30 ([▼])nM SR 120819A. The radioligand (80 pM) was incubated in a Krebs–Ringer buffer pH 7.4 for 1 h at 30°C in the presence of membranes (20 μg/assay) and compounds to be tested (Serradeil-Le Gal *et al.*, 1995).

3226, for Y1 receptors in this model (Figure 3A). Saturation experiments performed with $[^{125}I]$PYY in the human Y1 cell line demonstrated a full competitive interaction of SR 120819A with Y1 receptors yielding a K_i value of 15 nM (Figure 3B).

In terms of specificity, SR 120819A showed a highly selective profile *in vitro*. As illustrated in Table 1, this compound neither binds to Y2 receptors nor interacts with Y3 receptors when investigated in the contractile response of NPY in the Y3 rat colon model (Cadieux *et al.*, 1990; Dumont *et al.*, 1993a). Additional studies, performed with SR 120819A (1 μM) in more than 30 typical binding assays, showed no interaction of the compound with any other receptors.

Obviously, to investigate the profile of SR 120819A fully, the affinity of this compound for the recently cloned PP receptor, called PP1 (Lundell *et al.*, 1995) or Y4 (Bard *et al.*, 1995), has to be further explored.

8.3.2 SR 120819A as a selective Y1 tool for the characterization of NPY receptors

The following example illustrates both the complexity of NPY receptors and the usefulness of SR 120819A for the characterization and specific localization of Y1 receptors in tissues that express heterogeneous populations of NPY/PYY sites. Recently, the two radioiodinated PYY analogues, $[^{125}I][Leu^{31},Pro^{34}]$PYY and $[^{125}I]$PYY3–36, were developed as the first selective Y1 and Y2 receptor ligands, respectively (Dumont *et al.*, 1993b, 1994, 1995; Fournier *et al.*, 1993). Thus, we used these tools together with SR 120819A to investigate the presence and the distribution of NPY receptors in the rabbit kidney by the autoradiographic technique in slide-mounted sections. $[^{125}I]$PYY3–36 produced intense labeling both in the cortical and medullary regions, and clearly showed the massive presence of NPY Y2 receptors throughout the kidney (Plate 17A), as already previously described (Leys *et al.*, 1987 Sheikh *et al.*, 1989; Gimpl *et al.*, 1990; Michel *et al.*, 1992). As expected, the Y1 receptor ligand, SR 120819A, is almost ineffective in displacing $[^{125}I]$PYY3–36 bound to rabbit kidney sections. However, most interestingly, the Y1-described receptor ligand, $[^{125}I][Leu^{31},Pro^{34}]$ PYY, provides labeling of the medulla area and, to a lesser extent, of the cortex. This binding is highly specific, since it is totally displaced in both regions by incubating with 0.3 μM NPY. Intriguingly, only partial displacement of $[^{125}I][Leu^{31},Pro^{34}]$PYY binding could be obtained, even when challenged with high concentrations (up to 10 μM) of the selective Y1 receptor antagonist, SR 120819A (Plate 17B), although this compound has shown high efficacy at NPY Y1 receptors even in the rabbit (see Figure 5).

Firstly, our results demonstrated for the first time the significant presence of Y1 receptors in the kidney suggesting that both Y1 and Y2 receptors are involved in the control of the renal function, at least in the rabbit kidney. Secondly, $[^{125}I][Leu^{31},Pro^{34}]$PYY labeled not only Y1 receptors but also another site throughout the kidney, non-displaceable by SR 120819A. Thus, this radioiodinated ligand, and the subsequently unlabeled peptide, cannot be considered as selective tools for Y1 receptors. The characterization of this unknown site non-displaceable by SR 120819A, needs to be explored further using various reference NPY/PYY/PP-related peptides or fragments. It is worth noting that during the preparation of this manuscript, $[^{125}I][Leu^{31}, Pro^{34}]PYY$ sites resistant to high concentrations of another selective Y1-receptor antagonist, BIBP 3226, have also been reported in the rat brain (Dumont and Quirion, 1995). However, owing to the insufficiency of available data, no precise correlation between the two sites can be made at the moment.

8.4 *In vitro* functional studies with SR 120819A

The characterization of the *in vitro* pharmacological profile of SR 120819A is illustrated here in two relevant well-known Y1-receptor preparations: the human neuroblastoma SK-N-MC cell line (Fuhlendorff *et al.*, 1990; Feth *et al.*, 1991) and the rabbit vas deferens (Doods and Krause, 1991).

At the second messenger level, the Y1-receptor activation is linked to two main signaling mechanisms involving intracellular Ca^{2+} mobilization and adenylate cyclase inhibition. These transduction signals have been observed in several cell preparations, such as human erythroleukemia (HEL) cells (Michel, 1991), SK-N-MC (Feth *et al.*, 1991) or stably transfected cells with the Y1 receptor (Herzog *et al.*, 1992; Larhammar *et al.*, 1992). In order to determine the antagonist (or agonist) properties of SR 120819A, we examined its effects on NPY-induced inhibition of cAMP accumulation elicited by forskolin (0.5 μM). As shown in Figure 4, SR 120819A (1–1000 nM) dose-dependently antagonized the effect of NPY on adenylate cyclase activity with an IC_{50} value of 92 nM (66–140 nM, with a 95% confidence interval, $n = 3$) in good agreement with the previously described binding affinity of SR 120819A for human NPY Y1 receptors in SK-N-MC cells (Table 1 and Figure 3).

In rabbit vas deferens preparations, NPY and the Y1-receptor agonist, $[Leu^{31}, Pro^{34}]NPY$, produced a concentration-dependent inhibition of the electrically-induced twitch contraction (pD_2 value of 8.32 ± 0.03, $n = 6$). SR 120819A (0.1–1 μM) elicited a parallel rightward shift in the $[Leu^{31}, Pro^{34}]NPY$ dose–response. Schild-plot analysis of these data gave a pA_2 value of 7.2 ± 0.07 and a slope about unity, indicating a fully competitive antagonist profile for SR 120819A for the presynaptic Y1 receptors in the rabbit vas deferens *in vitro* (Figure 5).

In addition, even at high concentrations (1–10 μM), SR 120819A did not show any agonistic effects in both Y1-receptor preparations.

8.5 Pharmacological profile of SR 120819A *in vivo*

8.5.1 Cardiovascular studies

NPY is one of the most potent vasoconstrictor agents described so far that is active in several vascular beds, such as cerebral, coronary and renal vessels (Edvinsson *et al.*,

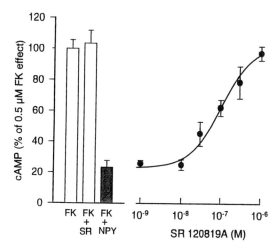

Figure 4 Inhibitory effect of SR 120819A on 10 nM NPY-induced cAMP inhibition in human SK-N-MC. Histograms represent the effect of 0.5 μM forskolin (FK) alone or in the presence of either 1 μM SR 120819A or 10 nM NPY. The results are expressed as a percentage of maximal 0.5 μM forskolin (FK) effect. Each point is the mean ± SEM of three independent experiments performed in triplicate.

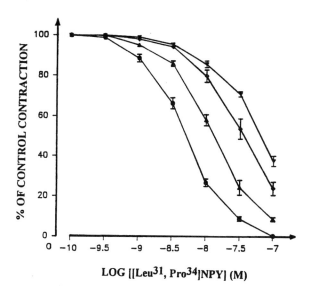

Figure 5 Inhibitory effect of SR 120819A on the electrically stimulated rabbit vas deferens. Cumulative concentration–response curves for [Leu^{31},Pro^{34}]NPY on the amplitude of twitch contractions elicited by electrical field stimulation were established in the absence (●) or in the presence of 0.1 (▲), 0.3 (◆) and 1 (▼) μM of SR 120819A. Results are expressed as a percentage of the twitch control responses measured after 45 min incubation with or without SR 120819A, and are the mean ± SEM of 5–6 experiments.

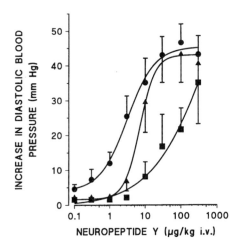

Figure 6 Effect of SR 120819A on the dose–response curve of NPY in pithed rats. Wistar rats were prepared as previously described (Serradeil-Le Gal et al., 1993). SR 120819A [100 (▲), 300 (■) μg kg^{-1} IV] or vehicle [control (●)] was injected 15 min before establishing the dose–response of NPY.

1987; Aubert et al., 1988). This peptide contributes to the cardiovascular regulation, and may also be directly and indirectly involved in the control of blood pressure. Several studies, using in particular Y1- and Y2-receptor reference agonist peptides, NPY, PYY, [Leu[31],Pro[34]]NPY and NPY13–36, have shown that NPY Y1 receptors mainly support the cardiovascular actions of NPY (for review, see Dermott et al., 1993). Accordingly, we investigated the effects of our selective NPY Y1-receptor antagonist, SR 120819A, on the arterial blood pressure in several *in vivo* pharmacological models.

A preliminary set of experiments was performed in pithed rats in which central blood pressure control is totally abolished. In this preparation, exogenous administration of NPY [0.1–300 μg kg^{-1} intravenously (IV)] dose-dependently increased diastolic blood pressure with ED_{50} (the dose inducing a half-maximal effect) and E_{max} (maximal effect) values of 2.2 ± 0.4 μg kg^{-1} IV and 45.3 ± 2.1 mmHg ($n = 6$), respectively. SR 120819A, injected at 100 and 300 μg kg^{-1} IV 15 min prior to NPY administration, shifted the dose–pressor response curve for NPY to the right without significantly modifying the NPY maximal hypertensive effect (Figure 6). This suggests full competitive antagonism. The apparent *in vivo* pA_2 value of 7.06 ± 0.24 ($n = 8$), calculated from these experiments, is consistent with the affinity and potency of SR 120819A at NPY Y1 receptors in various preparations *in vitro* (Table 1 and Figures 3 to 5).

Preliminary experiments performed in anesthetized guinea-pigs have shown that NPY, PYY and the Y1-receptor agonist, [Leu[31],Pro[34]]NPY, induced hypertension whereas the Y2-receptor agonist, NPY13–36, was totally inactive. This confirmed the Y1 nature of the observed *in vivo* response. As shown in Figure 7, repeated injections

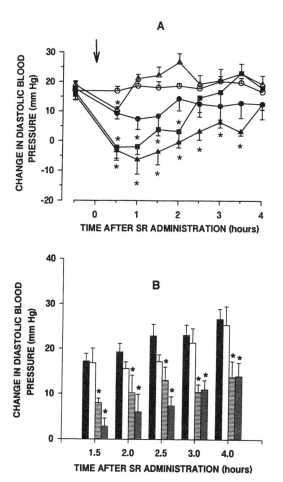

Figure 7 Time-course of the inhibitory effect of SR 120819A intravenously (A) and *per os* (B) on [Leu^{31},Pro^{34}]NPY (5 μg kg^{-1} IV)-induced hypertension in anesthetized guinea-pigs. Comparison with BIBP 3226 (1 mg kg^{-1} IV). Data are expressed as a change in diastolic blood pressure, observed after each [Leu^{31},Pro^{34}]NPY injection and represent the mean ± SEM of 5–11 determinations per group. Statistical analysis was performed using Anovarep followed by Dunnett's test and the level of significance (*) was taken as $P < 0.0.5$. (A) O, [L.P.]NPY 5 μg kg^{-1} IV ($n = 7$); ●, [L.P.]NPY+SR 120819A 0.1 mg kg^{-1} ($n = 6$); ■, [L.P.]NPY+SR 120819A 0.5 mg kg^{-1} ($n = 6$); ▲, [L.P.]NPY+SR 120819A 1 mg kg^{-1} ($n = 6$); △, [L.P.]NPY+BIBP 3226 1 mg kg^{-1} ($n = 6$). (B) ■, vehicle ($n = 11$); ☐, SR 120819A 1 mg kg^{-1} ($n = 5$); ▤, SR 120819A 5 mg kg^{-1} ($n = 5$); ▦, SR 120819A 10 mg kg^{-1} ($n=5$).

of [Leu^{31},Pro^{34}]NPY (5 μg kg^{-1} IV) at 30 min intervals induced a constant rise in diastolic blood pressure without observing tachyphylaxis. This convenient preparation was used for further studying the time-course of SR 120819A efficacy in preventing [Leu^{31},Pro^{34}]NPY-induced hypertension in anesthetized guinea-pigs. Using an IV

167

route, SR 120819A (0.1–1 mg kg^{-1}) produced a dose-dependent inhibition of the pressor response of [Leu^{31},Pro^{34}]NPY (Figure 7A). At the higher dose of 1 mg kg^{-1} IV, the effect lasted significantly more than 3 h whereas the other non-peptide Y1-receptor antagonist, BIBP 3226 (1 mg kg^{-1} IV), is almost inactive in producing only brief and slight protection at 30 min suggesting high metabolization and/or elimination for this compound (Figure 7A). More importantly, when given by an oral route, SR 120819A (5 and 10 mg kg^{-1}) significantly counteracted the hypertensive effects of the Y1-receptor agonist with a long duration of action ($>$4 h). In contrast, BIBP 3226 is totally inactive up to 10 mg kg^{-1} by mouth (not shown) showing that, despite the similar affinity and efficacy observed at NPY Y1 receptors *in vitro*, SR 120819A has a much better bioavailability than BIBP 3226.

Thus, SR 120819A is the first, selective Y1-receptor antagonist displaying significant oral efficacy. Moreover, the absence of agonist activity detected for SR 120819A in these *in vivo* models confirms the full antagonist profile of this compound at NPY Y1 receptors.

8.5.2 Central nervous system evaluations with SR 120819A

Further studies were designed to address the effects of SR 120819A on the main central nervous system (CNS) functions regulated by NPY and especially involving Y1 (or supposed Y1-like) receptors: hypothermia, food intake, anxiolysis, analgesia, epilepsia, etc. (Heilig *et al.*, 1993; Wettsein *et al.*, 1995).

Up to now, no significant effects can be reported with SR 120819A on NPY or [Leu^{31},Pro^{34}]NPY-induced CNS effects in the mouse when tested at 5 mg kg^{-1} intraperitoneally. We assume that this is the result of the low ability of SR 120819A to cross the blood–brain barrier. Thus, the poor CNS bioavailability observed for this compound has precluded further major investigation for identifying the role of NPY in the CNS, Y1-receptor function, the existence of potential NPY receptor subtypes and clinical developments with this prototype compound.

8.6 Conclusion

The present report demonstrates that SR 120819A is a potent, highly selective and competitive antagonist for Y1 receptors *in vitro* and *in vivo*. The most striking finding is the long-lasting *in vivo* activity observed for the first time for a synthetic compound regarding the exogenous NPY effects on arterial blood pressure. Moreover, these results provide convincing evidence of the cardiovascular role of NPY through Y1 receptors.

Even if there is a great number of endogenous peptides from different origins able to control blood pressure (Ganten *et al.*, 1991; Maish *et al.*, 1995), NPY could be considered as a potential target for new drugs in the cardiovascular area through interaction with Y1 receptors. At first sight, NPY is a potent vasoconstrictor *per se*, also able to potentiate the action of vasocontracting agents, especially on the small arteries of skeletal muscle that contribute largely to total peripheral resistance (Waeber et al., 1988). Although it seems unlikely that NPY controls basal arterial blood pressure under physiological state, this peptide could contribute to blood pressure dysfunctions in situations with aberrant expression of this hormone, such as exercise, cold stress, some forms of hypertension, congestive heart failure and in pheochromocytoma in which NPY high plasma levels are reported (Tabarin et al., 1992; Michel and Rascher, 1995; Takahashi et al., 1987).

In addition, NPY is well known for its severe vasospastic properties on coronary vessels in vitro and in vivo via Y1 receptors. This effect has been widely documented in several species, including man, with damaged coronary arteries, in which chest pain and myocardial ischemia are associated with NPY infusions (Clarke et al., 1987). Another study has clearly demonstrated an enhanced coronary response to NPY associated with increasing age and with hereditary hyperlipidemia in rabbits, which is consistent with an important role for NPY in vasospasm associated with coronary diseases (Corr et al., 1993). Indeed vasospasm is a complex phenomeon resulting from multifactorial synergic events involving vasoconstrictive agents (such as NPY), platelets, diseased coronary arteries with atheromatous lesions and proliferative vascular smooth muscle cells. All this rationale argues for testing the therapeutical relevance of Y1-receptor antagonists in pathologies, such as atherosclerosis, hypertension, congestive heart failure and in that respect, SR 120819A could be a relevant candidate.

Besides cardiovascular indications for Y1-receptor antagonists, strong interest is expressed in developing non-peptide antagonists and agonists directed towards the treatment of CNS diseases, such as eating disorders (i.e. bulimia, obesity/anorexia, cachexia), anxiety, depression, stress, pain, memory deficits, etc. (Heilig, 1993; Heilig et al., 1994; Chance et al., 1995; Kalra et al., 1995; Wettsein et al. 1995). As evidenced by the numerous reports in that field, NPY is a main target for new drugs to treat obesity. However, one question still remains open concerning the receptor involved in appetite (Y1-like) and probably will be fully understood with the cloning of this entity. Unfortunately, the poor ability of SR 120819A to cross the blood–brain barrier has hampered major investigations into the role of NPY in the CNS, the Y1-receptor contribution and characterization of potential receptor subtypes in the brain.

Since NPY triggers its multiple effects through at least six receptor subtypes defined either at the molecular level (Y1, Y2 and PP1 or Y4 are now cloned) or based on biochemical and pharmacological considerations, there is a crucial need for specific tools (agonists and antagonists) to establish an accurate classification, and to identify receptor types and their basic functions. Altogether, the results presented here on SR 120819A and the high degree of selectivity of this compound for Y1 receptors point out the usefulness of SR 120819A as a specific Y1-receptor probe in acutely discriminating NPY/PYY receptors and in localizing Y1 binding sites in complex tissues such as the kidney or the brain expressing a mixed population of NPY/PYY receptor subtypes. Thus, using SR 120819A, we report here for the first time the significant presence of Y1 receptors in the kidney.

In conclusion, SR 120819A represents the first generation of potent and highly selective NPY Y1-receptor antagonists with a remarkable *in vivo* intravenous and oral activity. In that respect, SR 120819A can be considered as a prototype for studying further NPY peripheral functions, its pathophysiological role and for developing future therapeutic agents.

Acknowledgements

I would like to acknowledge here the team of Sanofi Recherche involved in the design and the characterization of NPY receptor antagonists in Toulouse and Montpellier. Our thanks are extended to Dr B. Christophe from Bio-Pharma, Lab. J. Simon (B-1301 Wavre, Belgium) and to Dr G. Neliat from Cerep (Celle l'Evescault, France). We are grateful to M. Laborde and S. Sabattier for typing this work, and to A.J. Patacchini and K.J. Mulvaney for their helpful comments on the manuscript. We would like to thank H. Jaouy and his team for their helpful advice in preparing this manuscript.

References

Akabayashi, A., Wahlestedt, C., Alexander, J.T. & Leibowitz, S.F. (1994) Specific inhibition of endogenous neuropeptide Y synthesis in arcuate nucleus by antisense oligonucleotides suppresses feeding behaviour and insulin secretion. *Mol. Brain Res.* **21**, 55–61.

Allen, J., Novotny, J., Martin, J. & Heinrich, G. (1987) Molecular structure of mammalian neuropeptide Y: Analysis by molecular cloning and computer-aided comparison with crystal structure of avian homologue. *Proc. Natl Acad. Sci. USA* **84**, 2532–2536.

Aubert, J.F., Waeber, B., Rossies, B., Geering, K., Nussberger, J. & Brunner, H.R. (1988) Effects of neuropeptide Y on the blood pressure response to various vasoconstrictor agents. *J. Pharmac. Exp. Ther.* **246**, 1088–1092.

Bard, J.A., Walker, M.W., Branchek, T.A. & Weinshank, R.L. (1995) Cloning and functional expression of a human Y4 subtype receptor for pancreatic polypeptide, neuropeptide Y, and peptide YY. *J. Biol. Chem.* **270**, 26 762–26 765.

Bouali, S.M., Fournier, A., St-Pierre, S. & Jolicoeur, F.B. (1994) *In vivo* central actions of NPY(1–30), an N-terminal fragment of neuropeptide Y. *Peptides* **15**, 799–802.

Cadieux, A., Benchekroun, M.T., Fournier, A. & St Pierre, S. (1990) Pharmacological actions of neuropeptide Y and peptide YY in rat colon. *Ann. N. York Acad. Sci.* **611**, 372–375.

Chance, W.T., Balasubramaniam, A. & Fischer, J.E. (1995) Neuropeptide Y and the development of cancer anorexia. *Ann. Surg.* **221**, 579–589.

Chaurasia, C., Misse, G., Tessel, R. & Doudhty, M.B. (1994) Nonpeptide peptidomimetic antagonists of the neuropeptide Y receptor: benextramine analogs with selectivity for the peripheral Y2 receptor. *J. Med. Chem.* **37**, 2242–2248.

Cheng, Y. & Prusoff, W. (1973) Relationship between the inhibition constant (K_i) and the concentration of inhibitor which causes 50 per cent inhibition (I_{50}) of an enzymatic reaction. *Biochem. Pharmacol.* **22**, 3099–3108

Clarke, J.G., Kerwin, R., Larkin, S., Lee, Y., Yacoub, M., Davies, G.J., Hackett, D., Dawbarn, D., Bloom, S.R. & Maseri, A. (1987) Coronary artery infusion of neuropeptide Y in patients with angina pectoris. *Lancet*, 1057–1059.

Corr, L., Burnstock, G. & Poole-Wilson, P. (1993) Effects of age and hyperlipidemia on rabbit coronary responses to neuropeptide Y and the interaction with norepinephrine. *Peptides* **14**, 359–364.

Currie, P.J. & Coscina, D.V. (1995) Dissociated feeding and hypothermic effects of neuropeptide Y in the paraventricular and perifornical hypothalamus. *Peptides* **16**, 599–604.

Darbon, H., Bernassau, J.M., Deleuze, C., Chenu, J., Roussel, A. & Cambillau, C. (1992) Solution conformation of human neuropeptide Y by ^{1}H nuclear magnetic resonance and restrained molecular dynamics. *Eur. J. Biochem.* **209**, 765–771.

Dermott, B.J. Mc, Millar, B.C. & Piper, H.M. (1993) Cardiovascular effects of neuropeptide Y: receptor interactions and cellular mechanisms. *Cardiovas. Res.* **27**, 893–905.

Doods, H.N. & Krause, J. (1991) Different neuropeptide Y receptor subtypes in rat and rabbit vas deferens. *Eur. J. Pharmacol.* **204**, 101–103.

Dumont, Y. & Quirion, R. (1995) Possible Y1 receptor heterogeneity as revealed by using the newly developed non-peptide neuropeptide Y Y1 receptor antagonist, BIBP 3226. The Physiologist 38 (*Am. J. Physiol.*) *Abstr.* **4**, 16, A–248

Dumont, Y., Satoh, H., Cadieux, A., Taoudi-Benchekroun, M., Pheng, L.H., St-Pierre, S., Fournier, A. & Quirion, R. (1993a) Evaluation of truncated neuropeptide Y analogues with modifications of the tyrosine residue in position 1 on Y1, Y2 and Y3 receptors sub-types. *Eur. J. Pharmacol.* **238**, 37–45.

Dumont, Y., Fournier, A., St-Pierre, S. & Quirion, R. (1993b) Characterization of a selective neuropeptide Y/peptide YY, Y2 receptor radioligand: [^{125}I]PYY. *Soc. Neurosci. Abstr.* **19**, 726.

Dumont, Y., Cadieux, A., Pheng, L.H., Fournier, A., St-Pierre, S. & Quirion, R. (1994) Peptide YY derivatives as selective neuropeptide Y/peptide YY, Y1 and Y2 agonists devoided of activity for the Y3 receptor sub-type. *Mol. Brain Res.* **26**, 320–324.

Dumont, Y., Fournier, A., St-Pierre, S. & Quirion, R. (1995) Characterization of neuropeptide Y binding sites in rat brain membrane preparations using [^{125}I][Leu^{31},Pro^{34}]peptide YY and [^{125}I]Peptide YY3–36 as selective Y1 and Y2 radioligands 1. *J. Pharmacol. Exp. Ther.* **272**, 673–680.

Edvinsson, L., Hakanson, R., Wahlestedt, C. & Uddman, R. (1987) Effects of neuropeptide Y on the cardiovascular system. *Trends Pharmacol. Sci.* **8**, 231–235.

Erlinge, D., Edvinsson, L., Brunkwall, J., Yee, F. & Wahlestedt, C. (1993) Human neuropeptide Y Y1 receptor antisense oligodeoxynucleotide specifically inhibits neuropeptide Y-evoked vasoconstriction. *Eur. J. Pharmacol.* **240**, 77–80.

Eva, C., Oberto, A., Sprengel, R. & Genazzani, E. (1992) The murine NPY-1 receptor gene. Structure and delineation of tissue-specific expression. *FEBS Lett.* **314**, 285–288.

Feth, F., Rascher, W. & Michel, M.C. (1991) G-Protein coupling and signalling of Y1-like neuropeptide Y receptors in SK-N-MC cells. *Naunyn-Schmiedeberg's Arch. Pharmacol.* **344**, 1–7.

Fournier, A., Dumont, Y., St-Pierre, S. & Quirion, R. (1993) Autoradiographic distribution and characterization of [^{125}I]-[Leu^{31},Pro^{34}]PYY binding sites in rat brain: a selective Y1 radioligand. *Soc. Neurosci. Abstr.* **19**, 727.

Frankish, H.M., Dryden, S., Hopkins, D., Wang, Q. & Williams, G. (1995) Neuropeptide Y, the hypothalamus, and diabetes: insights into the central control of metabolism. *Peptides* **16**, 757–771.

Fuhlendorff, J., Gether, U., Aakerlund, L., Langeland-Johansen, N., Thogersen, H., Melberg, S.G., Olsen, U.B., Thastrup, O. & Schwartz, T.W. (1990) [Leu^{31},Pro^{34}]Neuropeptide Y: a specific Y1 receptor agonist. *Proc. Natl Acad. Sci. USA* **87**, 182–18.

Ganten, D., Paul, M. & Lang, R.E. (1991) The role of neuropeptides in cardiovascular regulation. *Cardiovas. Drugs Therapy* **5**, 119–130.

Gehlert, D.R. (1994) Subtypes of receptors for neuropeptide Y: implications for the targeting of therapeutics. *Life Sci.* **55**, 551–562.

Gerald, C., Walker, M.W., Vaysse, P.J.J., He, C., Branchek, T.A. & Weinshank, R.L. (1995)

Expression cloning and pharmacological characterization of a human hippocampal neuropeptide Y/peptide YY Y2 receptor subtype. *J. Biol. Chem.* **270**, 26 758–26 761.

Gimpl, G., Gerstberger, R., Mauss, U., Kotz, K.N. & Lang, R.E. (1990) Solubilization and characterization of active neuropeptide Y receptors from rabbit kidney. *J. Biol. Chem.* **265**, 18 142–18 147.

Gray, T.S. & Morley, J.E. (1986) Neuropeptide Y: anatomical distribution and possible function in mammalian nervous system. *Life Sci.* **38**, 389–401.

Grundemar, L. (1995) Will neuropeptide Y receptor antagonists offer new therapeutic approaches? *Exp. Opin. Ther. Patents* **5**, 1007–1013.

Grundemar, L. & Hakanson, R. (1994) Neuropeptide Y effector systems: perspectives for drug development. *Trends Pharmacol. Sci.* **15**, 153–159.

Heilig, M. (1993) Neuropeptide Y in relation to behaviour and psychiatric disorders. In *The Biology of Neuropeptide Y and Related Peptides* (eds Colmers, W.F. & Wahlestedt, C.), pp. 511–544. Totowa, NJ, Humana Press Inc.

Heilig, M. (1995) Antisense inhibition of neuropeptide Y (NPY)-Y1 receptor expression blocks the anxiolytic-like action of NPY in amygdala and paradoxically increases feeding. *Regul. Pept.* **59**, 201–205.

Heilig, M., McLeod, S., Brot, M., Heinrichs, S.C., Menzaghi, F., Koob, G.F. & Britton, K.T. (1993) Anxiolytic-like action of neuropeptide Y: mediation by Y1 receptors in amygdala, and dissociation from food intake effects. *Neuropsychopharmacology* **8**, 357–363.

Heilig, M., Koob, G.F., Ekman, R. & Britton, K.T. (1994) Corticotropin-releasing factor and neuropeptide Y: role in emotional integration. *Trends Neuro. Sci. Letters* **17**, 80–85.

Herzog, H., Hort, Y.J., Ball, H.J., Hayes, G., Shine, J. & Selbie, L.A. (1992) Cloned human neuropeptide Y receptor couples to two different second messenger systems. *Proc. Natl Acad. Sci. USA* **89**, 5794–5798.

Kalra, P.S., Bonavera, J.J. & Kalra, S.P. (1995) Central administration of antisense oligodeoxynucleotides to neuropeptide Y (NPY) mRNA reveals the critical role of newly synthesized NPY in regulation of LHRH release. *Regul. Pept.* **59**, 215–220.

Kirby, D.A., Boublik, J.H. & Rivier, J.E. (1993) Neuropeptide Y: Y1 and Y2 affinities of the complete series of analogues with single D-residue substitutions. *J. Med. Chem.* **36**, 3802–3808.

Kirby, D.A., Koerber, S.C., May, J.M., Hagaman, C., Cullen, M.J., Pelleymounter, M.A. & Rivier, J.E. (1995) Y1 and Y2 receptor selective neuropeptide Y analogues: evidence for a Y1 receptor subclass. *J. Med. Chem.* **38**, 4579–4586.

Knieps, S., Michel, M.C., Dove, S. & Buschauer, A. (1995) Non-peptide neuropeptide Y antagonists derived from the histamine H2 agonist arpromidine: role of the guanidine group. *Bioorg. Med. Chem. Lett.* **5**, 2065–2070.

Larhammar, D., Blomqvist, A.G., Yee, F., Jazin, E., Yoo, H. & Wahlestedt, C. (1992) Cloning and functional expression of a human neuropeptide Y/peptide YY receptor of the Y1 type. *J. Biol. Chem.* **267**, 10 935–10 938.

Leys, K., Schachter, M. & Sever, P. (1987) Autoradiographic localisation of NPY receptors in rabbit kidney: comparison with rat, guinea-pig and human. *Eur. J. Pharmacol.* **134**, 233–237.

Lundberg, J.M. & Tatemoto, K. (1982) Pancreatic polypeptide family (APP, BPP, NPY and PYY) in relation to sympathetic vasoconstriction resistant to α-adrenoceptor blockade. *Acta Physiol. Scand.* **116**, 393–398.

Lundell, L., Blomqvist, G., Berglund, M.M., Schober, D.A., Johnson, D., Statnick, M.A., Gadski, R.A., Gehlert, D.R. & Larhammar, D. (1995) Cloning of a human receptor of the NPY receptor family with high affinity for pancreatic polypeptide and peptide YY. *J. Biol. Chem.* **270**, 29 123–29 128.

Maisch, B., Brilla, C. & Kruse, T. (1995) Directions in antihypertensive treatment – our future from the past. *Eur. Heart J.* (Suppl. C) **16**, 74–83.

Michel, M.C. (1991) Receptors for neuropeptide Y: multiple subtypes and multiple second messengers. *Trends Pharmacol. Sci.* **12**, 389–394.

Michel, M.C. & Motulsky, H.J. (1990) He 90481: a competitive nonpeptidergic antagonist at neuropeptide Y receptors. *Annu. Rev. N. York Acad. Sci.* **611**, 392–394.

Michel, M.C. & Rascher, W. (1995) Neuropeptide Y: a possible role in hypertension? *J. Hypertens.* **13**, 385–395.

Michel, M.C., Gaida, W., Beck-Sickinger, A.G., Wieland, H.A., Doods, H., Dürr, H. *et al.* (1992) Further characterization of neuropeptide Y receptors subtypes using centrally truncated analogs of neuropeptide Y: evidence for subtype-differentiating effects on affinity and intrinsic efficacy. *Mol. Pharmacol.* **42**, 642–648.

Potter, E.K. (1988) Neuropeptide Y as an autonomic neurotransmitter. *Pharmacol. Ther.* **37**, 251–273.

Rose, P.M., Fernandes, P., Lynch, J.S., Frazier, S.T., Fisher, S.M., Kodukula, K., Kienzle, B. & Seethala, R. (1995) Cloning and functional expressing of a cDNA encoding a human type 2 neuropeptide Y receptor. *J. Biol. Chem.* **270**, 22661–22664.

Rudolf, K., Eberlein, W., Engel, W., Wieland, H.A., Willim, Entzeroth, A., Wienen, W., Beck-Sickinger, A.G. & Doods, H.N. (1994) The first highly potent and selective non-peptide neuropeptide Y Y1 receptor antagonist: BIBP3226. *Eur. J. Pharmacol.* **271**, R11–R13.

Sautel, M., Martinez, R., Munoz, M., Peitsch, M.C., Beck-Sickinger, A.G. & Walker, P. (1995) Role of a hydrophobic pocket of the human Y1 neuropeptide Y receptor in ligand binding. *Mol. Cell. Endocrinol.* **112**, 215–222.

Serradeil-Le Gal, C. (1996) Autoradiographic localization of vasopressin V_{1a} receptors in the rat kidney using [^{3}H]SR49059. *Kidney Int.* **50**, 499–505.

Serradeil-Le Gal, C., Wagnon, J., Garcia, C., Lacour, C., Guiraudou, P., Christophe, B., Villanova, G., Nisato, D., Maffrand, J.P., Le Fur, G., Guillon, G., Cantau, B., Barberis, C., Trueba, M., Ala, Y. & Jard, S. (1993) Biochemical and pharmacological properties of SR 49059, a new, potent, nonpeptide antagonist of rat and human vasopressin V_{1a} receptors. *J. Clin. Invest.* **92**, 224–231.

Serradeil-Le Gal, C., Valette, G., Rouby, P.E., Pellet, A., Villanova, G., Foulon, L., Lespy, L., Neliat, G., Chambon, J.P., Maffrand, J.P. & Le Fur, G. (1994a) SR 120107A and SR 120819A: two potent and selective orally-effective antagonists for NPY Y1 receptors. *Soc. Neurosci. Abst.* **20**, 907.

Serradeil-Le Gal, C., Raufaste, D., Marty, E., Garcia, C., Maffrand, J.P. & Le Fur, G. (1994b) Binding of [3H]SR49059, a potent nonpeptide vasopressin V_{1a} antagonist, to rat and human liver membranes. *Biochem. Biophys. Res. Commun.* **199**, 353–360.

Serradeil-Le Gal, C., Valette, G., Rouby, P.E., Pellet, A., Oury-Donat, F., Brossard, G., Lespy, L., Marty, E., Neliat, G., de Cointet, P., Maffrand, J.P. & Le Fur, G. (1995) SR 120819A, an orally-active and selective neuropeptide Y Y1 receptor antagonist. *FEBS Lett.* **362**, 192–196.

Sheikh, S.P., Sheikh, M.I. & Schwartz, T.W. (1989) Y2-type receptors for peptide YY on renal proximal tubular cells in the rabbit. *Am. J. Physiol.* **257**, F978–984.

Stanley, B.G. (1993) Neuropeptide Y in multiple hypothalamic sites controls eating behaviour, endocrine, and autonomic systems for body energy balance. In *The Biology of Neuropeptide Y and Related Peptides* (eds Colmers, W.F. & Wahlestedt, C.), pp. 457–509. Totowa, NJ, Humana Press Inc.

Tabarin, A., Minot, A.P., Dallochio, M., Roger, P. & Ducassou, D. (1992) Plasma concentration of neuropeptide Y in patients with adrenal hypertension. *Regul. Pept.* **42**, 51–61.

Takahashi, K., Toraichi, M., Keiichi, I., Masahiko, S., Ohneda, M., Murakami, O. *et al.* (1987) Increased plasma neuropeptide Y. Concentrations in phaeochromocytoma and chronic renal failure. *J. Hypertens.* **5**, 749–753.

Tatemoto, K. (1982) Neuropeptide Y: complete amino acid sequence of the brain peptide. *Proc. Natl Acad. Sci. USA* **79**, 5485–5489.

Tatemoto, K., Carlquist, M. & Mutt, V. (1982) Neuropeptide Y – a novel brain peptide with structural similarities to peptide YY and pancreatic polypeptide. *Nature (Lond.)* **296**, 659–660.

Waeber, B., Aubert, J.F., Corder, R., Evequoz, D., Nussberger, J., Gaillard, R. & Brunner, H.R.

(1988) Cardiovascular effects of neuropeptide Y. *Am. J. Hypertens.* **1**, 193–199.

Wahlestedt, C. & Reis, D.J. (1993) Neuropeptide Y-related peptidiques and their receptors – are receptors potential therapeutic drug targets. *Annu. Rev. Pharmacol. Toxicol.* **32**, 309–352.

Walker, P., Grouzmann, E., Burnier, M. & Waeber, B. (1991) The role of neuropeptide Y in cardiovascular regulation. *Pharmacol. Sci.* **12**, 111–115.

Walker, P., Munoz, M., Martinez, R. & Peitsch, M.C. (1994) Acidic residues in extracellular loops of the human Y_1 neuropeptide Y receptor are essential for ligand binding. *J. Biol. Chem.* **269**, 2863–2869.

Wettstein, J.G., Earley, B. & Junien, J.L. (1995) Central nervous system pharmacology of neuropeptide Y. *Pharmacol. Ther.* **65**, 397–414.

CHAPTER 9

BIBP 3226, A POTENT AND SELECTIVE NEUROPEPTIDE Y Y1-RECEPTOR ANTAGONIST. STRUCTURE–ACTIVITY STUDIES AND LOCALIZATION OF THE HUMAN Y1 RECEPTOR BINDING SITE

Klaus Rudolf, Wolfgang Eberlein, Wolfhard Engel, Annette G. Beck-Sickinger, Helmut Wittneben, Heike A. Wieland and Henri N. Doods

Table of Contents

9.1 Introduction

Neuropeptide Y is a 36-amino-acid peptide (Tatemoto, 1982), which belongs to a peptide family including peptide YY (PYY) and pancreatic polypeptide (PP). NPY is considered to be an important mammalian neuropeptide in the periphery and possibly the most abundant neuropeptide in the central nervous system (CNS). Because NPY has been shown to produce a variety of pharmacological effects, both in the periphery and in the CNS, it attracted widespread attention. Recent data clearly demonstrate the existence of at least four different NPY receptor types. The Y1 receptor possesses a high affinity for analogs of NPY or PYY, which possess a proline instead of glutamine in position 34, whereas the Y2 receptor exhibits a high affinity for C-terminal fragments of NPY or PYY, e.g. NPY13–36 and PYY3–36. The Y3 and Y4 receptor can be defined by their low affinity for PYY and high affinity for PP, respectively.

Neuropeptide Y and Drug Development
ISBN 0-12-304990-3

Despite the knowledge that currently at least four NPY receptor types exist and although it is well known that NPY exerts a multitude of biological effects, the precise physiological role of NPY could not be clearly revealed owing to the lack of appropriate NPY-receptor antagonists. In recent years peptide analogs, such as PYX-1 and PYX-2 (Tatemoto, 1992), [D-Trp^{32}]NPY (Balasubramaniam *et al.*, 1994), and non-peptide compounds, e.g. HE 90481 (Michel and Motulsky, 1990), Benextramine (Doughty *et al.*, 1990, 1992), PP56 (Edvinsson *et al.*, 1990) have been described as NPY antagonists, however, none of these compounds fulfilled the criteria of high affinity, specificity and competitiveness. Therefore, in order to elucidate the physiological role of the Y1 receptor, the development of a potent, selective and preferably non-peptide Y1 receptor antagonist was required. In this chapter we describe the design of BIBP 3226, a highly potent and selective non-peptide Y1 antagonist, and discuss its interaction with the human Y1 receptor based on structure–activity studies and receptor mutation work. Furthermore, the pharmacological properties of BIBP 3226 will be briefly summarized.

9.2 The design of the Y1-receptor antagonist BIBP 3226

Currently, two strategies for the discovery of low-molecular-weight neuropeptide receptor antagonists are commonly used: a random screening (Snider *et al.*, 1990; Clozel *et al.*, 1993) of an available compound library, or a rational mimetic strategy where the neuropeptide itself, derivatives or fragments thereof, serve as the initial lead structures (Horwell *et al.*, 1991; Jung and Beck-Sickinger, 1992). Within our drug discovery program, the latter approach turned out to be the most successful. The results of an alanine scan (Beck-Sickinger *et al.*, 1994) and further structure–activity work on peptidic NPY analogs (Beck-Sickinger and Jung, 1995) clearly suggested that the C-terminally located amino acids of NPY – especially Arg-35 and Tyr-36 – are of major importance for the interaction with the Y1 and the Y2 receptor. Extensive structural modifications of the C-terminal part of the NPY molecule indicated that the deletion of the C-terminally located carboxamide group afforded a peptide possessing nano-molar Y1- and Y2-receptor affinity and, most importantly, human Y1-antagonistic properties in an *in vitro* cell assay (Hoffmann *et al.*, 1996). Based on these results, a set of several hundred low-molecular-weight analogs mimicking the C-terminal part of the NPY molecule were synthesized, characterized and subsequently optimized with respect to their human Y1-receptor affinity.

This strategy eventually led to the identication of a highly selective and potent non-peptide Y1-receptor antagonist (Rudolf *et al.*, 1994; Doods *et al.*, 1995, Wieland *et al.*, 1995), code name BIBP 3226 ((R)-N^2- (diphenylacetyl)-N-[(4-hydroxyphenyl)methyl] argininamide: Figure 1).

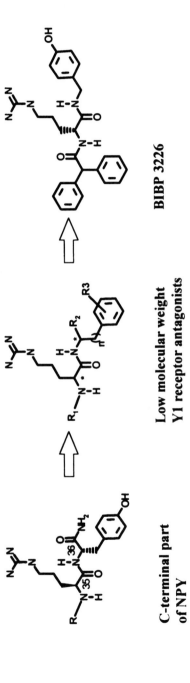

C-terminal part of NPY

Low molecular weight Y1 receptor antagonists

BIBP 3226

Figure 1 Strategy for the design of BIBP 3226.

9.3 The first structure–activity relationships

The efficient exploitation of this structural class of Y1-receptor antagonists required a simple, enantioselective route for the preparation of BIBP 3226 and its analogs. Starting with a commercially available (R)-arginine derivative, BIBP 3226, and its analogs were prepared in four steps (Figure 2) with >99.9% enantiomeric purity as confirmed by HPLC measurements.

Interestingly, highly stereospecific interaction of BIBP 3226 with the human Y1 receptor expressed in SK-N-MC cells could be shown by the drastically reduced receptor binding affinity (hY1, IC_{50}>10 000 nM) of the corresponding (S)-enantiomer of BIBP 3226.

In order to establish the first structure–activity relationships around our lead compound BIBP 3226, four arbitrarily selected structural elements (N-terminus, amino acid, C-terminus, backbone) were defined (Figure 3) and modified individually while keeping the rest of the molecule constant. First results of these structural variations are summarized below:

The hY1-receptor binding data established for the N-terminal variations (Figure 4) indicate that both aromatic rings present in the diphenylacetic acid moiety of BIBP 3226 are required for high hY1-receptor affinity. Furthermore, it is evident that the restriction of the two phenyl rings into one plane induces a significant loss in binding affinity.

The nature of the basic group and its distance (number of methylene groups) from the backbone is of importance for good receptor affinity as can be seen from the amino-acid modifications (Figure 5).

With respect to the C-terminal variations (Figure 6) one finds that the 4-hydroxy group as well as the correctly positioned aromatic system contribute to hY1-receptor binding.

Interestingly, this work also reveals the importance of the backbone part for hY1-receptor binding: variation of the backbone (Figure 7) with respect to stereochemistry as well as the orientation of the individual amide groups indicates that, within this structural class of hY1-receptor antagonists, the backbone moiety represents more than just scaffolding and participates directly in the binding to the hY1-receptor.

9.4 The receptor binding model of BIBP 3226

Subsequent to the identification of BIBP 3226, a question of general interest came up: does BIBP 3226 really mimic the C-terminal portion of the NPY molecule as suggested by our design strategy? In order to answer this rather fundamental question, a comparison has been made between the recently established (Walker *et al.*, 1994; Sautel *et al.*, 1995) mode of Y1-receptor binding of NPY and a hY1-receptor binding model of BIBP 3226. Thus, the interaction of [^{3}H]BIBP 3226 with the hY1-receptor has been experimentally elucidated using a series of single Ala-mutated hY1-receptors (Sautel *et al.*, 1996).

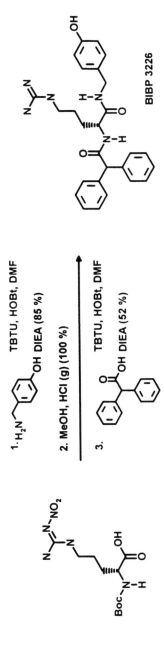

Figure 2 Enantioselective synthesis of BIBP3226. This synthetic route has also been used for the preparation of BIBP 3226 analogues. BIBP 3226 was prepared with >99.9% purity as determined by HPLC experiments. The (S)-configured analogs have been prepared by starting the synthesis with H-(S)-Arg(NO$_2$)-OH.

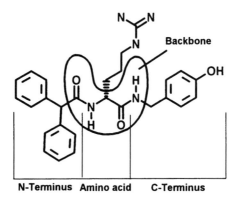

N-Terminus Amino acid C-Terminus

Figure 3 Dissection of BIBP 3226 into four structural elements, which were individually modified.

Alanine mutants at positions Y100, D104, W288 and H298 of the hY1-receptor showed no or significantly reduced binding for NPY, but were not affected in their ability to bind BIBP 3226 (Plate 18). Receptors with alanine mutations at positions W163, F173, Q219, N283, F286 and D287 showed reduced binding for both NPY and BIBP 3226. Mutations at other positions were tested (H105, S170, L174, V178, D200, D205, S206, H207, S210, T212, T280, T284, N289, H290, Q291) and did not affect the binding of NPY or BIBP 3226. The hY1-receptor mutant Y211A showed no affinity for BIBP 3226 but retained wild-type affinity for NPY. Based on these experimental results, summarized in Plate 18, a detailed model for the interaction of BIBP 3226 with the hY1-receptor was developed (Sautel *et al.*, 1996), using a Y1-receptor model and a three-dimensional model of BIBP 3226 (Plate 19).

In addition to the ionic interaction of the guanidino group present in BIBP 3226 with D287 of the hY1-receptor, a cation-π-interaction of the guanidino group of BIBP 3226 with F286 and a π–π-interaction of the benzene rings of the diphenylacetyl moiety of BIBP 3226 with the benzene rings of F173 and Y211 is suggested in this model. Moreover, the C-terminal segment of BIBP3226 might interact through a π–π interaction of the benzene ring of BIBP 3226 with W163 and via two hydrogen bonds: Q219(NH2) could interact with the 4-OH of the C-terminal 4-hydroxybenzylamid moiety of BIBP 3226 and N283(NH2) with the backbone carbonyl group of BIBP 3226. Interestingly, the only hY1-receptor mutant displaying no affinity for BIBP 3226 but high affinity for NPY binds, in this model, to the diphenylacetyl moiety of BIBP 3226, a structural element that is exclusively present in the non-peptide antagonist. A comparison of the hY1-receptor binding models of BIBP 3226 (Sautel *et al.*, 1996) and NPY (Sautel *et al.*, 1995) substantiates the notion that the non-peptide antagonist BIBP 3226 indeed mimics the C-terminal region of the native peptide ligand NPY and supports the validity of our design strategy for the development of this structural class of hY1-receptor antagonists.

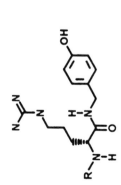

R-				
hY$_1$ IC$_{50}$, [nM]	5	370	10000	72

Figure 4 N-Terminal variations of BIBP 3226. The receptor affinity has been determined using human neuroblastoma cells (SK-N-MC), which constitutively express the Y1 receptor.

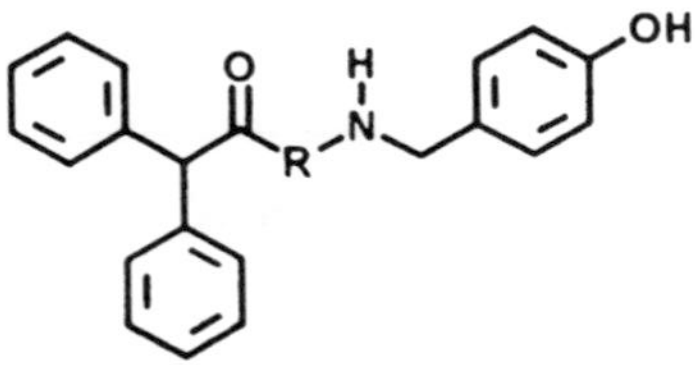

Figure 5 Amino acid variations of BIBP 3226. The receptor affinity has been determined using human neuroblastoma cells (SK-N-MC), which constitutively express the Y1 receptor.

-R-	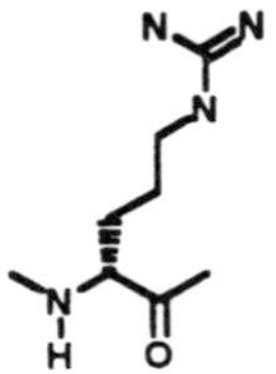	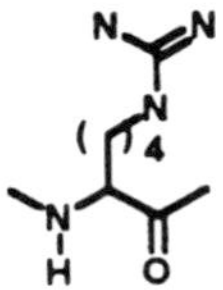	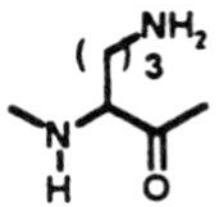	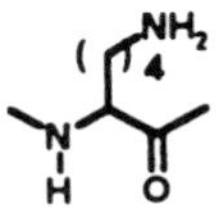
hY$_1$ IC$_{50}$, [nM]	5	220	> 10000	> 10000

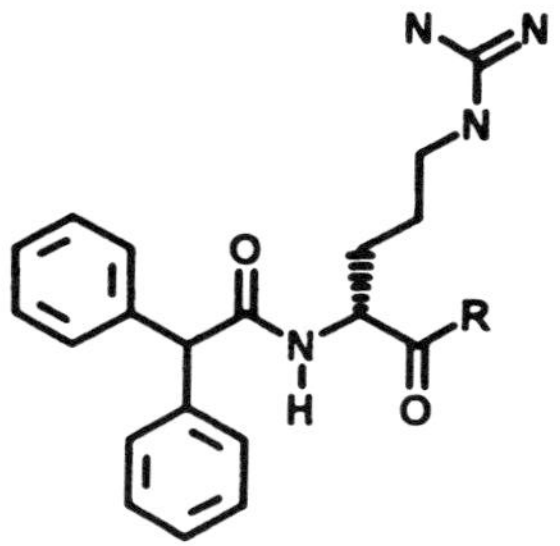

-R	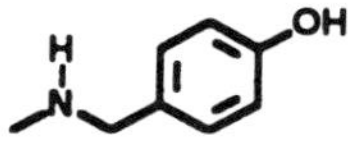	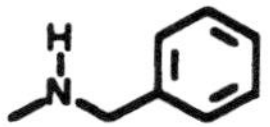	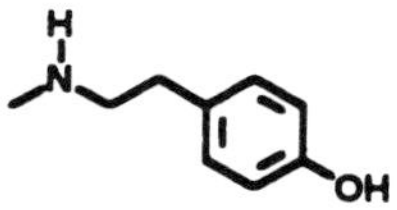	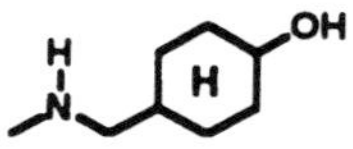
hY_1 IC_{50}, [nM]	5	70	290	9000

Figure 6 C-Terminal variations of BIBP 3226. The receptor affinity has been determined using human neuroblastoma cells (SK-N-MC), which constitutively express the Y1 receptor.

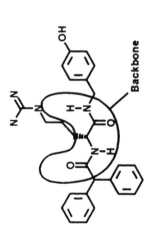

Backbone

Backbone	 	CH₃		
hY₁ IC₅₀, [nM]	5	25	> 10000	> 10000

Figure 7 Backbone variations of BIBP 3226. The receptor affinity has been determined using human neuroblastoma cells (SK-N-MC), which constitutively express the Y1 receptor.

9.5 The pharmacological profile of BIBP 3226

The affinity of BIBP 3226 for NPY receptor types has been investigated in a variety of tissues and cell lines. BIBP 3226 displayed K_i values of 5.1 and 6.8 nM for the human and rat Y1 receptors (Wieland et al., 1995) and virtually no affinity ($K_i > 10\,000$ nM) for Y2, Y3 and Y4 receptors (see Table 1; Wieland et al., 1995; Doods et al.,1996). In addition, no measurable affinity could be detected for a wide variety of other receptors or enzyme systems (see Table 2).

In the SK-N-MC cell the Y1 receptor is stimulatory to the release of intracellular calcium. As shown in Figure 8, BIBP 3226 caused a concentration-dependent rightward shift of the NPY concentration–response curve. The corresponding mean pK_b value was 7.3.

The selectivity of BIBP 3226 was also examined in functional in vitro experiments. For Y1 receptors the rabbit vas deferens (Doods and Krause, 1991; Doods et al., 1995), rat renal tissue (Entzeroth et al., 1994; Doods et al., 1995), guinea-pig vena cava (Doods et al., 1996) and human cerebral arteries (Abouander et al., 1995) were used. Besides this, Y2 receptors were examined using the rat vas deferens (Doods and Krause, 1991; Doods et al., 1995), Y3 receptors by employing the rat colon (Jacques et al., 1995) and Y4 receptors by using the rat vas deferens (Doods et al., 1996).

As listed in Table 1, the pK_b values of BIBP 3226 for Y1 receptors ranged from 7.0 to 8.5. Concentration up to 10 μM had no effect on Y2, Y3 and Y4 receptors. Summarizing the receptor data, it can be concluded that BIBP 3226 is a highly selective Y1 antagonist.

In order to investigate the NPY antagonistic properties in vitro, the ability of BIBP 3226 to antagonize the pressor response elicited by intravenous administration of NPY in the pithed rat was examined. A dose of approximately 0.1 mg kg^{-1} intravenously (iv) was necessary to inhibit the increase in blood pressure induced by 10 μg kg^{-1} (iv) NPY (Doods et al., 1995). In conscious spontaneously hypertensive-rats, BIBP 3226 in doses up to 5 mg kg^{-1} (iv) had no effect on basal blood pressure. However, BIBP 3226 (3 mg kg^{-1} iv bolus + 3 mg kg^{-1} h^{-1} infusion) reduced the pressor response induced by cold stress and normalized the cardiovascular changes, e.g. mesenteric vascular resistance, during the recovery phase (Zukowska-Grojec et al., 1996). These data clearly demonstrate that NPY and Y1 receptors play a significant role in the regulation of vascular tone during stress.

With respect to CNS effects of BIBP 3226, only limited data are available. Since BIBP 3226 does not penetrate the blood–brain barrier, it has been injected directly into the hypothalamus in order to observe the effect of this compound on NPY-induced feeding. However, we and others were not able to demonstrate unambiguously an effect of BIBP 3226 on feeding since after intracerebroventricular or paraventricular nucleus application, unwanted side effects, e.g. barrel rolling, occur.

Table 1 Affinity of BIBP 3226 for NPY receptor types in radioligand binding and functional studies

Type	Tissue/cell line	Radioligand	pK_i	Reference	Tissue	Agonist	pK_b	Reference
Y1	Human SK-N-MC	[¹²⁵I]NPY	8.3	a	Rabbit vas deferens	NPY	7.0	d
	Rat cortex	[¹²⁵I]NPY	8.2	a	Rat kidney	NPY	7.5	d
					Human cerebral artery	NPY	8.5	e
					Guinea-pig vena cava	NPY	7.6	b
					Rat vas deferens	NPY	<5	d
Y2	Human SMS-KAN	[¹²⁵I]NPY	<5	a				
	Rat hippocampus	[¹²⁵I]NPY	<5	a				
Y3	Rat brainstem	[¹²⁵I]NPY2–36	<5	b	Rat colon	NPY	<5	f
Y4	Human CHO	[¹²⁵I]PP	<5	c	Rat vas deferens	PP	<5	b

References: a, Wieland *et al.* (1995); b, Doods *et al.* (1996); c, Cloned Y4 receptor, unpublished data; d, Doods *et al.* (1995); e, Abounader *et al.* (1995); f, Jacques *et al.* (1995).

Receptor assays	Enzyme assays
Adenosine A_1	Acetyl CoA synthetase
Adenosine A_2	Calpain
α_1-Adrenergic	Carbonic anhydrase
α_2-Adrenergic	Cyclooxygenase
β-Adrenergic	Elastase
β_1-Adrenergic	HMG–CoA reductase
β_2-Adrenergic	Leukotriene A_4 hydrolase
Androgen	Leukotriene C_4 synthetase
Angiotensin II	Lipid peroxidase
Atrial natriuretic factor	5-Lipoxygenase
Benzodiazepine	15-Lipoxygenase
Bombesin	Neutral endopeptidase
Bradykinin	Phospholipase A_2
Calcitonin gene-related peptide	Protein kinase C
Calcium channels	EGF tyrosine kinase
Chloride channel	
Cholecystokinin A	
Cholecystokinin B	
Dopamine D_1	
Dopamine D_2	
Endothelin A	
Endothelin B	
Epidermal growth factor	
Excitatory amino acid	
Estrogen	
Kainate	
NMDA	
Quisqualate	
Galanin	
Histamine 1 (H_1)	
Histamine 3 (H_3)	
$GABA_A$	
Insulin	
Interleukin 1-α	
Leukotriene B_4	
Leukotriene D_4	
Muscarinic (M_1)	
Muscarinic (M_2)	
Muscarinic (M_3)	
Muscarinic (M_4)	
NK1	
Opiate	
Opiate (delta)	
Opiate (kappa)	
Opiate (mu)	
Phencyclidine	
Phorbol ester	
Platelet activating factor	
Potassium channels	
Progestin	
Serotonin (5-HT_1)	
Serotonin (5-HT_{1A})	
Serotonin (5-HT_2)	
Serotonin (5-HT_3)	
Sigma	
Sodium channel	
Somatostatin	
Thromboxane A_2	
Thyrotropin releasing hormone	
Tumor necrosis factor-α	
Vasoactive intestinal polypeptide	
Vasopressin	

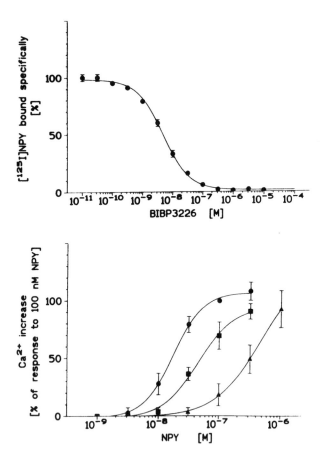

Figure 8 Displacement of specifically bound [^{125}I] Bolton Hunter NPY by BIBP 3226 in human Y1 receptor expressing SK-N-MC cells (top panel). Antagonism of the NPY-induced Ca^{2+} response in SK-N-MC cells by 0.1 μM (■) or 1 μM (▲) BIBP 3226 (lower panel). ●, solvent.

9.6 Conclusions

BIBP3226, a potent and selective NPY Y1-receptor antagonist has been designed by mimicking the C-terminal amino acids of the native ligand NPY. A hY1-receptor binding model of BIBP 3226 has been established, which indicates that the receptor binding sites of the native peptide NPY and the antagonist BIBP 3226 overlap. First structure–activity relationships indicate that all four structural elements (N-terminus, amino acid, C-terminus and backbone) of BIBP 3226 contribute to receptor binding. The pharmacological properties of BIBP 3226 characterize this compound as a competitive and highly selective Y1-receptor antagonist. Thus, BIBP 3226, together with the recently disclosed Y1-receptor antagonists SR120819A (Serradeil-Le Gal *et al.*,

1995) and 1229U91 (Daniels *et al.*, 1995) will be useful tools to elucidate the (patho)physiological role of NPY Y1-receptors. Further insight into the physiological role of NPY depends on the availability of, preferably non-peptide, receptor antagonists for all existing NPY receptor types.

References

Abounader, R., Villemure, J.G. & Hamel, E. (1995) Characterization of neuropeptide Y (NPY) receptors in human cerebral arteries with selective agonists and the new Y1 antagonist BIBP 3226. *Br. J. Pharmacol.* **116**, 2245–2250.

Balasubramaniam, A., Sheriff, S., Johnson, M.E., Prabhakarn, M., Huang, Y., Fischer, J.E. & Chance, W.T. (1994) [D-Trp32] Neuropeptide Y: A competitive antagonist of NPY in rat hypothalamus. *J. Med. Chem.* **37**, 811–815.

Beck-Sickinger, A.G. & Jung, G. (1995) Structure–activity relationships of neuropeptide Y analogues with respect to Y1 and Y2 receptors. *Biopolymers* **37**, 123–142.

Beck-Sinkinger, A.G., Wieland, H.A., Wittneben, H., Willim, K., Rudolf, K. & Jung, G. (1994) Complete L-alanine scan of neuropeptide Y reveals ligands binding to Y1 and Y2 receptors with distinguished conformations. *Eur. J. Biochem.* **225**, 947–958.

Clozel, M., Breu, V., Burri, K., Cassal, J.-M., Fischli, W., Gray, G.A., Hirth, G., Loeffler, B.-M., Mueller, M., Neidhart, W. & Ramuz, H. (1993) Pathophysiological role of endothelin revealed by the first orally active endothelin receptor antagonist. *Nature (Lond.)* **365**, 759–761.

Daniels, A.J., Matthews, J.E., Slepetis, R.J., Jansen, M., Viveros, O.H., Tadepalli, A., Harrington, W., Heyer, D., Landavazo, A., Leban, J.J. & Spaltenstein, A. (1995) High-affinity neuropeptide Y receptor antagonists. *Proc. Natl Acad. Sci. USA* **92**, 20, 9067–9071.

Doods, H.N. and Krause, J. (1991) Different neuropeptide Y receptor subtypes in rat and rabbit vas deferens. *Eur. J. Pharmacol.* **294**, 101–103.

Doods, H.N., Wienen, W., Entzeroth, M., Rudolf, K., Eberlein, W., Engel, W. & Wieland, H.A. (1995) Pharmacological characterization of the selective nonpeptide NPY Y1 antagonist BIBP 3226, *J. Pharmacol. Exp. Ther.* **275**, 136–142.

Doods, H.N., Wieland, H.A., Engel, W., Eberlein, W., Willim, K.D., Entzeroth, M., Wienen, W. & Rudolf, K. (1996) BIBP3226, the first highly selective NPY Y1 receptor antagonist: a review of its pharmacological properties, *Regul. Pept.* (in press).

Doughty, M.B., Chu, S.S., Miller, D.W., Li, K. & Tessel, R.F. (1990) Benextramine: A long-lasting neuropeptide Y receptor antagonist. *Eur. J. Pharmacol.* **185**, 113–114.

Doughty, M.B., Li, K., Hu, L., Chu, S.S. & Tessel, R. (1992) Benextramine-neuropeptide Y (NPY) binding site interactions: Characterization of 3H-NPY binding site heterogeneity in rat brain. *Neuropeptides* **23**(3), 169–180.

Edvinsson, L., Adamsson, M. & Jansen, I. (1990) Neuropeptide antagonistic properties of D-myo-inositol-1,2,6-triphosphate in guinea-pig basilar arteries. *Neuropeptides* **17**, 99–105.

Entzeroth, M., Wieland, H.A., Wienen, W. & Doods, H.N. (1994) The increase in renal perfusion pressure by neuropeptide Y is mediated via receptors of the Y1 subtype, *Can. J. Physiol. Pharmacol.* **72** (Suppl. 1), 170.

Hoffmann, S., Rist, B., Videnov, G., Jung, G. & Beck-Sickinger, A.G. (1996) Structure–affinity studies of C-terminally modified analogs of neuropeptide Y led to a novel class of peptidic Y1 receptor antagonists, *Regul. Pept.* (in press).

Horwell, D.C., Hughes, J., Hunter, J., Pritchard, M., Richardson, R., Roberts, E. & Woodruff, G. (1991) Rationally designed 'dipeptoid' analogues of CCK. Alpha-methyltryptophan derivatives as highly selective and orally active gastrin and CCK-B antagonists with potent anxiolytic properties, *J. Med. Chem.* **34**, 404–414.

Jacques, D., Cadieux, A., Dumont, Y. & Quirion, R. (1995) Apparent affinity and potency of BIBP 3226, a non-peptide neuropeptide Y antagonist, on purported neuropeptide Y Y1, Y2 and Y3 receptors, *Eur. J. Pharmacol.* **278**, R3–R5.

Jung, G. & Beck-Sickinger, A.G. (1992) Multiple peptide synthesis methods and their applications. *Angew Chem. (Int. Ed)* **31**, 367–383.

Michel, M.C. & Motulsky, H.J. (1990) HE 90481: A competitive nonpeptidergic antagonist at neuropeptide Y receptors. *Ann. N. York Acad. Sci.* **611**, 392–394.

Rudolf, K., Eberlein, W., Engel, W., Wieland, H.A., Willim, K.D., Entzeroth, M., Wienen, W., Beck-Si⬤nger, A.G., Doods, H.N. (1994) The first highly potent and selective non-peptide neuropeptide Y1 receptor antagonist: BIBP3226, *Eur. J. Pharmacol.* **271**, R11–R13.

Sautel, M., Martinez, R., Munoz, M., Peitsch, M.C. & Beck-Sickinger, A.G. (1995) Role of hydrophobic residues of the human Y1 neuropeptide Y receptor in ligand binding, *Mol. Cell Endocrinol.* **112**, 215–222.

Sautel, M., Rudolf, K., Wittneben, H., Herzog, H., Martinez, R., Munoz, M., Eberlein, W., Engel, W., Walker, P. & Beck-Sickinger, A.G. (1996) Neuropeptide Y and the non-peptide antagonist BIBP3226 share an overlapping binding site at the human Y1 receptor. *Mol. Pharmacol.* **50**, 285–292.

Serradeil-Le Gal, C., Valette, G., Rouby, P.E., Pellet, A., Oury-Donat, F., Brossard, G., Lespy, I., Marty, E., Neliat, L., De Cointet, P., Maffrand, J.-P. & Le Fur, G. (1995) SR 120819A, an orally-active and selective neuropeptide Y Y1 receptor antagonist. *FEBS Lett.* **362**, 192–196.

Snider, R.M., Constantine, J.W., Llowe, J.A., Longo, K.P., Lebel, W.S., Woody, H.A., Drozda, S.E., Desai, M.C., Vinick, F.J., Spencer, R.W. & Hess, H. (1990) A potent nonpeptide antagonist of the substance P (NK1) receptor. *Science* **251**, 435–437.

Tatemoto, K. (1982) Neuropeptide Y: Complete amino acid sequence of the brain peptide, *Proc. Natl Acad. Sci. USA* **79**, 5485–5489.

Tatemoto, K. (1992) Synthesis of receptor antagonists of Neuropeptide Y. *Proc Natl Acad. Sci. USA,* **89**, 1174–1178.

Walker, P.M., Munoz, M., Martinez, R. & Peitsch, M.C. (1994) Acidic residues in extracellular loops of the human Y1 neuropeptide Y receptor are essential for ligand binding. *J. Biol. Chem.* **269**, 2863–2869.

Wieland, H.A., Willim, K.D., Entzeroth, M., Wienen, W., Rudolf, K., Eberlein, W., Engel, W. & Doods, H.N. (1995). Subtype selectivity and antagonistic profile of the nonpeptide Y1 receptor antagonist BIBP 3226. *J. Pharmacol. Exp. Ther.* **275**, 143–149.

Zukowska-Grojec, Z., Dayao, E., Karwatowska-Prokopczuk, E., Hauser, G.J. & Doods, H.N. (1996) Stress induced mesenteric vasoconstriction in rats is mediated by neuropeptide Y Y1 receptors. *Am. J. Physiol.* **270**(2), H796–H800.

_____ CHAPTER 10 _____

DISCOVERY OF NEUROPEPTIDE Y RECEPTOR ANTAGONISTS

Aleksandr Rabinovich, Anatoly Mazurov, Galina Krokhina, Anthony Ling, Nurit Livnah, Yufeng Hong, Eileen Valenzuela, Vlad Gregor, Robert Feinstein, Alexander Polinsky, John M. May, Cristin Hagaman and Marvin Brown

Table of Contents

10.1 Introduction

The history, physiology and pharmacology of neuropeptide Y (NPY) and NPY receptors are discussed in other chapters in this book. Our goal has been to discover NPY receptor antagonists for use in the treatment of obesity and cardiovascular disease. The cardiovascular actions of NPY (vasoconstrictor) are mediated by the Y1 receptor present on vascular smooth muscle cells (Grundemar *et al.*, 1993). Current evidence suggests that NPY effects on feeding are mediated by a Y1-like receptor with a pharmacology that differs from the cardiovascular Y1 receptor (Stanley, 1993). An NPY receptor type that mediates the action of NPY to stimulate feeding is rumoured to have been cloned; however, no publication has yet appeared to confirm this speculation. In this report we will confine discussion to our efforts to discover selective Y1 receptor antagonists.

To discover NPY receptor antagonists we have followed three different strategies: (1) design and synthesis of peptide or peptide-like NPY receptor antagonists based on

Neuropeptide Y and Drug Development
ISBN 0-12-304990-3

the analysis of structural analogs of NPY; (2) design and synthesis of non-peptide NPY receptor antagonists based on pharmacophore information derived from the analysis of peptide or peptide-like NPY receptor antagonists; and (3) identification of non-peptide NPY receptor antagonists through the screening of combinatorial libraries.

10.2 Design and synthesis of peptide or peptide-like NPY receptor antagonists based on the analysis of structural analogs of NPY

Our initial efforts utilized a computational approach to guide the design of peptide and peptide-like Y1 receptor antagonists. An artificial intelligence-based pattern recognition system, Alanet-I, was developed to detect features critical for receptor binding. Alanet-I was trained on a set of available peptide analogs of known affinity and the extracted features were then used to predict the activity of novel molecules prior to their synthesis, thus facilitating the design of more active analogs. After new analogs were synthesized and tested, the system was retrained to take advantage of new structural information contained in those analogs.

Alanet-I applications to our NPY project resulted in the synthesis of the NPY receptor antagonists shown in Table 1. Both antiparallel dimeric (AXC00216, AXC00232, AXC00148) and monomeric (AXC00018) cyclic peptides demonstrated high affinity and selectivity for the Y1 receptor present on SK-N-MC cells (Table 1). The greater activity of the dimeric forms of these peptides may result from incorporation of additional receptor and non-receptor contact points or through stabilization of a more favourable conformation. A representative example of these peptides, AXC00232, was found to be a competitive antagonist of Y1 receptors and this is illustrated in Figure 1. The receptor specificity of AXC00232 was tested through its evaluation in several different G-protein coupled receptor binding assay systems (Table 2). Of interest, AXC00232 exhibited high specificity for the Y1 receptor when compared to other G-protein-coupled receptors tested, except for rat forebrain somatostatin receptors.

These and other studies support the conclusion that tyrosine and arginine present in the C-terminus of NPY confer those elements necessary for binding to the Y1 reeptor (Beck-Sickinger *et al.*, 1990; Perlman *et al.*, 1987) Attainment of high-affinity Y1-receptor binding of C-terminal fragments of NPY has been achieved through modification of the C-terminal backbone or through the introduction of constrained cyclic structures (Daniels *et al.*, 1995).

In rodent studies, several of these peptide NPY receptor antagonists given intravenously produced a lowering of arterial pressure that was prevented by prior administration of the histamine H1-receptor antagonist, diphenhydramine. NPY and NPY analogs have also previously been demonstrated to elicit histamine release and to lower arterial pressure by a histamine H1-receptor-dependent mechanism (Feinstein *et al.*, 1992; Grundemar *et al.*, 1994). In animals pre-treated with diphenhydramine, AXC00216 produced a dose-dependent inhibition of NPY-induced increase of arte-

Table 1 Structures and binding affinities of peptide NPY receptor antagonists

Compound	Chemical structure	Affinity (nM)		Selectivity
		Y1	Y2	Y2/Y1
AXC00216	(–Pmp-dArg-dTyr-Arg-dPen-NH$_2$)$_2$	5	>3000	600
AXC00232	(–Pmp-dArg-dTyr-Arg-dCys-NH$_2$)$_2$	12	>1000	>80
AXC00148	(–Pmp-dArg-dCys-dArg-pl-Phe-NH$_2$)$_2$	32	>1000	>30
AXC00018	Pmp-dArg-dCys-dArg-pl-Phe-NH$_2$	150		
AXC00254	Pmp-dArg-dTyr-Arg-dCys-NH$_2$	>1000	>1000	
AXC02632	DPAA-dArg-Tyr-NH$_2$	4	32000	8000

Pen, penicillamine; Pmp, β–mercapto-β,β-cyclopentamethylene-propionic acid; DPAA, diphenylacetic acid.

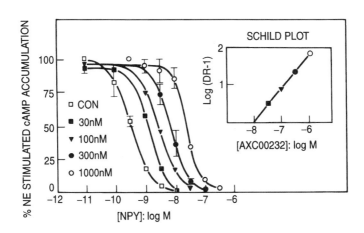

Figure 1 Competitive antagonism of Y1 receptors by AXC00232. Norepinephrine (10 μM) was used to stimulate the formation of cAMP in SK-N-MC cells, and this stimulation was inhibited by the addition of NPY. Pre-incubation of the cells with AXC00232 produced parallel rightward shifts in the NPY dose–response curves. The Schild transformation of the data is shown in the inset. Schild analysis yielded a slope of 1.08 and a calculated K_b of 10 nM.

rial pressure (Figure 2). These peptide NPY receptor antagonists did not consistently affect arterial pressure in spontaneously hypertensive rats, which were pre-treated with diphenhydramine. These observations do not support a role of NPY in regulating arterial pressure; however, participation of NPY in regulating regional organ blood flow, cardiac contractilty or electrical conduction has not been assessed. The results of these studies are in agreement with studies in which BIBP3226 did not influ-

Table 2 AXC00232 and AXC01018 binding to different G-protein-coupled receptors

Receptor	AXC00232 IC$_{50}$(nM)	AXC01018 IC$_{50}$(nM)
NPY	12	150
Somatostatin	300	200
Substance K	2000	1000
Neurotensin	>10000	>10000
Substance P	>10000	>10000
CRF$_1$	>10000	>10000
CRF$_2$	>10000	>10000
Bradykinin	>10000	>10000
GLP-1	>10000	>10000

CRF=Corticotropin releasing factor
GLP-1=Glucagon-like peptide 1

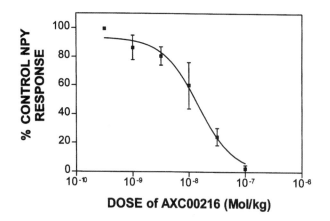

DOSE of AXC00216 (Mol/kg)

Figure 2 Blockade of NPY-induced pressor responses in diphenhydramine-treated, urethane-anesthetized rats by AXC00216. Intravenous injections of 0.3 nmol kg-1 NPY were made at 5 min intervals. The initial 2–3 injections were used to determine the baseline response. AXC00216 was injected intravenously, and the animals were challenged with NPY 5 mins later. The data are normalized to the initial response to NPY in the absence of an antagonist.

ence arterial pressure when administered to spontaneously hypertensive rats (Doods, *et al.*, 1995). To determine the possible effects of Y1-receptor antagonism on feeding in rats, peptides were administered into the lateral cerebroventricle. In the final analysis, each of these peptides administered into the central nervous system produced behavioral changes that precluded evaluating their ability to block NPY-induced feeding.

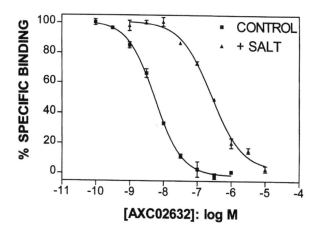

Figure 3 Effects of cations on the binding of AXC02632 to SK-N-MC cell membranes. AXC02632 showed different potencies in displacing the binding of $[^{125}I]$PYY from membrane homogenates, depending on whether or not sodium and calcium were present at physiological concentrations. Magnesium was present at 2 mM in all experiments. The IC_{50} values for AXC02632 were: control, 6 nM; +salt, 290 nM.

In an attempt to develop peptidic antagonists with a lower molecular weight, libraries of modified small peptides and pseudopeptides were synthesized and tested for their ability to bind to Y1 receptors. The diphenylacetyl-dipeptide, AXC02632, was found to have high binding affinity and selectivity for the Y1 receptor (Table 1). Although highly active in a salt-free assay system, AXC02632 exhibited a much lower affinity when assayed in the presence of physiological concentrations of sodium and calcium (see Figure 3), or when tested on intact cells. AXC02632 is structurally similar to BIBP3226 (Rudolf *et al.*, 1994); however, the latter compound is equally active in both salt-free and saline containing systems. Consistent with the lower potency of AXC02632 in physiological buffers, the compound was not active as an antagonist of NPY *in vivo*. None of the other compounds listed in Table 1 exhibited such sensitivity to the ionic composition of the assay media. An explanation for this salt sensitivity is not readily apparent.

10.3 Design and synthesis of non-peptide NPY receptor antagonists based on pharmacophore information derived from the analysis of peptide or peptide-like NPY receptor antagonists

This approach was based on the application of the pharmacophore analysis software, Alanet-II, developed at Alanex. This software was designed to deal specifically with flexible molecules, so that peptide or peptide-like analogs of up to ten amino acids in length could be analyzed. The high flexibility of peptide-like structures presented a challenge both for performing efficient conformational analysis, and for deducing pharmacophore hypotheses. The conformational search was accelerated in Alanet-II through the use of an extensive database of stable conformations of amino acids and their mimics, with potential energy surfaces around those conformations pre-calculated and stored on disk. A simplified force field was also used to calculate long-range interactions. The deduction of viable pharmacophore hypotheses was complicated by the fact that the pharmacophoric elements of a set of active molecules can be superimposed with each other in a very large number of ways. In addition to the commonly used geometric criteria to characterize the quality of the superposition of those elements in different molecules, Alanet-II analyzed the shape of the whole molecule to predict where the hypothetical surface of the receptor could be. The superpositions where such surfaces were not consistent with all active molecules were rejected, which allowed for substantial pruning of the list of generated pharma-cophore hypotheses.

The output of Alanet-II was a list of putative pharmacophore hypotheses that required purchase and/or synthesis of multiple non-peptide compounds to test each hypothesis. Information obtained from the identification of an active compound was then used to retrain the system and proceed to the next round of hypothesis genera-tion and synthesis. A number of pharmacophore hypotheses were generated using a set of active peptide analogs and their derivatives listed in Table 1. These hypotheses were used to select several non-peptide structures from Alanex's compound collection for screening. These compounds exhibited selective binding to the Y1 receptor (Table 3). Among this group of structures, the bis-dihydrotriazine class of compounds was further optimized, and exhibited high affinity and competitive binding to the Y1 receptor (Table 4, Figure 4). The structure–activity relationship for the bis-dihydro-triazines shown in Table 4 demonstrate that the replacement of the central *m*-disub-stituted phenyl in AXC01829 for the para analog (AXC01018) did not have significance on either the binding affinity or selectivity. Comparison of AXC01018 with AXC01020 indicates that the desmethoxy analog AXC01020 was two times less selective for Y1 over Y2 than the corresponding methoxy analog AXC01018 owing to the lack of the neutral H-bond acceptor methoxy groups. The superposition of one of the peptide analogs used to generate the hypothesis with one of the bis-dihydrotri-azine analogs is shown in Figure 5. Similar to the peptide antagonists of NPY, one of these bis-triazine NPY receptor antagonists exhibited significant affinity for the rat forebrain somatistatin receptor (Table 2). Owing to undesirable side effects in animal studies, the bis-triazine class of compounds have not been pursued further.

Several potential problems should be kept in mind when trying to use peptide phar-macophore information in the design of non-peptide ligands:

1. Peptides interact with receptors through multiple contact points that can be spread over a considerable space, thus leading to non-peptide structures of a large size.

2. Most of the contact points of peptides could be on the membrane surface rather than in the transmembrane region, while high-affinity small molecule ligands typi-cally have contact points in the hydrophobic transmembrane region of the receptor.

3. In many biologically active peptides, arginines play a critical role in binding to

Table 3 Structures and NPY binding affinities of three non-peptides

Compound	Chemical structure	Binding affinity (nM)		Selectivity
		Y1	Y2	Y2/Y1
AXC00181		150	>100 000	>650
AXC01494		400	>100 000	>250
AXC01006		2777	9107	3

Table 4 Structures and NPY binding affinities of three series of optimized bis-dihydrotriazines

Compound	Chemical structure	Binding affinity (nM)		Selectivity
		Y1	Y2	Y2/Y1
AXC01829		117	1555	13
AXC01018		150	1725	12
AXC01020		230	1475	6

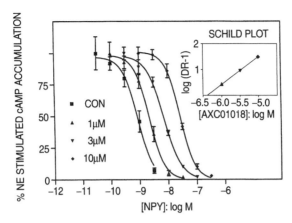

Figure 4 Competitive antagonism of Y1 receptors by AXC01018. The NPY-induced inhibition of norepinephrine-stimulated cAMP accumulation in SK-N-MC cells was antagonized by pre-treating the cells with AXC01018. Analysis of the Schild plot shown in the inset gives a slope of 0.88 and K_b of 400 nM.

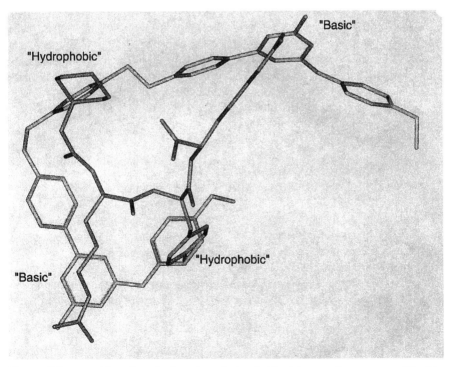

Figure 5 Superposition of two basic and two hydrophobic pharmacophore centers of the bis-dihydrotriazine derivative, AXC01018 and a peptide analog, AXC00092 (cHexAc-dArg-dTyr-Arg-NH$_2$, IC$_{50}$=3.6 μM, cHexAc=cyclohexylacetic acid), corresponding to one of the pharmacophore hypotheses.

Table 5 NPY receptor binding affinity of ligands discovered using combinatorial chemistry

Compound	Y1 IC_{50} (nM)	Y2 IC_{50} (nM)	Y2/Y1
AXC03916	3000		
AXC04166	174	10 300	60
AXC04141	30	2 400	80

the receptor. This may lead to pharmacophore hypotheses and, consequently, to compounds that contain a guanidino group, which may not always be a desirable moiety in a drug. While in some cases this group can be easily replaced with other basic moeities, in other cases the replacement of guanidino groups without compromising activity can be very difficult.

4. A set of active analogs used for the pharmacophore hypothesis generation must include related but structurally diverse, preferably constrained, molecules. This requirement could be a difficult task to achieve, especially when all known active analogs represent trivial variation around a structurally common theme that does not provide sufficient diversity.

5. Because of the flexibility of most peptide-like analogs, even with extensive methods to prune the list of pharmacophore hypotheses the number of reasonably good candidates is usually large. This represents a significant synthetic challenge, because a number of non-peptide molecules fitting the putative pharmacophore must be evaluated. Carefully designed combinatorial libraries can be used to test multiple pharmacophore hypotheses simultaneously.

10.4 Identification of non-peptide NPY receptor antagonists through the screening of combinatorial libraries

We developed combinatorial chemistry technology, Pharmacophore Directed Parallel Synthesis, as a method to generate large numbers of compounds to test and exploit rapidly pharmacophore hypotheses. Our combinatorial chemistry also explores unbiased libraries for the identification of NPY ligands unrelated to preconceived requirements for binding. Alanex combinatorial chemistry technology produces small molecule libraries of three to ten thousand individual compounds per library, using either solution or solid-phase synthesis (Polinsky *et al.*, 1996).

This approach has by far been the most successful means for the rapid identification of diverse and drug-like structures that bind to the NPY receptor. Table 5 shows the binding affinities of several of our initial hits identified using this combinatorial chemistry and high throughput screening approach. AXC04141 exhibits high affinity and selectivity for the Y1 receptor and is currently being optimized further.

Identification of small molecule agonists or antagonists for one or more of the known NPY receptor types represent an exciting opportunity in drug discovery. Presently, the receptor type and biological target on which a viable drug candidate will be based remains controversial. Application of combinatorial chemistry and the availability of relevant receptor types will lead to the identification of novel structures devoid of the undesirable chemical features contained in the past generations of NPY receptor ligands.

References

Beck-Sickinger, A.G., Jung, G., Gaida, W., Köppen, H., Schnorrenberg, G. & Lang, R. (1990) Structure-activity relationships of C-terminal neuropeptide Y peptide segments and analogues composed of sequence 1–4 linked to 25–36. *Eur. J. Biochem.* **194**, 449–456.

Daniels, A.J., Matthews, J.E., Viveros, O.H., Leban, J.J., Cory, M. & Heyer, D. (1995) Structure–activity relationship of novel pentapeptide neuropeptide Y receptor antagonists is consistent with a noncontinuous epitope for ligand-receptor binding. *Mol. Pharmacol.* **48**, 425–432.

Doods, H.N., Wienen, W., Entzeroth, M., Rudolf, K., Eberlein, W., Engel, W. & Wieland, H.A. (1995) Pharmacological characterization of the selective nonpeptide neuropeptide Y Y1 receptor antagonist BIBP 3226. *J. Pharmacol. Exp. Ther.* **275**, 136–142.

Feinstein, R.D., Boublik, J.H., Kirby, D., Spicer, M.A., Craig, A.G., Malewicz, K., Scott, N.A., Brown, M.R. & River, J. E. (1992) Structural requirements for neuropeptide Y18-36-evoked hypotension: a systematic study. *J. Med. Chem.* **35**, 2836–2843.

Grundemar, L., Sheikh, S.P. & Wahlestedt, C. (1993) Characterization of receptor types for neuropeptide Y and related peptides. In *The Biology of Neuropeptide Y and Related Peptides* (eds Colmers, W.F. & Wahlestedt, C.), pp. 197–239. Totowa, NJ, Humana Press.

Grundemar, L., Krstenansky, J.L. & Håkanson, R. (1994) Neuropeptide Y and truncated neuropeptide Y analogs evoke histamine release from rat peritoneal mast cells. A direct effect on G Proteins? *Eur. J. Pharmacol.* **258**, 163–166.

Perlman, M.O., Perlman, J.M., Adamo, M.L., Hazelwood, R.L. & Dyckes, D.F. (1987) Binding of C-terminal segments of neuropeptide Y to chicken brain. *Int. J. Pept. Protein Res.* **30**, 153–162.

Polinsky, A., Feinstein, R.D., Shi, S. & Kuki,. A. (1996) LiBrain: Software for automated design of exploratory and targeted combinatorial libraries. In *Molecular Diversity and Combinatorial Chemistry: Libraries for Drug Discovery* (eds Chaiken, I. & Jauda, K). ACS Symposium Series.

Rudolf, K., Eberlein, W., Engel, W., Wieland. H.A., Willim, K.D., Entzeroth, M., Wienen, W., Beck-Sickinger, A.G. & Doods, H.N. (1994) The first highly potent and selective non-peptide neuropeptide Y Y1 receptor antagonist: BIBP3226. *Eur. J. Pharmacol.* 271, R11–R13.

Stanley, B.G. (1993) Neuropeptide Y in multiple hypothalamic sites controls eating behavior, endocrene, and autonomic systems for body energy balance. In *The Biology of Neuropeptide Y and Related Peptides* (eds Colmers, W.F. & Wahlested, C.), pp. 457–509. Totowa, NJ, Humana Press.

Index

Index

Index

DATE DUE
